THE TEACHING NURSING HOME
A New Approach to Geriatric Research, Education, and Clinical Care

The Teaching Nursing Home

A New Approach to Geriatric Research, Education, and Clinical Care

Senior Editor

Edward L. Schneider, M.D.

Deputy Director, National Institute on Aging
National Institutes of Health, Bethesda, Maryland

Associate Editors

Carroll J. Wendland, Ph.D.

Executive Director, The Beverly Foundation
South Pasadena, California

Anne Wilder Zimmer, M.S., Noel List, M.D., Marcia Ory, Ph.D., M.P.H.

National Institute on Aging
National Institutes of Health, Bethesda, Maryland

Raven Press ∎ New York

Raven Press, 1140 Avenue of the Americas, New York, 10036

Made in the United States of America

Library of Congress Cataloging in Publication Data
Main entry under title:

The Teaching nursing home.

Based on the proceedings of a conference held in Washington, D.C., Mar. 25–27, 1984.
Includes bibliographies and index.
1. Teaching nursing homes—United States—Congresses.
2. Geriatrics—Study and teaching—United States—
Congresses. 3. Geriatrics—Research—United States—
Congresses. 4. Nursing home care—United States—
Congresses. I. Schneider, Edward L. [DNLM: 1. Geriatric
Nursing—education—congresses. 2. Geriatrics—education
—congresses. 3. Nursing Homes—congresses. 4. Teaching
—methods—congresses. WT 18 T2526 1984]
RA997.A15T43 1984   618.97′007′1073   84-42863
ISBN 0-88167-060-X
ISBN 0-88167-061-8 (pbk)

Preface

In this book, a new and exciting concept is explored—the teaching nursing home (TNH). Although teaching and research have been conducted for many years in a few nursing homes, these activities have increased enormously in the last few years. This is the result of several public and private sector programs which have brought together the talents of the academic community and chronic care facilities.

The initial section of this book reviews the epidemiologic, social, economic, and financial reimbursement aspects of long-term care. Particular emphasis is given to the role of TNHs within the continuum of long-term care. Since teaching and research are equally important components of the TNH concept, major sections are devoted to each of these topics. To reflect the multidisciplinary nature of TNHs, educational issues are discussed from the perspective of physicians, nurses, and other health professionals, while research approaches are examined from biomedical, social, and behavioral perspectives.

Different models of TNHs have been developed by the public and private sectors, which vary in orientation and emphasis. Several models are presented as examples, including one that is primarily research-oriented and involves multiple disciplines, and another that concentrates on a specific discipline with research, teaching, and clinical care components.

A section is reserved for those broad issues that concern all disciplines and activities in TNHs: values and ethics, management and administration, and assessment. A most important chapter in this section portrays the often neglected view of the nursing home resident. A section devoted to the specific issues of importance to TNHs complements the sections on general issues. Issues examined include dementia, nutrition, rehabilitation, mental health, urinary incontinence, drug therapy, communication disorders, mobility, and physical environment.

The book concludes with two thoughtful perspectives about the future of TNHs. The view from the public sector is discussed by the Director of the National Institute on Aging, T. Franklin Williams, and that of the private sector by the President of Beverly Enterprises, David Banks.

November 1, 1984   EDWARD L. SCHNEIDER, M.D.

Contents

Contributors

Senior Editor: Edward L. Schneider, M.D.
Deputy Director, National Institute on Aging
National Institutes of Health, Building 31, Room 2C-06
9000 Rockville Pike, Bethesda, Maryland 20205

Associate Editors

Carroll J. Wendland, Ph.D.
Executive Director, The Beverly Foundation
1445 Huntington Drive, South Pasadena, California 91030

Anne Wilder Zimmer, M.S.
Special Assistant to the Director, National Institute on Aging
National Institutes of Health, Building 31, Room 2C-02
9000 Rockville Pike, Bethesda, Maryland 20205

Noel D. List, M.D.
Medical Officer, Geriatrics Branch
Biomedical Research and Clinical Medicine, National Institute on Aging
National Institutes of Health, Building 31, Room 5C-21
9000 Rockville Pike, Bethesda, Maryland 20205

Marcia G. Ory, Ph.D., M.P.H.
Health Scientist Administrator, Behavioral Sciences Research
National Institute on Aging
National Institutes of Health, Building 31, Room 4C-32
9000 Rockville Pike, Bethesda, Maryland 20205

Linda H. Aiken, R.N., Ph.D.
Vice-President
Robert Wood Johnson Foundation
PO Box 2316
Princeton, New Jersey 08540

David R. Banks
President
Beverly Enterprises
873 South Fair Oaks Avenue
Box 90130
Pasadena, California 91109

Richard W. Besdine, M.D.
Director, Geriatric Fellowship
Training, and Assistant Professor of
Medicine
Harvard Medical School
and Director, Geriatric Education

Hebrew Rehabilitation Center for the
Aged
1200 Center Street
Boston, Massachusetts 02131

Elaine M. Brody, M.S.W.
Director, Department of Human
Services and Senior Researcher
Philadelphia Geriatrics Center
5301 Old York Road
Philadelphia, Pennsylvania 19141

Jacob A. Brody, M.D.
Associate Director for Epidemiology,
Demography and Biometry
National Institute on Aging
National Institutes of Health
Federal Building, 7550 Wisconsin
Avenue
Bethesda, Maryland 20205

Stanley J. Brody, J.D., M.S.W.
Professor of Social Planning
Hospital of the University of
  Pennsylvania
3400 Spruce Street, Box 590
Philadelphia, Pennsylvania 19104

Ewald W. Busse, M.D., Sc.D.
Professor of Psychiatry and Dean
  Emeritus
Medical Center
Duke University, Box 2948
Durham, North Carolina 27710

Robert N. Butler, M.D.
Professor and Chairman
Department of Geriatrics and Adult
  Development
Mt. Sinai Medical Center
Annenberg Building, Room 1330
One Gustave L. Levy Place
New York, New York 10029

Christine K. Cassel, M.D.
Assistant Professor
Department of Geriatrics and Adult
  Development
Mt. Sinai Medical Center
Annenberg Building, Room 1330
One Gustave L. Levy Place
New York, New York 10029

Gene D. Cohen, M.D.
Chief, Center for Study of the Mental
  health of the Aging
National Institute of Mental Health
National Institutes of Health
Parklawn Building, Room 11A16
Rockville, Maryland 20852

Carl Eisdorfer, Ph.D., M.D.
President
Montefiore Medical Center
111 East 210th Street
Bronx, New York 10467

Henry Erle, M.D.
Member, Supportive Care Team
Department of Medicine
Cornell University Medical College
1300 York Avenue, Room E-515
New York, New York 10021

Daniel J. Foley
Statistician
Epidemiology, Demography, and
  Biometry

National Institute on Aging
National Institutes of Health
Federal Building, 7550 Wisconsin
  Avenue
Bethesda, Maryland 20205

Marsha D. Fretwell, M.D.
Director, Geriatrics Education
Assistant Professor of Medicine
Southeastern New England Long-
  Term Gerontology Center
Brown University, Box G
Providence, Rhode Island 02912

Harriet Goodman, M.S W.
Member, Supportive Care Team
Departments of Pharmacology and
  Medicine
Cornell University Medical College
1300 York Avenue, Room E-515
New York, New York 10021

Geri Gray, R.N., Ph.D.
The New York Hospital
525 East 68th Street
New York, New York 10021

Evan C. Hadley, M.D.
Chief, Geriatrics Branch
Biomedical Research and Clinical
  Medicine
National Institute on Aging
National Institutes of Health
Building 31, Room 5C-21
9000 Rockville Pike
Bethesda, Maryland 20205

Tom Hickey, Ph.D.
Professor and Director of Health
  Gerontology Program
School of Public Health
University of Michigan
Ann Arbor, Michigan 48109

Carol C. Hogue, R.N., Ph.D.
Associate Professor, School of Nursing
and Assistant Professor, School of
  Medicine
and Senior Fellow, Center for the
  Study of Aging and Human
  Development
Duke University
Durham, North Carolina 27710

Linda Kaeser, R.N., A.C.S.W., Ph.D.
Program Director for Oregon Teaching Nursing Home Program
Oregon Health Sciences University
3181 S. W. Sam Jackson Park Road
Portland, Oregon 97201

Sidney Katz, M.D.
Associate Dean of Medicine
Brown University Program in Medicine and Director, South Eastern New England Long-Term Care Gerontology Center
Box G
Providence, Rhode Island 02912

Robert Katsman, M.D.
Professor and Chair
Department of Neuroscience
School of Medicine (M024)
University of California, San Diego
La Jolla, California 92093

Rosanne M. Leipzig, Ph.D., M.D.
Fellow
Departments of Pharmacology and Medicine
Cornell University Medical College
1300 York Avenue, Room E-515
New York, New York 10021

Leslie S. Libow, M.D.
Clinical Director and Vice Chairman
Department of Geriatrics and Adult Development
Mt. Sinai Medical Center, and Chief of Medical Services
The Jewish Home and Hospital for the Aged
Annenberg Building, Room 1330
One Gustave L. Levy Place
New York, New York 10029

Joan E. Lynaugh, R.N., Ph.D., F.A.A.N.
Associate Director, Robert Wood Johnson Foundation Teaching Nursing Home Program
University of Pennsylvania School of Nursing
Nursing Education Building/S2
Philadelphia, Pennsylvania 19104

George L. Maddox, Ph.D.
Director, Center for the Study of Aging and Human Development
Medical Center, Box 3003
Duke University
Durham, North Carolina 27710

Robert B. McGandy, M.D.
Professor of Nutrition
USDA–Human Nutrition Research Center on Aging at Tufts University
711 Washington Street
Boston, Massachusetts 02111

Mathy D. Mezey, R.N., Ed.D., F.A.A.N.
Director, Robert Wood Johnson Foundation Teaching Nursing Home Program
University of Pennsylvania School of Nursing
Nursing Education Building/S2
Philadelphia, Pennsylvania 19104

Anna Morgan-Fisher, B.A.
Doctoral Student
Callier Center
University of Texas
1966 Inwood Road
Dallas, Texas 75235

George Moushegian, Ph.D.
M. F. Jonsson Professor in Human Development
Callier Center
University of Texas
1966 Inwood Road
Dallas, Texas 75235

Adrian M. Ostfeld, M.D.
Lauder Professor
Laboratory of Epidemiology and Public Health
School of Medicine
yale University
60 College Street
New Haven, Connecticut 06510

Joseph G. Ouslander, M.D.
Assistant Professor of Medicine
Division of Geriatric Medicine
University of California, Los Angeles
10833 LeConte
A671 Factor Building
Los Angeles, California 90024

Leon A. Pastalan, Ph.D.
Professor of Architecture and
  Chairman of the Doctoral Program
  in Architecture
and Co-Director of the National
  Housing Center
Department of Architecture
University of Michigan
Ann Arbor, Michigan 48109

Larry J. Pipes, Ph.D.
Director of New Program
  Development
Beverly Enterprises
873 South Fair Oaks Avenue
Box 90130
Pasadena, California 92209

Marcus M. Reidenberg, M.D.
Head of Division of Clinical
  Pharmacology
Department of Medicine
Cornell University Medical College
1300 York Avenue, Room E-515
New York, New York 10021

Matilda White Riley, D.Sc.
Associate Director for Behavioral
  Sciences Research
National Institute on Aging
National Institutes of Health
Building 31, Room 4C-32
9000 Rockville Pike
Bethesda, Maryland 20205

John W. Rowe, M.D.
Director, Geriatric Research
  Education Clinical Center
Veterans Administration Outpatient
  Clinic
and Director, Division on Aging and
  Associate Professor of Medicine
Harvard Medical School
1200 Center Street
Boston, Massachusetts 02131

Anne R. Somers, D.Sc.(Hon.)
Adjunct Professor of Environmental
  and Community Medicine

University of Medicine and Dentistry
  of New Jersey
Rutgers Medical School
Piscataway, New Jersey 08854
and Lecturer at Woodrow Wilson
  School of Public and International
  Affairs
Princeton University
31 Scott Lane
Princeton, New Jersey 08540

Gwen C. Uman, M.N., G.N.P.
School of Education
University of Southern California
3113 Nichols Canyon Road
Los Angeles, California 90046

Mitchell M. Waife
Executive Vice-President
Jewish Home and Hospital for Aged
120 West 106th Street
New York, New York 10025

Thelma J. Wells, Ph.D.
Associate Professor of Nursing
School of Nursing
University of Michigan
Medical-Surgical Nursing Area
400 North Ingalls
Ann Arbor, Michigan 48109

Carter Williams, A.C.S.W., CSW
(formerly social worker with Jewish
  Home and Infirmary Day Services,
  Reformation Lutheran Church, and
  consultant to Social Work
  Departments in Nursing Homes,
  Monroe County, New York)
5202 West Cedar Lane
Bethesda, Maryland 20814

T. Franklin Williams, M.D.
Director
National Institute on Aging
National Institutes of Health
Building 31, Room 2C-02
9000 Rockville Pike
Bethesda, Maryland 20205

The Teaching Nursing Home, edited by Edward
L. Schneider et al. © 1985 The Beverly
Foundation. Raven Press, New York.

Introduction

Edward L. Schneider

*National Institute on Aging for Biomedical Research and Clinical Medicine, National
Institutes of Health, Bethesda, Maryland 20205*

The increased longevity that we have experienced this century is expected
to continue in the next century (see Epidemiologic Considerations by Brody
and Foley). Perhaps the most significant impact of this additional longevity
will be in the group aged 85 and above, which is now the fastest growing
age group in America. It is in the ninth decade of life that chronic diseases
and disorders take their greatest toll. This statistic is reflected by the average
age of a nursing home resident, which is 82. The impending growth of the
over 85-year-old group, which may triple in the next 50 years, will severely
test our health resources. It is therefore timely that we explore ways of
preventing the chronic diseases and disorders that disable our elderly. We
cannot accept the chronic diseases of old age as a necessary part of aging
any more than we could accept acute diseases such as typhoid fever and
cholera. We must search for the causes of chronic diseases and for ways of
improving the functioning of older persons with these disorders.

The successful conquest of many diseases has been facilitated in part by
research conducted in the fertile environment of teaching hospitals affiliated
with academic medical centers. However, gains in our knowledge of chronic
diseases have not kept pace with the impressive advances that have been
made in the prevention and treatment of acute illnesses. The chronic diseases that result in the need for long-term care (LTC) are frequently seen
in the nursing home, a location both geographically and intellectually removed from the academic medical center.

The concept of a teaching nursing home (TNH) is offered as one means
of promoting attention to research, teaching, and clinical care issues related
to the diseases and disorders of the elderly. It is not a new concept. Teaching
LTC facilities have flourished under the direction of Libow, Williams, and
others (1,2). However, the momentum toward developing teaching nursing
homes has been accelerated by the seminal article by Butler in the *Journal
of the American Medical Association* (3) and the Teaching Nursing Home
grant programs initiated by the Robert Wood Johnson Foundation, the National Institute on Aging (NIA), and Beverly Enterprises (4).

1

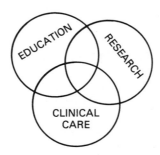

FIG. 1

This book was conceived to provide a discussion of approaches to developing TNHs, not solely to present the NIA view or the Beverly Enterprises view. The success of teaching hospitals has been partially attributed to the synergistic interaction of clinicians, teachers, and researchers. In Fig. 1, the mixture of research, teaching, and clinical care that should comprise a TNH is conceptualized. The NIA Teaching Nursing Home Program comprises only part of the research component—biomedical, social, and behavioral research, and a smaller part of the educational component—research training (Fig. 2). The Robert Wood Johnson Teaching Nursing Home Program involves part of the education component—nursing education, part of the clinical care component—nursing care, and part of the research component—nursing research (Fig. 3). The Beverly Enterprises model also covers parts of the research, education, and research components (Fig. 3). Clearly, there are many important areas that have not been covered by these programs.

The teaching hospital model cannot be directly applied to the problems of LTC. For example, the emphasis on diagnosis and cure needs to be replaced in a TNH with assessment and functional improvement. I do not wish to suggest that accurate diagnosis and cure of reversible diseases are

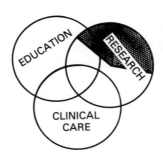

FIG. 2

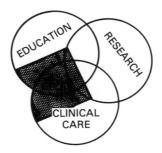

FIG. 3

not important in the nursing home, since timely recognition of conditions such as drug-induced dementias is crucial. However, we must not neglect the importance of even small gains in functioning to the older individual with a chronic disease.

Few nurses and fewer physicians set foot in a nursing home during their training. Since the demand for acute care hospital beds is declining and the demand for nursing home beds continues to increase, it is timely that medical and nursing schools, which traditionally have had strong affiliations with acute care hospitals, develop affiliations with LTC institutions. Physicians and nurses are treating increasing numbers of older patients. It is therefore urgent that they receive part of their training in LTC in an appropriate setting, the TNH.

Long-term care, in contrast to acute hospital care, is provided largely by the private sector. The majority of nursing homes are proprietary. Therefore, it is appropriate that this book as well as other efforts related to new approaches to LTC be collaborative ventures between public and private organizations.

This book has been organized to include multidisciplinary views of TNHs, since LTC in any setting is best delivered by an interdisciplinary team. Thus, in the organization of this book, suggestions have been solicited from several disciplines, including medicine, nursing, behavioral science, social work, and nursing home administration. It is hoped that this book will stimulate these disciplines to turn their attention to LTC through collaborative ventures such as TNHs.

REFERENCES

1. Williams TF, Izzo AJ, Steel RK: Innovations in teaching about chronic illness and aging in a chronic disease hospital, in Clark DW, Williams TF (eds): *Teaching of Chronic Illness and Aging*. Bethesda, Fogarty International Center, National Institutes of Health, 1976, pp. 21–30.
2. Libow L: A geriatric medical residency program: a four-year experience. *Ann Int Med* 1976;85:641–647.
3. Butler R: The teaching nursing home. *JAMA* 1981;245:1435–1437.
4. Schneider E: The teaching nursing home. *N Engl J Med* 1983;308:336–337.

PART I
Background—Health and Aging

The *Teaching Nursing Home*, edited by Edward
L. Schneider et al. © 1985 The Beverly
Foundation. Raven Press, New York.

Introduction

Carroll J. Wendland

The Beverly Foundation, South Pasadena, California 91030

For us to give meaning to the advent of the teaching nursing home
(TNH)—and its future—we should have an understanding of the circumstances that preceded its conception. The conditions and events that form
this backdrop are historical, social, financial, and technical. Significant
changes are occurring in each of these areas. Particularly dramatic are the
demographic and economic shifts and the transforming characteristics of
aging adults as a group.

The elderly to which we refer were born between 1880 and 1920, and they
are living longer than anyone had foreseen. In fact, in large numbers they
have defied the statistics, and now they are upward of 65, 80, even 100 years
old.[1] A burgeoning population, these older adults are pioneering the new
age of a senior citizen culture. More than this, they are forming a geron-
tocracy. By virtue of their numbers, intelligence, and voice, they are becoming united and active in their own behalf.

These erstwhile elders are experienced survivors. Their years were buf-
feted by world wars, the Great Depression, astounding inventions, and the
most dramatic social changes in history. They survived respiratory infections, kidney diseases, childbirth, polio, and the crippling accidents of an
industrial society. Clearly, they benefited from the advancements of medical
technology, but only to face a different specter: chronic disease. Here, too,
they were expected to be resigned to physical, mental, and social decline
in old age. But phrases such as "life-span development," "life quality," "disease prevention," and "health promotion" are becoming part of their vo-
cabulary and, some say, their "just due."

Similarly, long-term care (LTC) is now expected to provide "quality of
care," "maximum functioning," a "continuum of care," and multidisciplinary care via a team approach; in other words, a comprehensive, coordinated system of quality care, practices, and services. Although this concept

---

[1] The Census of April 1, 1980 reported that 32,000 people in the United States had given
their age as 100 years or older. But the Social Security Administration reported that only 15,258
people as of that date were over 100 years. Spokespeople for the Census Bureau suggest that
the Social Security Administration's figure is probably more accurate, as people have a tendency
to overreport their age, particularly in the Southern States (1).

7

is widely accepted in the health community, we have yet to fully develop the ways, and means, for making it happen.

It is in LTC that these issues are being raised for study. And it is in the TNH, designated as a center for training and research, that answers will be found to many questions, including these:

1. What will be the impact on care-giving practices as the findings of research in TNHs become known and as on-site training takes effect?
2. How can the TNH be used to augment the continuum-of-care chain?
3. What incentives will there be to develop programs that least hinder and best promote the maximum functioning of disabled elderly whose handicaps force them to depend on others for assistance?

In these first chapters we consider the factors already in place that will influence the directions we take in LTC and the decisions we make about the role of professional education and research in the nursing home setting.

REFERENCES

1. Hines W: Many of nation's old-timers aren't as old as they say. *Chicago Sun-Times*, December 16, 1982.

The Teaching Nursing Home, edited by Edward L. Schneider et al. © 1985 The Beverly Foundation. Raven Press, New York.

Epidemiologic Considerations

Jacob A. Brody and Daniel J. Foley

Epidemiology, Demography, and Biometry Program, National Institute on Aging, National Institutes of Health, Bethesda, Maryland 20205

Significant demographic changes have occurred this century, and even more impressive shifts are anticipated in the future. As the number of elderly persons in our population increases, plans for geriatric research, education, and care become even more pressing. The teaching nursing home concept marks a turning point in acknowledging the health care implications of these demographic precedents. Demographic trends and future population projections based on changing morbidity and mortality patterns are summarized in this chapter. Specific epidemiologic considerations to be addressed include projections of the number of nursing home residents to the year 2050, a review of available data on nursing homes and trends in nursing home care, a discussion of the limitations of current data, and a description of new data on nursing home use that will be collected in the 1985 National Nursing Home Survey.

DEMOGRAPHIC CHARACTERISTICS

Age

The population in the United States aged 65 and over has been increasing steadily during the 20th century both in absolute numbers and as a percentage of the total population. In 1900, about 4% of our population was aged 65 and over, representing approximately 3 million persons, whereas by 1980 this proportion had risen to 11% and now represents about 25 million persons. During this same period the percentage of people aged 85 and over had risen from 0.2% to 1.1% (1). Perhaps a better way to dramatize the influence of changing mortality patterns is to point out that in 1900 approximately 25% of the population could expect to live more than 65 years, and less than 4% could expect to survive until age 85. However, in 1980, about 70% of the population will live to be 65 and over, and 17% will survive to age 85 (2). Fairly conservative projections to the year 2050 suggest that at least 50% of the population will survive to their 85th birthday, and in that year the population aged 85 and over will constitute at least 15 million people. The obvious social and medical challenge as well as the impact on long-

9

TABLE 1. *Population 65 years and over by race and sex, 1982 (numbers in thousands)[a]*

Age (years)		Total	White	Black	Other races
Total	65 to 74	16,129	14,531	1,380	218
	75 to 84	8,239	7,495	646	98
	85 and over	2,466	2,272	169	24
Male	65 to 74	6,996	6,318	576	102
	75 to 84	3,053	2,761	245	47
	85 and over	728	664	55	9
Female	65 to 74	9,133	8,213	804	116
	75 to 84	5,186	4,734	400	52
	85 and over	1,738	1,609	114	15

[a] Source: Bureau of the Census (3).

term care services implicit from these data and trends will require our utmost dedication and wisdom (3).

Recent data on age, race, and sex for 1982 are presented in Table 1. There were approximately 10.7 million people over age 75, of whom 2.4 million were 85 and over. About 175,000 people survived 95 years or more. The proportion of the elderly (65 years of age and over) who were 75 and over was about 40% in 1982 and will rise to 50% by the year 2000 or sooner (3).

Sex

Throughout the 20th century, age-specific mortality rates were consistently higher for males than females, resulting in greater life expectancy for females. This female survival advantage is also increasing with time in spite of the fact that both sexes are living longer. In 1940 life expectancy at birth for females exceeded that for males by about 4 years (males 60.9, females 65.3), and by 1980 the difference was about 8 years (males 69.8, females 77.5). Consequently, females increasingly predominate in the elderly population of the United States. Of the 25 million people aged 65 and over, about 15 million are females. Expressed in another way, there are 137 females per 100 males in the age group 65 to 74, increasing to 224 females per 100 males in the population aged 85 and over.

Living arrangements are heavily influenced by discrepancies in sex-related survivorship. Most persons 65 and over live in families typically consisting of an elderly married couple with no children or other relatives residing in their homes. In 1978, only 15% of males but 36% of females were living alone. For those aged 75 and over, half the female population was living alone in 1978 as compared to about one-fifth of the male group. In terms of numbers, about 5.5 million women and 1.5 million men over age 65 lived alone (6). With such disproportionate numbers of females to males, it appears that long-term care services will need to focus more on the special needs of aged females than on those of males.

Race

Among the population 65 and over, whites constitute 87.9%, a slightly higher figure than for the entire U.S. population. This varied by age group, increasing from 87.9% for the 65- to 69-year-olds to a high of 91.4% among the 75- to 79-year-olds and declining to 87.8% for those 85 and over. Differences in life expectancy at birth between "whites" and "all others" (85% black) have decreased substantially since 1940. At age 65 the differences in life expectancy between the races were small even in 1940 and have remained so for years. Death rates for the "all other" population were higher than those for whites for all adult age groups up to age 75, but lower for persons aged 75 and over. Although there may be some methodological biases operating here, this crossover effect occurred for both males and females and has been observed both in previous years' mortality data and in other studies involving comparisons among races (7).

Geographic Distribution

Although the population 65 and over for the United States was somewhat greater than 11%, eight states had under 9% in this age range: Alaska, Colorado, Hawaii, Maryland, Nevada, New Mexico, South Carolina, and Wyoming. In four states the population was over 13%: Florida, Iowa, Missouri, and South Dakota. Although Florida had the highest percentage of people aged 65 and over (17.3%) in 1980, two states, California and New York, had more elderly people than Florida, each in excess of 2 million individuals. In addition to Florida, the four states of Pennsylvania, Texas, Illinois, and Ohio each had more than a million elderly people. Thus, 46% of all elderly people in the 50 states lived in the seven states of California, New York, Florida, Pennsylvania, Texas, Illinois, and Ohio (8).

PROJECTED NUMBER OF NURSING HOME RESIDENTS

With the anticipated surge in the number of elderly people, the demand for nursing home care will increase. If conservative population projections and the most recent age and sex prevalence rates of nursing home residents are used, the total increase in nursing home use by 2050 and the considerable excess of females are apparent (Fig. 1). Total females aged 65 and older in nursing homes now number over 800,000 and will increase to an estimated 2.9 million in 2030 and over 4 million in 2050. Similar numbers for males are currently about 300,000 and will rise to an estimated 900,000 in 2030 and over 1.2 million in 2050.

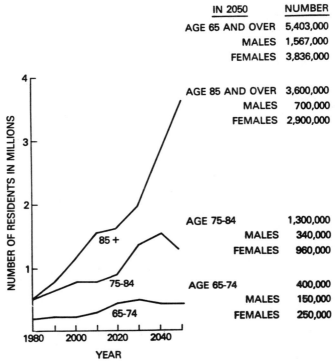

IN 2050	NUMBER
AGE 65 AND OVER	5,403,000
MALES	1,567,000
FEMALES	3,836,000

AGE 85 AND OVER	3,600,000
MALES	700,000
FEMALES	2,900,000

AGE 75-84	1,300,000
MALES	340,000
FEMALES	960,000

AGE 65-74	400,000
MALES	150,000
FEMALES	250,000

FIG. 1. Projected number of nursing home residents in the United States by age: 1980–2050.

SOURCES AND QUALIFICATIONS OF NATIONAL NURSING HOME DATA

Since 1963, the National Center for Health Statistics has utilized two types of surveys to gather nursing home data—universe surveys and sample surveys. The universe surveys, which include all known nursing homes in the United States, consist of questionnaire mailouts eliciting basic information on the facilities such as number of beds, number of residents, type of ownership, and type of care provided. These universe surveys are known as the National Master Facility Inventory and have been conducted in 1963, 1967, 1969, 1971, 1973, 1976, 1978, 1980, and most recently in 1982 (9).

Sample surveys, in which personal interviews are conducted, elicited information in greater detail than the mailout surveys. Sample surveys were completed in 1963, 1964, 1969, 1973–1974, and most recently in 1977. The universe used in drawing the sample for these surveys has in each case been the most recent National Master Facility Inventory listing with newly opened nursing homes added to the list. Consequently, these sample survey data can be no more representative of the establishments in the United

States than the National Master Facility Inventory listing from which the sample was selected (10).

The first three samples were called the Resident Places Surveys (RPS-1, -2, -3). These surveys provided the framework for the development of the National Nursing Home Survey series, which consists of the latter two samples. The next National Nursing Home Survey is tentatively scheduled to begin in March of 1985 and will have some new features that are described at the end of this chapter.

For the earlier Resident Places Surveys no commonly held definitions for the various types of nursing homes were generally held, and, therefore, criteria for classifying homes were developed by the National Center for Health Statistics. These criteria were based on the types of service provided in the home rather than on state licensure laws or on what the home was called. The three classification levels used in the analysis of the Resident Places Surveys data are summarized as follows:

1. A *Nursing Care Home* was defined as one in which 50% or more of the residents received nursing care during the week prior to the survey in the home, with an RN or LPN employed.
2. A *Personal Care with Nursing Home* was defined as one in which either
    (a) over 50% of the residents received nursing care during the week prior to the survey but there were no RNs or LPNs on the staff; or
    (b) some, but fewer than 50%, of the residents received nursing care during the week prior to the survey regardless of the presence of RNs or LPNs on the staff, but one or more of the following conditions were met:
        (i) medications and treatments were administered in accordance with physicians' orders;
        (ii) supervision over self-administered medications was provided;
        (iii) three or more personal services were routinely provided.
3. A *Personal Care Home* was defined as one in which residents routinely received personal care, but no residents received nursing care during the week prior to the survey, and medications and treatments were administered in accordance with physician's orders and supervision over medications, which may be self-administered, was provided (11).

By the late 1960s and early 1970s, the Medicare and Medicaid programs were fully enacted with set standards and criteria for reimbursement. Thus, nursing homes were capable of being further classified by certification status. Certification now refers to a facility's certification by the Medicare or Medicaid program or by both. A skilled nursing facility provides the most intensive nursing care available outside a hospital. Skilled nursing facilities certified by the Medicare program provide posthospital care to eligible Medicare enrollees. Facilities certified by the Medicaid program as skilled nursing facilities provide intensive nursing care on a daily basis to individuals eligible for Medicaid benefits. An intermediate care facility is certified by the Medicaid program only and provides health-related services on a regular basis to persons eligible for Medicaid who do not require hospital or skilled nursing facility care but do require institutional care above the level of room and board (12). Since the National Master Facility Inventory was begun prior to the passage of Medicare and Medicaid legislation, the National Center for Health Statistics criteria for classification of nursing homes according to the type of service provided do not correspond exactly to the criteria for certification under Medicare and Medicaid standards. Furthermore, the 1973–1974 National Nursing Home Survey marks the first time in which the certification status of a facility was ascertained.

INCREASED UTILIZATION AND DEMOGRAPHIC CHANGES

The rate of nursing home use increased dramatically in the past 20 years, fueled primarily by the enactment of the Medicare and Medicaid programs in the mid-1960s. Some of the change may also be related to the policy of deinstitutionalization in mental institutions. Table 2 shows that in 1963 only 2.5% of the nation's elderly resided in nursing homes, comprising about one-half million residents. By 1969, the number of elderly residents in nursing homes had risen to 700,000, or 3.7% of the elderly population. This proportion reached 4.5% by 1974, and the most recent figure from the 1977 National Nursing Home Survey was 4.8% of the elderly population or 1.1 million residents aged 65 and over. At present, one in 20 persons aged 65 and over resides in one of the estimated 19,000 nursing homes across the country.

Table 3 shows the distributions by age and sex of nursing home residents surveyed in 1963, 1969, 1973–1974, and 1977. During these years the number of nursing home residents more than doubled from about one-half million to 1.3 million residents, and changes occurred in the age and sex composition of the nursing home residents. The most notable trend was the increase and then decline in the proportion of very old residents aged 85 and over. This proportion increased by 31% between 1964 and 1973–1974, from 29 to 38%, and then declined to 35% in 1977. This recent decline corresponds to a decrease in utilization since 1973–1974 by those aged 85 and over (Table 2). Although no attempt has been made to fully explain this recent decline in utilization by the 85 and over age group, it seems likely that the rapid expansion of alternative long-term care community services throughout the 1970s has influenced this shift.

During the time in which the proportion of very old residents declined, the proportion of residents under age 65 grew from 11% to 14%, reflecting greater use by a younger cohort. This coincides with a sharp increase in utilization by blacks since 1973–1974, particularly for those aged 65 to 74, whose prevalence increased by 54% (Table 2).

TABLE 2. *Percent of the elderly population in nursing homes, by age, race, and sex: United States, 1963, 1969, 1973–74, and 1977*

| | | Sex | | | Race | |
| | | | | | | Black and other | |
Age and year	Total	Male	Female	White[a]	Total	Black
1963						
65 years and over	2.5	1.8	3.1	2.7	1.0	—
65–74 years	0.8	0.7	0.9	0.8	0.6	—
75–84 years	4.0	2.9	4.8	4.2	1.4	—
85 years and over	14.8	10.6	17.5	15.8	4.2	—
1969						
65 years and over	3.7	2.5	4.6	3.9	1.8	1.8
65–74 years	1.2	1.0	1.3	1.2	1.0	1.0
75–84 years	5.2	3.6	6.2	5.4	2.3	2.2
85 years and over	20.3	13.1	24.8	22.2	5.2	5.2
1973–74[b]						
65 years and over	4.5	3.0	5.6	4.7	2.2	2.2
65–74 years	1.2	1.1	1.3	1.3	1.1	1.1
75–84 years	5.9	4.1	7.1	6.2	3.0	4.0
85 years and over	25.4	18.0	29.0	26.9	9.1	9.6
1977						
65 years and over	4.8	3.1	6.0	5.0	3.0	3.1
65–74 years	1.5	1.3	1.6	1.4	1.7	1.7
75–84 years	6.8	4.7	8.1	7.1	3.9	4.2
85 years and over	21.6	14.0	25.2	22.9	10.2	10.7

[a] Includes persons of Hispanic origin.
[b] Excludes residents in personal care homes.
From ref. 17, with permission.

The difference in life expectancy between males and females continues to increase. Consequently, whereas the proportion of females in the nursing home population rose from 65% in 1963 to 71% in 1977, the proportion of males in the 85-and-over age group dropped from 28% to 20% during this period. During this 14-year period, greater utilization of nursing homes occurred for women than men, the former increasing 7% annually, and the latter 5% annually.

Increased utilization was also evidenced by increases in the number of nursing home admissions. During the interviews with facility administrators, the question was asked: "How many persons were admitted to the facility during the previous calendar year?" Based on the responses to this question, the number of admissions was aggregated for each survey year as displayed in Table 4. The ratio of admissions to beds for each year indicated a sharp increase per 100 beds from about 70 admissions in 1963 to about 111 admissions in 1969 and 98 admissions in 1977.

During this time in which the nursing home population approximately doubled, the number of people aged 65 and over grew by 32% from 17.8

TABLE 3.   *Number and percent of nursing home residents by sex and age: United States, 1963, 1969, 1973–74, and 1977[a]*

	1963		1969		1973–74		1977	
Sex and age	Number	%	Number	%	Number	%	Number	%
Both sexes								
Total	505,200	100	815,100	100	1,075,800	100	1,303,100	100
65 and over	445,500	88	722,200	89	961,500	89	1,126,000	86
65 to 74	89,600	18	138,500	17	163,100	15	211,400	16
75 to 84	207,200	41	321,800	39	384,800	36	464,700	36
85 and over	148,700	29	261,900	32	413,600	38	449,900	35
Males								
Total	173,100	100	251,900	100	318,100	100	375,300	100
65 and over	141,000	81	207,100	82	265,800	84	294,000	78
65 to 74	35,100	20	52,200	21	65,200	20	80,200	21
75 to 84	65,200	38	90,800	36	102,300	32	122,100	33
85 and over	40,700	24	64,100	25	98,300	31	91,700	24
Females								
Total	332,200	100	563,300	100	757,700	100	927,800	100
65 and over	304,500	92	515,200	91	695,800	92	832,000	90
65 to 74	54,500	16	86,300	15	98,000	13	131,200	14
75 to 84	142,000	43	231,500	41	282,500	37	342,600	37
85 and over	108,000	33	197,800	35	315,300	42	358,200	39

[a] Data from National Center for Health Statistics (20,25,26,27).

million in 1963 to 23.5 million in 1977 (Table 4), which changed the proportion of elderly in the total population from 9.4% in 1963 to 10.9% in 1977 (13,14). The increased number of elderly people in the population combined with the expansion of public financing via Medicaid and Medicare have led to striking increases in the size of the facilities and in the level of care provided by the nursing home industry.

INCREASED FACILITY SIZE AND INTENSITY OF CARE

From 1963 to 1973, the average nursing home nearly doubled in size from approximately 40 beds to about 75 beds. An estimated 13,000 facilities provided about one-half million beds in 1963, whereas by 1977 the number of

TABLE 4.   *Number of persons 65 and over in the population, number of nursing home beds, and admissions: United States, 1963, 1969, 1973–74, and 1977[a]*

	1963	1969	1973–74	1977
Population aged 65 and over	17,778,000	19,365,000	21,346,000	23,494,000
Nursing home beds	510,180	854,910	1,174,800	1,402,400
Nursing home admissions	358,480	946,020	1,110,800	1,367,400

[a] Data from refs. 10, 11, 13, 14, 20, 28.

beds almost tripled to 1.4 million, but only 6,000 more new facilities were in operation, representing a 46% increase in facilities and a remarkable 180% increase in beds (Table 4).

During this same period, the intensity of care offered in nursing homes also changed. Just over one-half of the nursing homes in 1963 were classified as nursing home care (53%), and another 30% as personal care homes with some nursing care. The remaining 17% were classified as personal care homes only. In just 6 years (1969), the proportion of facilities classified as nursing care homes increased 10% to reach 63% of all nursing homes, and the proportion of facilities classified as personal care with some nursing care dropped from 30% to 20%. This decrease in personal care homes with some nursing care most likely represented an upgrading of facilities to nursing home care to meet the standards for Medicare and Medicaid reimbursement (15). The proportion of facilities offering exclusively personal care remained fairly constant at about 17%.

The changing care offered in nursing homes is also reflected by the certification status of nursing homes. In 1973, just 15% of all nursing homes were certified for both skilled and intermediate care. In response to incentives provided by the Medicare and Medicaid programs, more facilities began to offer both skilled and intermediate levels of care, so that by 1977, 24% of all facilities were certified for both skilled and intermediate care. This was accompanied by a compensatory shift in which the proportion of homes classified as exclusively skilled nursing facilities dropped from 34% to 19%, presumably to offer a wider range of services (16).

Nursing care, physician visits, and therapy services also increased in nursing homes over the years. Since 1963, the proportion of residents receiving nursing care rose from 60% of all residents to 85% in 1977, and the proportion having seen a physician within the last month increased from 39% to 66%. In 1973, 28% of the residents received one or more therapeutic services, a figure that grew to 35% by 1977 (17).

EPIDEMIOLOGIC CONSIDERATIONS

Two broad trends in nursing home care have been maintained over the past 20 years: increased prevalence of nursing home residents in much larger facilities and a substantial improvement in the level of care provided to these residents. These trends are highly visible when the summary data from each survey year are compared. More specific and detailed analyses of changes in health characteristics of the users of nursing homes are hampered by the numerous caveats in the data when comparisons are made over time, particularly regarding the definition of terms. Furthermore, these data on samples of current residents are biased because of a systematic overrepresentation of long-stay residents versus short-stay residents in nursing homes (18,19). As early as 1963, when the first sample survey was conducted, the notion that nursing homes provided for two distinct groups of users, short-stay and long-stay residents, was addressed in a Vital and Health Statistics Series report (20). On the basis of estimates of admissions and discharges from interviews with facility administrators, the following observation was made:

> Although over 60% of the 1962 admissions were discharged before the end of the calendar year, average length of stay of residents in the institutions at the time of the survey was 3 years. This indicates that many residents stay short periods as well as long periods of time (10).

Descriptive trends based on current resident data reflect changes over time for only a subset of users, the long-stay residents. Statistical inferences are further compromised since estimates derived from the sample of current residents cannot predict the total length of stay for these residents. In order to provide information on completed episodes of care in nursing homes, the 1977 National Nursing Home Survey included data on a nationally representative sample of discharges. However, this results in new problems, since these estimates produce a bias with overrepresentation of short-stay residents (18). More than 50% of the discharges had a length of stay of under 3 months in 1976, as compared to only 15% of the current residents (20). Discharge data, however, are believed to be a more useful indication of the dynamics of nursing home users. They are more likely to approximate the ideal but costly longitudinal data derived from a sample of nursing home admissions followed over time (19,21). Data collection from a sample of nursing home admissions is currently being pretested for inclusion in the next National Nursing Home Survey. This may provide a valid basis for subsequent longitudinal analysis.

Table 5 highlights differences in selected characteristics between the data from the 1977 sample of residents, which are weighted toward the long-stay population, and the 1976 sample of discharges. Discharges are more likely to be male, 36% compared to 29% among current residents; more likely to be married, 23% compared to 12%; and more likely to be younger, 70% of the discharges are under 85 years of age compared to only 65% of the residents. The short-stay bias in the sample of discharges was also highlighted by the greater proportion of discharges whose medical records indicate Medicare as the primary source of payment. Medicare reimbursement in 1976 allowed for a maximum of 100 days of skilled nursing care. Seventeen percent of the discharged residents in 1976 had Medicare listed on the discharge record as the primary source of payment as compared to only 2% of the records for the sample of current residents in 1977. Current residents may have originally entered the nursing home under Medicare coverage but converted to another source of payment, such as Medicaid, on expiration of Medicare coverage. This conversion rate can be established accurately in a prospective study of nursing home admissions. A review of these data suggests that short-stay residents form a large subpopulation

TABLE 5. *Differences in Selected Characteristics of Discharges in 1976 and Residents in 1977*

Characteristic	Proportion of discharges (%)	Proportion of residents (%)
Married	23	12
Male	36	29
Older than 85	30	35
Diagnoses and conditions		
Mental disorders and senility	12	22
Heart disease	45	43
Fractures	10	3
Cancer	8	2
Bedfast	22	5
Continence difficulties	49	45
Source of support		
Medicare	17	2
Medicaid	35	48
Median length of stay	75 days	597 days

From ref. 20, with permission.

whose characteristics more closely resemble those of the noninstitutional-ized population. It has been estimated that whereas 5% of those 65 and over are in nursing homes on any given day (prevalence), the annual rate for total nursing home use would probably be 8 to 9% of the elderly population (22). At present, there are no national estimates of incidence rates for ad-mission to nursing homes.

NURSING HOME RESIDENTS VERSUS ELDERLY NONINSTITUTIONALIZED PERSONS

The following section contrasts the demographic characteristics of the current residents and those of the elderly noninstitutionalized population aged 65 and over. The magnitude of the differences between nursing home residents and the community-based elderly may be influenced by the long-stay bias in the 1977 sample of current residents referred to above. These figures do, however, represent the 5% minimum population of elderly re-siding in nursing homes.

Age and Marital Status

Advancing age increases the likelihood of residence in a nursing home. In 1977, about 5% of the population aged 65 and over resided in nursing homes, and this figure increased to 20% for those aged 85 and over (Table 2). The median age for current residents was 81, whereas the median age for the total population aged 65 and over is slightly less than 72 years. In the noninstitutionalized elderly population aged 65 and over only about 9%

TABLE 6. *Number of nursing home residents and the noninstitutionalized population aged 65 years and over and percent distribution by age, sex, race, and marital status: United States, 1977[a]*

Age, sex, race, and marital status	Nursing home residents	Noninstitutionalized population
Age		
65 to 74 years	18.8	64.0
75 years and over	81.2	36.0
Sex		
Male	26.1	41.3
Female	73.9	58.7
Race		
White[b]	93.3	90.6
Black and other	6.7	9.4
Marital status		
Married	12.1	53.2
Widowed	69.3	36.4
Divorced or separated	4.5	4.2
Never married	14.2	6.2

[a] Data are expressed as percent of total population, i.e., of 1,126,000 nursing home residents and 22,100,000 noninstitutionalized elderly people.
[b] Includes persons of hispanic origin.
From ref. 17, with permission.

were aged 85 and above in 1977, whereas among nursing home residents aged 65 and over, 40% were in this age group.

Living alone is another frequently cited antecedent for nursing home stays, and this is evident in the comparison of marital status between the nursing home residents aged 65 and over and the elderly noninstitutionalized population aged 65 and over. About 69% of the residents were widowed, compared to only 36% of the noninstitutionalized elderly, and over 14% of the residents had never married, compared to 6% of the noninstitutionalized elderly (Table 6).

Sex Differences

Because of the seven-year difference in life expectancy between males and females, there are substantial differences in age and marital status between male and female nursing home residents. In general, the male population (29%) is younger, averaging 74 years of age, as compared to 80 years for the female residents. Only 78% of the male residents are aged 65 and over compared to 90% of the females (Table 3). Because females are more likely to be older, they are also more likely to be widowed. Seventy-two percent of female residents are widowed as compared to 38% of male residents. Conversely, a larger proportion of males were married (23%) than females (7%) (17).

TABLE 7. *Number of females per 100 males in the noninstitutionalized population and the nursing home resident population for selected age groups, 1977[a]*

Age group	Noninstitutionalized	Nursing home residents
65 and over	141	283
65 to 74	130	164
75 to 84	159	281
85 +	189	391

[a] Data from refs. 14, 17.

The ratio of females to males is greater in the nursing home population than in the comparable noninstitutionalized population. Table 7 compares the ratio of females to males for selected age groups over 65 for the nursing home population and the noninstitutionalized population aged 65 and over in 1977. Among the noninstitutionalized elderly aged 65 and over there are about 141 females per 100 males, whereas among the residents in nursing homes aged 65 and over there are about 283 females per 100 males. These figures increased to 189 and 391, respectively, for the group 85 and over.

Racial Differences

The nursing home population is predominantly white (92%), with only 6% of the residents being black as compared to 11.7% in the total U.S. population and about 1% Hispanic as compared to approximately 6.5% in the total U.S. population (20,23).

CHRONIC CONDITIONS AND FUNCTIONAL HEALTH

Nursing home residents are plagued with multiple chronic conditions and require considerable assistance in activities of daily living. Nearly all residents had one or more chronic conditions: the most prevalent was arteriosclerosis (48%), followed by heart trouble (34%), senility (32%), arthritis and rheumatism (25%), hypertension (21%), and diabetes (15%). The prevalence of each of these conditions increased with age (17).

Functional health within the nursing home population was measured by the performance in the activities of daily living. Of the six activities, bathing, dressing, using the toilet room, mobility, incontinence, and eating, the proportion requiring assistance was over 50% in five of the six activities, the exception being eating. Fully one-fourth of the elderly nursing home residents were dependent in all six activities of daily living, increasing from 18% for those aged 65 to 74 to 24% and 28% for those aged 75 to 85 and 85 and over, respectively.

Figure 2 highlights the predominance of required assistance in five of the six activities of daily living within the elderly nursing home population in 1977 as compared to the noninstitutionalized elderly population in 1979.

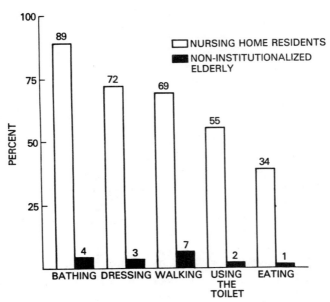

FIG. 2. Percent of elderly persons aged 65 and over requiring assistance in the activities of daily living among nursing home residents and the noninstitutionalized elderly.

Several studies on factors influencing nursing home admissions have shown that requiring assistance in the performance of an activity of daily living contributes significantly in the decision to admit a person to a nursing home (24). By comparison, about 89% of elderly nursing home residents require assistance in bathing as compared to about 4% of elderly nonresidents; 72% compared to 3% for dressing, 69% compared to 7% for walking, 55% compared to 2% for using the toilet, and 34% compared to less than 1% for eating. Fully 93% of the elderly nursing home residents were dependent in at least one activity of daily living as compared to about 9% for the elderly noninstitutionalized population.

THE 1985 NATIONAL NURSING HOME SURVEY

The next National Nursing Home Survey will once again establish a data base on nursing homes and nursing home residents. New data components will be pretested and evaluated for possible inclusion in this major national survey. The inclusion of these components depends on the degree of success experienced and the costs of collecting these new data in the pretest, particularly since support for these new items are from federal agencies other than the National Center for Health Statistics.

The nursing staff component, supported by the Bureau of Health Professions, collects detailed information from a sample of registered nurses about topics associated with job retention. With the demand for geriatric nursing increasing, these data will provide valuable information on the turnover of skilled nursing staff in nursing homes.

The family component, supported by the National Institute on Aging and the National Center for Health Statistics, collects information by means of a telephone survey of patients' families on the demographic and social background of residents in nursing homes. These data will provide valuable information on the characteristics of the institutionalized elderly, particularly with respect to the presence of family and any changes in health status and household composition just prior to institutionalization. Questions will also be asked about other nursing home stays.

The National Institute of Mental Health is supporting a Current Resident Interview and Examination Component to collect health status information from the patient by means of a brief physical examination and mental functioning measures. This effort will provide data on a national level for assessing the magnitude of mental dysfunction within the nursing home population, a very difficult figure to establish from the previous surveys.

The admission component, supported by the Health Care Financing Administration and the National Institute on Aging, collects information at four different times approximately 3 months apart on a sample of admissions to produce information on the patterns of use of various nursing home reimbursement mechanisms and the transitions into and out of nursing homes. Thus far, only discharge data have been analyzed to study the users of nursing homes by providing information on completed durations of stay. These discharge data indicate that the numbers and the health and social characteristics of the short-stay users differ considerably from the long-stay users. Additionally, many users have multiple stays over a relatively short period of time, and this can only be quantified by prospective study of a representative cohort of admissions. Longitudinal data will yield new information on multiple admissions and probabilities for reentering a nursing home within the year. With funds permitting, there will be the opportunity for extension of the surveillance period so that we may more fully know the morbidity and mortality outcomes of the range of nursing home users, particularly by age and sex categories.

CONCLUSION

The role of long-term care will surely broaden as more people reach their 65th birthday. For now, the most pressing issue in long-term care seems to be overwhelming costs and who pays them. Fifty-seven percent of nursing home costs are paid by public funds. The remaining 43% is paid for by direct personal out-of-pocket payments by the residents and their families. Hospitalization costs are split the same as nursing home costs with regard to public and private expenditures. However, private insurance plans cover about 75% of the private expenditures on hospital care but less than 2% of private expenditures on nursing home care.

Further knowledge of the size and composition as well as the morbidity and mortality patterns among the users of nursing home care will aid in the development of comprehensive long-term health care policies in both the private and public sectors. The studies currently proposed to follow admission cohorts in a longitudinal fashion and to pursue the nature of the relationships among nursing home residents and available family and other community support should contribute to the understanding of the dynamics of nursing home use. Moreover, the teaching nursing home model is expected to bring about a salutary forum to improve health care for the elderly. Still, the challenge to define the requirements of current and future elderly people in terms of overall long-term care needs, which include institutionalized as well as noninstitutionalized mechanisms, still looms before us.

REFERENCES

1. Brody JA, Brock DB: Epidemiologic and statistical characteristics of the United States elderly population, in Finch CE, Schneider EL (eds): *Handbook of the Biology of Aging*. New York, Van Nostrand Reinhold, 1984 (in press).
2. Brody JA: Life expectancy and the health of older people. *J Am Geriatr Soc* 1982;30:681–683.
3. US Bureau of the Census: *America in Transition: An Aging Society. Current Population Reports, Series P-23-No. 128*. Washington, DC, US Government Printing Office, 1983.
4. Siegel JS: Recent and prospective demographic trends for the elderly population and some implications for health care, in *Proceedings of the Second Conference on the Epidemiology of Aging*. Washington, DC, US Government Printing Office, 1980, pp. 289–314.
5. Brotman HB: Every ninth American. Report prepared for *Developments in Aging*, 1980, Special Committee on Aging, United States Senate.
6. US Bureau of the Census: *Marital Status and Living Arrangements: March 1978. Current Population Reports. Series P-20-No. 338*. Washington, DC, US Government Printing Office, 1979.
7. Brock DB, Brody JA: Statistical and epidemiologic characteristics of the United States elderly population, in Andres R, Bierman EL, Hazzard WR (eds): *Principles of Geriatric Medicine*. New York, McGraw-Hill, 1984 (in press).
8. US Bureau of the Census: *Social and Economic Characteristics of the Older Population 1978. Current Population Reports. Series P-23-No. 85*. Washington, DC, US Government Printing Office, 1979.
9. Sirrocco A: *Employees in Nursing Homes in the United States: 1977 National Nursing Home Survey*. Hyattsville, MD, National Center for Health Statistics, 1981.
10. Bryant E, Taube C: *Utilization of Institutions for the Aged and Chronically Ill, United States: April–June 1963*. Hyattsville, MD, National Center for Health Statistics, 1966.
11. Gagnon R: *Selected Characteristics of Nursing Homes for the Aged and Chronically Ill, United States: June–August 1969*. Hyattsville, MD, National Center for Health Statistics, 1974.
12. Foley DJ: *Nursing Home Utilization in California, Illinois, Massachusetts, New York, and Texas: 1977 National Nursing Home Survey*. Hyattsville, MD, National Center for Health Statistics, 1980.
13. US Bureau of the Census: *Estimates of the Population of the United States, by Age, Sex, and Race: April 1, 1960 to July 1, 1973. Current Population Reports, Series P-25-No. 519*. Washington, DC, US Government Printing Office, 1975.
14. US Bureau of the Census: *Estimates of the Population of the United States by Age, Sex, and Race: 1970 to 1977. Current Population Reports, Series P-25-No. 721*. Washington, DC, US Government Printing Office, 1978.

15. Ingram D: *Measures of Chronic Illness Among Residents of Nursing Homes, United States: June–August 1969.* Hyattsville, MD, National Center for Health Statistics, 1974.
16. Bloom B: *Utilization and Financial Characteristics of Nursing Homes in the United States: 1977 National Nursing Home Survey.* Hyattsville, MD, National Center for Health Statistics, 1981.
17. Hing E: *Characteristics of Nursing Home Residents, Health Status, and Care Received: 1977 National Nursing Home Survey.* Hyattsville, MD, National Center for Health Statistics, 1981.
18. Hing E, Zappolo A: A comparison of data availability and population differences using two approaches to measure characteristics of nursing home patients. *Am Stat Assoc Proc Soc Stat Sect* 1978;173–178.
19. Liu K, Manton KG: The characteristics and utilization pattern of an admission cohort of nursing home patients. *Gerontologist* 1983;23:92–98.
20. Van Nostrand JF, Zappolo A, Hing E, et al: *The National Nursing Home Survey: 1977 Summary for the United States.* Hyattsville, MD, National Center for Health Statistics, 1979.
21. Keeler EB, Kane RL, Solomon DH: Short- and long-term residents of nursing homes. *Med Care* 1981;19:363–369.
22. Liu K, Palesch YY: The nursing home population: Different perspectives and implications for policy. *Health Care Financ Rev* 1981;3:15–23.
23. The 1980 Census of Population: *General Population Characteristics for the United States. Summary, PC80-1-B1.* Washington, DC, US Government Printing Office, 1980.
24. Branch LG, Jette AM: A prospective study of long-term care institutionalization among the aged. *Am J Public Health* 1982;17:1373–1378.
25. Zappolo A: *Characteristics, Social Contacts, and Activities of Nursing Home Residents.* Rockville, Maryland, National Center for Health Statistics, 1977.
26. Mathis ES: *Characteristics of Residents in Nursing and Personal Care Homes.* Rockville, Maryland, National Center for Health Statistics, 1973.
27. Wunderlich GS: *Characteristics of Residents in Institutions for the Aged and Chronically Ill.* Washington, DC, National Center for Health Statistics, 1965.
28. Sutton JF: *Utilization of Nursing Homes.* Hyattsville, Maryland, National Center for Health Statistics, 1977.

The Teaching Nursing Home, edited by Edward L. Schneider et al. © 1985 The Beverly Foundation. Raven Press, New York.

The Social Aspects of Nursing Home Care

Elaine M. Brody

Philadelphia Geriatrics Center, Philadelphia, Pennsylvania 19141

If efforts to maintain or improve the health and functioning of nursing home residents are not to be sabotaged, attention to the psychosocial aspects of care is a practical necessity as well as an ethical responsibility. Several decades of gerontological research have led to a firm consensus that social needs and health needs are inextricably linked. The accumulated knowledge points unequivocally to the reciprocal dependence of mental and physical health on each other and on social and environmental factors. Those interrelationships are no less valid when older people live in nursing homes than when they live in the community. In fact, health professionals must attend even more to the psychosocial aspects of care for those who are institutionalized. Nursing home residents have experienced numerous and severe psychological and social losses. Their capacities to replenish the psychosocial supplies they need have been sharply reduced and they are vulnerable to additional assaults.

In that context, if a goal of teaching nursing homes (TNHs) is to strive for excellence in the education of health professionals who are responsible for the care of nursing home residents, TNHs should teach a psychological/social/medical/environmental model of care and treatment. If a parallel goal is to increase knowledge about the health of nursing home residents through research, that research should include psychosocial and environmental as well as biomedical investigations.

The psychosocial needs of different groups of nursing home residents vary to some extent because of their diversity. Two and one-half million people are in nursing homes in the course of a given year, and 23% to 38% of all people who are 65 years of age or over will spend time in such a facility at some point in their lives (1). These residents differ in the reasons for which they are admitted: 50% stay less than 3 months, having been admitted for terminal care or for time-limited rehabilitation or convalescence; others will make the nursing home their home for many years (1).

The nursing home population is heterogeneous in many other ways. It includes men and women; some "young" old though most are the "old" old; the economically well off and the indigent; those with mental or physical problems and those with both; those who are severely disabled and those who

27

function comparatively well; and those who are rich in family ties as well as those who have none. They have varied personalities, life-styles, and backgrounds—religious, cultural, ethnic, educational, and social. Some residents have experienced lifelong deprivations or disturbances; the problems of others are primarily age related. And some have been institutionalized most of their adult lives, though most were admitted in old age.

Despite their heterogeneity, nursing home residents share certain needs and values with all human beings. It is accepted that residents need quality maintenance services that preserve biological life (such as adequate shelter, environmental safety, food, and sanitation), health services to help them achieve maximum health and functional capacities (such as medical and nursing care, physical medicine and rehabilitation, nutritional programs, and others), and personal care (such as feeding, dressing, toileting, grooming, and bathing).

All taxonomies of human needs go beyond survival, subsistence, and medical maintenance to include needs for interpersonal contacts and relationships, love, affection, belongingness, self-esteem and the esteem of others, gratifying recreational and occupational activities, maintenance of roles, a sense of mastery and autonomy, and some degree of self-determination or control of one's own life (2). Older people in nursing homes share these needs.

Recently, in his Kleemeier lecture, Lawton conceptualized "the good life" as having four sectors: behavioral competence, psychological well-being, perceived quality of life, and objective environment. He translated these into the social goals of health, happiness, satisfaction with daily life, and a good environment (3).

There is no "perfect life," of course, and nursing home residents have a smaller chance than most other people of having a good life. But research and clinical practice have developed a considerable body of information about the ways in which nursing homes can foster or impede achievement of "the good life"—that is, how nursing homes meet (or fail to meet) needs that speak to the residents' psychological and social well-being.

CHARACTERISTICS OF NURSING HOME RESIDENTS

Social factors are critical determinants of why older people become residents of nursing homes. The surveys and epidemiological studies reviewed in the previous chapter (J. A. Brody and D. J. Foley, *this volume*) identified the demographic and health predictors of admissions. It merits reemphasis that such data do not fully explain why residents are in nursing homes, since they are outnumbered in a two-to-one ratio by equally old and impaired people who are not in institutions. Compared with the total elderly population, fewer of the institutionalized are married (14% vs. 56%). Fewer residents have at least one living adult child (half vs. 82% of all older people). More of those with children have only one child rather than two or more, and they have fewer daughters (4). When seriously impaired older people live in the community, they live with their families (5).

It is obvious that surviving spouses of institutionalized residents are likely to be in advanced old age. Adult children are often in late middle age or early old age. Catastrophic illnesses or deaths among these aging children often precipitate institutionalization of the parent (6). Other children may live at a geographic distance. Though most residents have some family ties, 10% are without anyone at all to name as "next-to-kin" (7), and the family resources of others are very slender.

Among the most salient characteristics shared by nursing home residents, then, is that virtually all have experienced multiple interpersonal losses as well as losses of physical and mental function, losses of roles, and economic losses. Many of the sources of supplies they need for "the good life"—supplies such as opportunities for nurturance, love, intimacy, and social support—have been depleted.

DECISION MAKING AND RELOCATION

Decisions for admission to nursing homes are made reluctantly by older people and their families. A consistent body of research has emphatically refuted the myth of "dumping." The relationships of older people with their families are strong and viable. Families (daughters, in particular) provide the vast majority of health and social services to the noninstitutionalized elderly. Older people prefer to live separately from their adult children and, in the main, share households with them when economic need or needs for care make such arrangements necessary. Most families of those who are institutionalized have endured prolonged and unrelenting strain in attempting to avoid such placement.

When institutionalization of an older person is necessary, the painful decision almost invariably precipitates severe emotional upset in the older person and the family. But such people rarely are offered counseling help. Moreover, the decisions occur in the context of social policies that set eligibility criteria and reimbursement for various types of facilities and therefore determine whether beds are available. The eligibility criteria, in the main, are linked to medical needs, omitting consideration of the social situations that so often cause the need for admission.

When nursing home placement is being considered, the individuals concerned are involved in making major and dramatic changes in their lifestyles. They face separation from family, home and possessions, and community. Some are deprived abruptly of the cherished traditions and customs of the ethnic context in which they have lived. Some are placed inappropriately. They often are anxious, fearful, and feel abandoned or rejected; psychologically, placement has overtones of death. Family members may suffer from feelings of grief and guilt.

In the main, knowledge about appropriate admission procedures has not been applied. Despite the universal professional emphasis on the importance of functional assessment and multidisciplinary professional evaluation, these rarely occur. Though participation of the elderly person in the decision-making process and careful preparation for admission are predictors of adjustment and well-being, such processes most often do not take place. The medical certification of need by a physician is generally a *pro forma* paper review. Although most of the older people have mental diagnoses, the vast majority of them enter nursing homes without having had any contact at all with any part of the mental health system (8).

Many of the negative effects that are often attributed to living in an institution have been shown to occur during the waiting period for admission (9,10). The move to a nursing home is often preceded by several other moves made in rapid succession—to and among the homes of family members, into and out of hospitals, from hospitals to nursing homes, and from one nursing home to another (7,10–12). Multiple moves continue even after admission—to hospitals and back to the same or another nursing facility, and from one room to another within the same facility in response to changing care needs, which may reflect artificial criteria for reimbursement. The net result is that those who are most vulnerable to the negative psychological and physical effects that can occur when old people are moved are constantly on the move nonetheless (4,13–16).

The debate about the phenomenon known as the relocation effect (that is, the possible negative effects of moving older people, such as mortality and morbidity) has escalated to the proportions of a feud. Undoubtedly, the perfect study remains to be done. But the fact that some participants in the controversy persist in focusing on the "mortality hypothesis" (the assertion that relocation results in a higher death rate) obscures other issues.

Depending on a variety of conditions, relocation can have positive or negative outcomes in terms of the psychological and emotional effects on the movers. For example, older people improve when they choose to move or when they move to better environments. But when mentally or physically frail old people are moved involuntarily without careful preparation or participation in the decision-making process, there often are negative effects such as depression, withdrawal, agitation, and anxiety. Even under optimum conditions, such symptoms may take several months to subside (17). The characteristics of the institutionalized are precisely those of the groups that have been identified as most vulnerable to such effects: the physically ill, the depressed, the confused and disoriented, and those who are moved involuntarily.

In short, the processes of decision-making, admission, and orientation are critical to the well-being of residents. Yet very few of the older people who are constantly being moved receive the kinds of services shown by research to mitigate those effects: opportunities for choice, participation in the decision-making process, individual preparation through counseling, and pre- and postmove orientation to the receiving facility.

Some moves are necessary and in the older person's best interests, of course, but others are not—notably, frequent and frenetic moves made in response to changing reimbursement criteria.

As matters stand, then, the decision-making and relocation processes operate to produce what Lawton calls "the polar opposite" of the "good life," that is, "the bad life" (3).

THE EFFECTS OF LIVING IN AN INSTITUTION

Reviews of the extensive literature on the consequences of living in an institution yield a litany of negative effects such as depression, poor adjustment, unhappiness, negative self-image, apathy, docility, withdrawal, unresponsiveness, and feelings of insignificance and impotence (18–22). These have been attributed to such factors as lack of privacy, restricted mobility, separation from society and family, routinization, depersonalization, desexualization, loss of self-determination, lack of productive or enjoyable activity, and the surrender of the control of one's own life to nursing home staff.

Although some factors that contribute to the level of well-being of nursing home residents may be preexisting population differences and experiences, the psychosocial qualities of the institutional environment are also influential. Research suggests that residents decline in emotionally cold, dehumanized, dependency-fostering environments (23). On the other hand, improvement is seen in facilities that treat people with warmth and positive attitudes, encourage autonomy and independence, foster personalization (i.e., privacy and respect), encourage access to the outside world and social interaction, and do not expect docility and passivity (23,24).

Residents who try to continue their preadmission life-styles are affected by the extent to which such continuation is permitted by the institution (25). Congruence between individual needs and environmental opportunity (mainly for privacy and impulse expression) are important to adjustment (26).

Overall, research data and clinical evidence indicate that positive effects accrue when the institutional environment is modified in the direction of being less "total," that is, when the institution is deinstitutionalized. Attention to that psychosocial component of the "good life" is a necessity if the decline induced by fitting nursing residents into procrustean beds is to be avoided (27).[1]

---

[1] Procrustes, a legendary highwayman of Attica, tied his victims on an iron bed and stretched or cut off their legs to adapt them to its length.

SPECIAL TREATMENT PROGRAMS

Over the years, a number of special psychosocial programs have been designed to improve the functioning of institutionalized older people. The inventory includes various milieu therapies, therapeutic communities, special group activities, occupational and social therapeutic techniques, reality orientation, remotivation, behavior therapy, individualized treatment of "excess disabilities," resocialization, and a long list of activity therapies based on productive, creative, or diversional pursuits. Some of the programs were evaluated by research; others are simply presented as case studies (19,20,28). Several common themes emerging from the literature can be identified:

1. All programs, whether clinical or experimental, report successful outcomes. It is probable that these programs did achieve some success for some people. The poverty of many institutional environments in relation to the psychosocial programs makes it likely that residents responded favorably to the various efforts to enrich their lives.

2. Programs are most successful when they (a) are geared to realistic goals that attend to the particular mental and/or physical disabilities of the target population and (b) take into account the residents' individual interests, skills, preferences, and culture.

3. Staff attitudes are central to the residents' well-being. Negative, disrespectful, or belittling attitudes increase dependency and confusion, whereas permissive, friendly attitudes, positive expectations, and encouragement of competent behavior are beneficial. Many research evaluations of experimental treatments state explicitly that the success of the treatment may have resulted as much from the increased contact of staff with residents and the favorable staff attitudes fostered as from the specific treatment itself.

4. Since most of the residents' psychosocial disabilities, like their physical and mental disabilities, are chronic, gains often disappear when the treatment is withdrawn. This does not indicate failure; rather, the expectation of "cure" for chronic problems may be inappropriate.

In the face of the accumulated evidence, however, social policy pays only token attention to providing for the psychosocial programming that contributes to the "good life": requirements and reimbursement for appropriate staff are minimal at best. Moreover, there is a tendency for institutions to allocate fewer psychosocial treatment resources to people who are least able to obtain such supplies on their own—those who are room bound or "problem" residents, for example (29). Inaccurate notions about residents' ability to benefit from programs may result in those who need more getting less.

FAMILIES OF THE INSTITUTIONALIZED

The myth of the dumping of old people into institutions has generated another myth—that once institutionalization has taken place, families sever their ties with their elderly relatives.

In contrast to the major research that has addressed the family relationships of noninstitutionalized elderly, research is sparse with respect to the family relationships of nursing home residents and the effects of those relationships on the residents' well-being. There has been even less attention to the well-being of the families themselves as it is affected by the institutionalization of the elderly family member. Some information is available, however.

Data from the Survey of Institutionalized Persons (7) indicated that the vast majority of nursing home residents who had a spouse, a child, or a grandchild received (at the least) weekly visits. They also had much more social contact outside the institution than those without next of kin. Family members were active in ways other than providing affective support: nine out of 10 were in touch with nursing home personnel; they managed the residents' money as the need arose, and some (17%) contributed financially to the residents' support.

These data do not speak to the qualitative aspects of the families' activities. Important neglected issues include the content of family visits to the residents and their contacts with staff, how admission affects the relationships of the older person and family, the effects family members experience from having institutionalized relatives and from visiting them, and how they perceive their roles and activities.

The continuity of family relationships with elderly nursing home residents has been described by a number of practitioners. In addition, some small-scale research studies have dealt with some of the relevant issues. The older person's and family's well-being depend to a significant extent on their mutual relationships after admission. That fact, well known to clinicians (30–35), has been supported by research findings. One study, for example, found that the well-being of residents in nursing and old-age homes is vitally affected by their receiving attention and assistance not from just anyone but from one or more preferred members of the family or a devoted friend (36).

A study of institutionalized women with senile dementia found that their emotional investment in family had become relatively more important to them in old age (37). Two other studies similarly indicated that families continue to be involved with their older relatives after nursing home admission and visit regularly (38,39).

Another investigation (40), which examined the consequences of institutionalization on the quality of family relationships, noted beneficial effects in more than half of the cases. Renewed closeness and strengthening of ties was attributed to the alleviation of preadmission stress, improved physical and/or mental status of the parent, an opportunity to spend time together in recreational and interpersonal activities rather than care-taking ones, and the parent's involvement with other residents in the institution. The facility in which the study was carried out provided a high quality of care, encouraged the involvement of families, and made family members feel welcome and comfortable. If this had not been so, the outcome on relationships might have been different.

There are many descriptive reports of the benefits that occur when facilities convey welcoming attitudes, when staff attitudes toward families are positive, and when there are family-focused approaches and special services to families (32,41). Unfortunately, many institutional facilities do little to sustain family relationships.

It is interesting to note that after nursing home placement, family members sustain the very roles that are most valued by the noninstitutionalized elderly—specifically, affective support and money management (42). They also continue to play the role of advocate and mediator with the formal system of care, though the "system" has become the microsystem of the nursing home rather than the social/health macrosystem in the community (42). This role is ambiguous; its active enactment by family members may elicit criticism from staff, who feel that such family members are complainers or are "interfering." Conversely, passivity or absence of family members may be interpreted as a lack of concern.

The importance of families to residents' well-being underlines the fact that there are residents without family, whose families are not close at hand geographically, or who are alienated from their families. They require special attention for feelings of loss, loneliness, or abandonment and need special services such as those usually given by family members to help them achieve some measure of a "good life."

THE RESIDENT "MIX"

Segregation versus integration on residents is a perennial issue, often phrased in terms of whether people with senile dementia should share living quarters with those who are cognitively intact. Experience indicates that segregation into different living areas of those with moderate to severe senile dementia and those who are intact cognitively (32,43,44) is a means of fostering the "good life" for both groups.

Those residents whose mental impairment is associated with behavioral problems—that is, those who babble, are incontinent, smear feces, wander, or rummage in other people's closets or bureau drawers—are extraordinarily distressing to their intact peers. Lawton's survey of staff and families at the Philadelphia Geriatric Center overwhelmingly indicated a preference for segregation (45).

Older people with functional mental disorders may, in some instances, share quarters with those who are "normal" when the decision is made carefully on a case-by-case basis. Obviously, such a mix is not advisable when such residents are dangerous to themselves or others, have acute or severe psychoses requiring special care, or exhibit behavior that is distressing to others.

A different integration versus segregation issue concerns the mix of short-stay and long-stay residents. In the course of a year, over a million people are admitted for terminal care or for rehabilitation or convalescence. They are the short-stayers, leaving within 3 months. In general, they share rooms and living areas with their long-stay peers who will remain in the facilities for the rest of their lives, often years. The effects of such integration have received virtually no attention at all.

THE PHYSICAL ENVIRONMENT

There has been increasing recognition of the importance of the physical environment as a component of quality care that affects the functioning of the residents and contributes to "the good life." Considerable attention has been given to designing nursing homes in order to help residents' enhance their ability to perceive their environment, negotiate its space, and derive some esthetic and affective benefits (46).

Though prosthetic and therapeutic design approaches positively affect the residents' well-being, Lawton (46) argues that in general older people are passive in the design process and should be more assertively involved in choosing among environmental alternatives, expressing their preferences, and (in many cases) creating their own environments. Despite impaired functioning, "for every level of competence . . . there is some range within which active behavior may become facilitated, with a resulting increment in self-esteem and psychological well-being." Moreover, he states, the person needs challenge as well as support, and serving as an expert is a powerful means of enhancing self-esteem. Growth-producing challenge may be enhanced by engaging the older person in affecting the environment. The resident can be encouraged to choose furniture, decor, or spatial arrangements, to make decisions about priorities in construction of the personal milieu, and to share evaluations of what is and is not functional in the environment.

The Weiss Institute of the Philadelphia Geriatric Center is an example of a careful process of planning a nursing home. The building, designed specifically for residents with senile dementia, was constructed after considerable research. The overall strategy was to compensate to the fullest possible extent for the disorientation, memory loss, and loss of social skills and sense of self that are typical of that population. The Weiss Institute aimed to eliminate architectural barriers to functioning, to support orientation by color-coding, installation of clocks, clear identification of rooms and spaces, to provide prosthetic aids such as grab bars, and to avoid the long institutional corridors. Research evaluation of the building indicated that residents spent more time in the "social space" and less time in bedrooms. There was less crowding, more participation in enriching activities, and more signs of interest in the physical surroundings. Staff and relatives overwhelmingly favored the new environment, and family visiting increased (45,47).

Another environmental consideration is the location of facilities. It is generally agreed that the old-fashioned practice of locating institutions away from residential areas is inappropriate. In fact, in the majority of cases (57%), a facility is selected because of its geographic proximity to family members. Most spouses (90%), children (70%), and grandchildren (74%) who were named as next of kin by nursing home residents live within 24 miles (7). When facilities are embedded in local communities, it is easier for family and friends to visit and be visited by the institutionalized older people. Such locations also foster integration of institutions with the community to the fullest possible extent by encouraging visits from schools, religious groups, other organizations, and volunteers.

THE INSTITUTIONAL SYSTEM

A basic issue about what constitutes a "good life" for nursing home residents is what the organization and atmosphere of nursing homes should be like. Unquestionably, a significant share of the responsibility for psychosocial well-being belongs to the social and physical attributes of the facilities themselves.

Nursing homes are not intrinsically "bad" places; they do have the potential and capability to be different and better. Although there is no doubt that any kind of institution is vulnerable to abuse, it has been demonstrated time and again that nursing homes can have different and "better" qualities that are in turn associated with improvement in the residents' well-being (28).

It bears repetition that the favorable institutional environment is the one that is less "total." Such an institution permits a life-style more similar to the natural one of a person's own home, fosters independence rather than dependence, encourages control over one's own life, offers privacy, respect, and personalization, treats residents with warmth and positive attitudes, does not regard the passive or docile individual as the "good" patient, and is congruent with individual needs.

Beyond those basic attributes that nursing homes should have, the evidence is that a "good life" for residents depends on their lives having dignity, meaning, and enjoyment. It is important for nursing homes to exploit the potentially healthy areas of functioning: residual strengths, self-determination, humor, assertiveness, creativity, capacity for enjoyment, gratification of work, meaningful personal relationships, and the continuity of past roles and development of new ones. Achievement of such goals relies on creative and varied social and recreational programming.

The discrepancy between what nursing homes should be like and what actually exists results in part from the historical roots of nursing homes, which increased rapidly without a thoughtful approach to developing a new and appropriate model. Among the "ancestors" of current long-term care facilities are institutions that were designed for other purposes—the county home, the convalescent home, and the acute general or psychiatric hospital, for example. The net result of relying for directions on those institutions is that nursing homes are a patchwork of borrowed identities.

The concept of "home" should be key to the nursing home setting to the fullest possible extent. There should be an orientation to the normal rhythm of life rather than routines that are set for the convenience of the provider. The predominant model at present is based heavily on the acute-care medical hospital in architecture, staffing patterns, organization of services, medical orientation, and overall atmosphere. The medical emphasis on "patient compliance" pervades every aspect of life for the residents. Yet research demonstrates that it is assertiveness and participation that are in the residents' best interests rather than the passivity and surrender of control that characterize the individual described as a "good patient." One recent study found that the quality of life of aged residents of institutions is directly related to the degree of influence of the "medical model" and the degree of "institutional totality" (48).

The strictly medical focus and the primacy of physicians in long-term care facilities are also questioned by physicians themselves. To quote a physician-authored article in the *New England Journal of Medicine*:

> The goals of long-term care and of acute care may be irreconcilable. The fundamental concern in the former is quality of life and restoration of function; in the latter it is treatment and cure of medical illness. Commitment to the chronically ill entails attending to social and emotional as well as physical needs. . . . It [a long-term care institution] should not be remade in the image of the hospital. . . (49).

The hospital-like characteristics of nursing homes are reinforced by social policies that link reimbursement to medical/nursing needs and the life-safety code but have only token requirements for meeting psychosocial needs. Status as full-time "patients" in the acute care sense is grossly inappropriate in view of the fact that one-third of the long-stay residents have been in the facilities in which they live for 1 to 3 years and another third have been there for 3 years or more (50). More than 20% of them have lived there for more than 5 years (7).

The argument often advanced to justify the medical atmosphere and routines is that the resident population is "sick." This is undoubtedly true, and the need for sophisticated medical and nursing services is unquestioned. Residents' ailments are primarily chronic rather than acute, however, and actual medical care uses only a small fraction (2.1%) of staff time (51). Another explanation offered for the routinization and lack of regard for individuality is that it is impossible to do otherwise in an institution. The difficulties of effecting change too often are used as a rationale for the failure to make efforts to do so.

MENTAL HEALTH CARE

Major factors in the provision of quality care in institutions are the existence, orientation, skills, attitudes, and appropriateness of staff. Some progressive facilities have staff psychiatrists, professional social workers, and activity therapists. In the main, however, such professionals are underrepresented or entirely absent. It is unlikely that that situation will be remedied unless their presence is federally mandated.

It is a shocking fact that there are no Federal standards for mental health care in nursing homes. This is especially inappropriate in light of the fact that a minimum of 50 to 60% of nursing home residents suffer from senile dementia. An additional 17% have either functional mental disorders or retardation (50), and "hordes" of residents show "obvious evidence of full-blown clinical depression" (8). The survey by the American Psychiatric Association (APA) points out that the general practitioners who provide most of the medical care rarely call for consultations from psychiatrists, who, in turn, are inexperienced in dealing with an aged population (8). The Social Security Act's Conditions of Participation (405.1130 Social Services) gives a token nod to social work and activity therapy but does not require that such staff be professionally trained.

The Long-Term Care Facility Study (8) made a searing indictment of the lack of attention to psychosocial services in nursing homes. It pointed out that in most facilities there was very limited understanding of the importance of psychosocial services. The goal of enriching the residents' daily environment was frequently cited in policies but rarely implemented. Personnel were not oriented to psychosocial needs or rehabilitation concepts. Fewer than half of the patients had any psychosocial data at all on their charts. Similarly, fewer than half (49.2%) of the facilities had any social work staff, and when they did, there were no requirements that such staff be professionally trained or be full time employees. About one-quarter of the facilities (26.3%) had a full-time social worker. A similar pattern obtained with respect to activities personnel. Psychologists and other behavioral scientists are virtually absent.

The bulk of resident care is given by nonprofessional, untrained staff. The APA survey found that within nursing homes, including those certified for Medicare and Medicaid, the necessity for pretraining the aides was ignored for all practical purposes despite some lip service to Federal regulations. Thus, tens of thousands of "patient care" personnel are largely, if not totally, ignorant of the particulars of caring for sick old people, and in-service programs have been of very limited scope (8).

THE CHALLENGE TO THE TEACHING NURSING HOME

Older people, their families, and society as a whole have expressed in unmistakable terms the value that living in one's own home is vastly preferable to living in an institution. This has given rise to the view of the nursing home as the feared last resort when all else fails and helps to explain the constellation of negative emotions that accompanies the process of admission and the call for "alternatives." "Home" means all those things of which the resident is deprived—privacy, control over one's life-style, ownership of one's own corner of physical space, freedom and self-determination, the opportunity to exercise choice, and being surrounded by one's own family and one's own possessions.

Barring major biomedical breakthroughs that would prevent or cure chronic ailments such as senile dementia, there is no doubt that the number of nursing home beds will increase (see J. A. Brody and D. J. Foley, *this volume*). The TNH experiments are a significant effort to bring knowledge and professionalism to bear on the situation. However, there is a more profound challenge.

Are the various TNHs teaching and conducting research on models of care that put available knowledge to work? Or does what is taught reflect the orientation of a particular profession, the goals of a particular provider, the perceptions of third-party payers as to the functions to which they key reimbursement, or the values of the historical ancestor institutions? Do the TNHs continue to rely for their developmental directions on the personalities of such institutions rather than evolving as a new model with a unique personality and identity? Whose values determine what life in a nursing home is like and what the TNH teaches?

In short, are the TNHs iteratively teaching old, inappropriate, models? Is any TNH experiment moving innovatively toward the creation of a new model—one that is shaped by a coherent concept synthesizing the needs and the perspectives of the people it is designed to serve? Surely, a major task of the TNH is to move toward the creation of nursing home environments that attend to all sectors of well-being or the "good life" and blends them creatively.

OLDER PEOPLE WHO CANNOT OBTAIN NURSING HOME CARE

Although this chapter has focused on the social aspects of care for those older people who are residents of nursing homes, a word is in order about those impaired older people who should be residents but are being denied admission.

Increasing costs of institutional care for the aged have occasioned a variety of government cost containment measures. People with senile dementia of the Alzheimer's types (SDAT) who need nursing home care the most and who constitute the majority of long-stay residents will be the principal group to suffer from cutbacks. Research at the Philadelphia Geriatric Center documents what nursing home personnel know well—that such people require more staff time and more direct care than those who are physically ill with an absence of SDAT.

Those who suffer from SDAT require heavy care, yet they are the ones most likely to be Medicaid dependent and eligible for the Intermediate Care Facility reimbursement rate, which is lower than the Skilled Nursing Facility rate. This situation inadvertently provides nursing homes with incentives to prevent admissions (52). At the same time, community services to aid overburdened caregivers are sparse. Costs to other parts of the health systems are increased by backups in acute hospitals when nursing home beds cannot be found. Medicaid eligibility and SDAT are the principal causes of such "administratively necessary" backup days, but Diagnosis Related Groups will close even that temporary resource. Since all avenues of care for SDAT patients are shrinking, society appears to be making a statement to the effect that they are not a public responsibility.

THE TEACHING NURSING HOME AND SOCIAL POLICY

Finally, if it is to be ultimately effective in improving the quality of care for older people in nursing homes, the TNH must communicate what it knows about the social policy constraints on its efforts. It is important to identify policies (such as grossly inadequate reimbursement) that make nursing home beds unavailable to those who need them most, that do not reimburse for assessment, that compel unnecessary and mismanaged moves, that do not take psychosocial and mental health needs into account either in admission criteria or in reimbursable services after admission, and that do not foster interdisciplinary approaches. Such advocacy is a significant part of the TNH's responsibility. If that role is abdicated, the TNH undermines the very purpose of its existence.

REFERENCES

1. Liu F, Palesch Y: The nursing home population: Different perspectives and implications for policy. *Health Care Financ Rev* 1981;3:15–23.
2. Maslow AH: *Motivation and Personality*. New York, Harper & Row, 1954.
3. Lawton MP: Environment and other determinants of well-being in older people, Robert W. Kleemeier Memorial Lecture. *Gerontologist* 1983;23:349–357.
4. Brody EM: The formal support network: Congregate treatment settings for residents with senescent brain dysfunction, in Miller NE, Cohen GD (eds): *Aging, Vol. 15: Clinical Aspects of Alzheimer's Disease and Senile Dementia*. New York, Raven Press, 1981, pp 301–331.
5. Brody SJ, Poulshock SW, Masciocchi CF: The family care unit: A major consideration in the long-term support system. *Gerontologist* 1978;18:556–561.
6. Brody EM: The aging family. *Gerontologist* 1966;6:201–206.
7. U.S. Bureau of the Census: *1976 Survey of Institutionalized Persons. Current Population Reports, Special Studies, Series P-23, No. 69*. Washington, DC, Bureau of the Census, 1978.
8. Glasscote RM: *Old Folks at Homes: A Field Study of Nursing and Board-and-Care Homes*. Washington, American Psychiatric Association and the National Association for Mental Health, Joint Information Service, 1976.

9. Lieberman MA, Prock VN, Tobin SS: Psychological effects of institutionalization. *J Gerontol* 1968;3:343–353.
10. Brody EM: Follow-up study of applicants and non-applicants to a voluntary home. *Gerontologist* 1969;9:187–196.
11. Friedsam HJ, Dick HR: Decisions leading to institutionalization of the aged. Unpublished Final Report, Social Security Administration, Cooperative Research and Demonstration Grant Program, Project 037 (C1) 20-031, 1963.
12. Townsend P: The effects of family structure on the likelihood of admission to an institution in old age: The application of a general theory, in Shanas E, Streib GF (eds): *Social Structure and the Family: Generational Relations*. Englewood Cliffs, NJ, Prentice Hall, 1965, pp 163–187.
13. Epstein L, Simon A: Alternatives to state hospitalization for the geriatric mentally ill. *Am J Psychiatry* 1968;124:955–961.
14. Stotsky B: Nursing home or mental hospital: Which is better for the geriatric mental patient? *J Genet Psychol* 1967;3:113–117.
15. Stotsky B: A systematic study of therapeutic interventions in nursing homes. *Genet Psychol Monogr* 1967;76:257–320.
16. Brody EM, Johnsen PT, Fulcomer MC, et al: Women's changing roles and help to the elderly: Attitudes of three generations of women. *J Gerontol* 1983;38:597–607.
17. Brody EM, Kleban MH, Moss M: Measuring the impact of change. *Gerontologist* 1974;14:299–305.
18. Lieberman MA: Institutionalization of the aged: Effects on behavior. *J Gerontol* 1969;24:330–340.
19. Bennett R, Eisdorfer C: The institutional environment and behavior change, in Sherwood S (ed): *Long-Term Care: A Handbook for Researchers, Planners and Providers*. New York, Spectrum Publications, 1975, pp 391–454.
20. Gottesman LE, Brody EM: Psycho-social intervention programs within the institutional setting, in Sherwood S (ed): *Long-Term Care: A Handbook for Researcher, Planners, and Providers*. New York, Spectrum Publications, 1975, pp 455–510.
21. Lawton MP: Institutions for the aged: Theory, content, and methods for research. *Gerontologist* 1970;10:305–312.
22. Lawton MP, Nahemow L: Ecology and the aging process, in Eisdorfer C, Lawton MP (eds): *The Psychology of Adult Development and Aging*. Washington, DC, American Psychological Association, 1973, pp 619–674.
23. Lieberman MA, Prock VN, Tobin SS: Psychological effects of institutionalization. *J Gerontol* 1968;3:343–353.
24. Marlowe RA: Effects of environment on elderly state hospital relocatees. Paper presented at 44th annual meeting of the Pacific Sociological Association, 1973.
25. Bennett R, Nahemow L: A two-year followup study of the process of social adjustment in residents in a home for the aged, in Lawton MP, Lawton FG (eds): *Mental Impairment in the Aged*. Philadelphia, Philadelphia Geriatric Center, 1965, pp 88–105.
26. Kahana E: Effects of matching institutional environments and needs of the aged. Paper presented at Annual Meeting of the Gerontological Society, Houston, TX, 1971.
27. Brody EM: A million procrustean beds. *Gerontologist* 1973;13:430–435.
28. Brody EM: The aging of the family. *Ann Am Acad Pol Soc Sci* 1978;438:13–27.
29. US DHEW, PHS, Office of Nursing Home Affairs: Long-Term Care Facility Improvement Study: Introductory Report, July 1975.
30. Brody EM, Spark G: Institutionalization of the aged: A family crisis. *Fam Process* 1966;5:76–90.
31. Spark G, Brody EM: The aged are family members. *Fam Process* 1970;9:195–210.
32. Brody EM: *Long-Term Care of Older People: A Practical Guide*. New York, Human Sciences Press, 1977.
33. Safford F: *Developing a Training Program for Families of the Mentally Impaired Aged*. New York, Isabella Geriatric Center, undated.
34. Locker R, Rublin A: Clinical aspects of facilitating relocation. *Gerontologist* 1974;14:295–299.
35. Dobrof R, Litwak E: *Maintenance of Family Ties of Long-Term Care Patients: Theory and Guide to Practice*. Washington, DC, USDHEW, NIMH, 1977.

36. Harel Z, Noelker L: The impact of social integration on the well-being and survival of institutionalized aged. Paper presented at Annual Meeting of the Gerontological Society, Dallas, TX, 1978.
37. Kleban MH, Brody EM: Prediction of improvement in mentally impaired aged: Personality ratings by social workers. *J Gerontol* 1972;27:69–76.
38. Moss M, Kurland P: Family visiting with institutionalized mentally impaired aged. *J Gerontol Soc Work* 1979;1:271–278.
39. York JL, Caslyn RJ: Family involvement in nursing homes. *Gerontologist* 1977;17:500–505.
40. Smith KF, Bengtson VL: Positive consequences of institutionalization: Solidarity between elderly parents and their middle-aged children. *Gerontologist* 1979;19:438–447.
41. Lewis K: Services for families of the institutionalized aged. *Aging* 1980; July–August, Nos 309–310:15–19.
42. Brody EM: The role of the family in nursing homes: Implications for research and public policy. Paper presented at Conference on Mental Illness in Nursing Homes: An Agenda for Research. Rockville, MD, NIMH, 1983.
43. Ablowitz M: Pairing rational and demented patients in long-term care facilities [Letter to the Editor]. *J Am Geriatr Soc* 1983;31:627.
44. Gang R, Ackerman JO: Pairing rational and demented patients in long-term care facilities [Letter to the Editor]. *J Am Geriatr Soc* 1983;31:627–628.
45. Liebowitz B, Lawton MP, Waldman A: Designing for confused elderly people: Lessons from the Weiss Institute. *Am Inst Architect J* 1979;68:59–61.
46. Lawton MP: A theoretical view of the person in a health care environment. Paper presented at Symposium on Social Supports and the Health of the Future Aged, International Symposium on Aging 2000: Our Health Care Destiny. Texas Research Institute of Mental Sciences, Texas Department of Mental Health and Retardation, Houston, TX, 1983.
47. Lawton MP: Institutions and alternatives for older people. *Health Social Work* 1978;3:109–134.
48. Bowker LH: *Humanizing Institutions for the Aged.* Lexington, MA, DC Heath, 1982.
49. Gillick MR: Is the care of the chronically ill a medical prerogative? *N Engl J Med* 1984;310:190–193.
50. U.S. National Center for Health Statistics: *Advance Data, An Overview of Nursing Home Characteristics: Provisional Data from the 1977 National Nursing Home Survey.* Washington, DC, USDHEW, PHS, 1978.
51. Gottesman LE, Bourestom NC: Why nursing homes do what they do. *Gerontologist* 1974;14:501–506.
52. US General Accounting Office: *Medicaid and Nursing Home Care: Cost Increases and the Need for Services are Creating Problems for the State and the Elderly.* Washington, DC, US Government Printing Office, 1983.

The Teaching Nursing Home, edited by Edward L. Schneider et al. © 1985 The Beverly Foundation. Raven Press, New York.

Long-Term Care for the Elderly: Policy and Economic Issues

Anne R. Somers

Environmental and Community Medicine, University of Medicine and Dentistry of New Jersey, Rutgers Medical School, Piscataway, New Jersey 08854

There is no universally accepted definition of good long-term care (LTC). For our purpose, the term will be used to refer to services required to improve or maintain the health and functioning of patients with chronic disease and disability involving significant functional impairment or to permit death to occur as painlessly as possible. The goal of such care should always be the maximum functional independence (MFI) of which the patient is capable.

The patient's needs may be affected by episodes of acute illness, sometimes requiring hospitalization, but the primary continuing need is for less intensive care, generally lasting at least 6 months, sometimes years,[1] and usually involving a combination of medical (physical and mental) and social services. Both institutional and community- or home-based care are included. Although our focus is on formal care, i.e., care that is paid for in one way or another, there is no intention to deprecate the value of informal or unpaid care. On the contrary, good LTC envisions maximum realistic use of family, neighbors, and other volunteers. Nor does the goal of MFI imply professional failure in the case of a dying patient. At times, patient autonomy in the choice of where and how to die may constitute MFI and hence should be facilitated.

It may be objected that this is the definition of an ideal goal rather than the existing situation. This may be true. However, agreement on some goal is essential as a yardstick against which to evaluate the rapidly evolving programs, institutions, and personnel, which constitute the "long-term care industry," and for appraisal of the different financial incentives implicit in different methods of paying for such care.

---

[1] There is no agreement on the definition of "long term" in LTC. The American Hospital Association defines a "long-term hospital" as one where the average length of stay exceeds 30 days. The National Center for Health Statistics defines a "chronic condition" as any condition lasting 3 months or more or one of a specific list of conditions—heart disease, cancer, stroke, etc.—regardless of duration (1). This paper concentrates primarily on conditions requiring at least 6 months' care.

In sharp contrast to the comprehensive, coordinated system contemplated in the above definition, LTC in the United States is highly fragmented and directed far more to "custodial" than to preventive or rehabilitative care. These characteristics were implicit in the historical development of LTC in this country. Although the general concept of LTC has emerged only in the past decade, separate elements have long been present in the American health care scene. These include mental hospitals, institutions for the mentally retarded, tuberculosis (TB) and other chronic disease hospitals, portions of the Veterans Administration (VA) medical system, domiciliary or "old folks" homes, and some forms of public health nursing. The common denominator for most of these programs was their remoteness from the mainstream of American medicine: different patients, different objectives, different institutions, different types of manpower, and different methods of financing. The general acceptance of this difference was clearly expressed and set in legislative concrete in the Medicare law, which prohibited payment for "custodial" care (Social Security Act, Sec. 1862).

However, the American health care scene is dynamic. No sooner had the Medicare capstone been placed on this professional and financial Iron Curtain separating acute from chronic care than efforts were begun to tear it down. Many state mental institutions were closed or drastically reduced in size. Some short-term patients were admitted to community hospitals, where they could qualify for Medicare or private insurance. Many long-term patients were simply dumped on the community or transferred to nursing homes and Medicaid support. Tuberculosis hospitals were closed or transformed into institutions for general chronic diseases with some hope of obtaining Medicare, or at least Medicaid, reimbursement. Even the tightly closed VA system began to contract out with some community services.

The major assault on the whole hopeless, incurable, "custodial" approach grew out of the "geriatric imperative" with its insistent demand for better and more relevant LTC (2), a demand that led to emergence of the exciting new fields of gerontology and geriatrics and the concept that inspired this book. Among the major factors involved in this change of public and professional interest were the increasing life expectancy of the elderly, the growing proportion of elderly in the population, the shift from acute to chronic disease and disability as the major causes of morbidity, the "shrinking" American family, reduced sources of informal LTC, and the escalating costs of all types of health care, especially for the elderly.

By the early 1980s, the demand for reform of LTC had become one of the major health concerns of the nation, probably second only to cost controls. The problem was made doubly difficult, however, by the vastly changed economic and political environment. Whereas the great expansion of funding and other resources for acute care came during the period of unprecedented affluence following World War II, the need for LTC emerged in a period of drastic financial retrenchment. New benefits, which might have been added, almost automatically, to Medicare, Medicaid, or private health insurance in the 1960s, are now subjected to intense critical and frequently hostile scrutiny, especially on financial grounds. The whole question of financial incentives, largely ignored in the 1960s, has become a major preoccupation of third-party payers and policymakers. It is now virtually impossible to discuss, let along enact, any significant reform of LTC benefits or systems without carefully considering the financial arrangements.

The purpose of this chapter is (a) to identify some of the major policy and financial issues involving LTC; and (b) to suggest some implications for the teaching nursing home (TNH). Most of the issues are presented as dichotomies, deliberately oversimplified in order to emphasize the existing polarity of views. Appropriate public policy probably lies somewhere in the broad middle ground between those extremes. However, it is helpful to understand the extremes in order to arrive at a viable compromise.

MAJOR POLICY AND ECONOMIC ISSUES

Appropriate LTC Population: Age-Based or Needs Based?

Some reasonable definition of the target population for a national LTC program is essential. The definition must both meet the need and be financially and politically viable. Should all those 65 and over be considered potential candidates? Or only those over 75? Or 85? Or should only those elderly, however defined, who meet certain criteria regarding physical, functional, and/or socioeconomic dependency be considered? Or should dependency, however defined, rather than age be the major factor, thus opening the program to the younger disabled and closing it to nondependent elders?

In 1982, 26.8 million Americans were 65 or over, a figure that is expected to rise to 32 million in 1990 and 35 million by 2000 (3). With regard to the total disabled population, a Department of Health and Human Services (DHHS) Long-Term Care Task Force estimated in 1980 that about six million were "substantially disabled," either physically or mentally, and represented the "hard core of the LTC population" (4). Although it is not known how many of these six million were over 65, two facts are known: (a) the elderly currently dominate the LTC population; (b) young people who are mentally ill, retarded, or physically disabled are increasing and obviously require more services over a lifetime than those whose problems begin in old age (4).

As the enormity of the potential population at risk becomes clearer, the old debate over "age" versus "need" as the primary criterion for eligibility to public health care programs has reemerged (5) with persuasive arguments on both sides. In favor of "need" as the primary criterion is the argument that not all those over any given age, even 85, will, in fact, need LTC. In a time of financial stringency, granting eligibility to those with lesser needs may result in inadequate benefits for those most in need. It also probably means higher taxes or premium costs.

Opponents of "need" as the principal criterion point to the numerous drawbacks involved in any form of individual means testing: high administration costs, arbitrary definitions or cutoff points, frequent incentives to fraud, and political opposition. Age, they say, is a good presumptive measure of need, far easier to administer, more acceptable politically, and more compatible with the basic goal of LTC—maximum functional independence.

This is an issue that has concerned policymakers for decades. In general, we have resolved it in typical American fashion by recognizing both criteria simultaneously. We have age-based Social Security backed up by needs-based Supplemental Security Income (SSI); age-based Medicare backed up by needs-based Medicaid. The current Administration appears ideologically committed to the needs approach but has not been able to dismantle the age-based programs because of their popularity. Still, the serious financial problems facing both Social Security and Medicare systems suggest that some modification is inevitable.

As a practical matter, the issue with respect to LTC amounts to a choice between the Medicare model or the Medicaid model. In sharp contrast to Medicare's near universal coverage of the elderly and seriously disabled, Medicaid eligibility involves a means test. Coverage is limited to the very poor, who in most states constitute only 5 to 10% of the elderly. Aside from gross regional inequities, the result is discrimination against patients with long-term illness and disability, a situation that many consider totally inconsistent with the central role of chronic illness and disability in our society.

I have previously suggested that basic Medicare eligibility be extended to LTC benefits, the additional costs to be met by transfer of Medicaid funds now used for LTC to Medicare, fixed prices on all Medicare benefits, acute and long term, and reasonable cost-sharing for all patients (6). Others disagree with this approach (7). Almost certainly, it would be more expensive in the first few years. Over the long run, however, the opposite should prove true. To meet the short-run problem, eligibility might be limited, say for the first decade, to those 75 and over and to those disabled adults of any age who currently qualify for Medicare. Using 1982 figures, the result would have been about 13.5 million eligibles, some 10.5 million over 75 (3) and 3 million younger disabled on Medicare (Department of Health and Human Services, Health Care Financing Administration, *personal communication*). If elderly eligibility were limited to those over 85, about 2.5 million, the total would have been only 5.5 million. Cost estimates based on these and other projections are essential to the development of any viable program.

Basic Goal of LTC: Cure Versus Care?

This dichotomy is generally stated as "medical model versus social model," which emphasizes the alleged turf battle between physicians and nonphysicians for control of the LTC field. Such a conflict, however, goes far beyond any such interprofessional competition and involves a basic difference in philosophy and objectives.

The arguments against the "cure" model for LTC are well known and persuasive. First, by definition, chronic disease is generally incurable. High-technology medicine is ill-suited to the long-term, often discouraging demands of chronic illness; and the aversion of most physicians to nursing-home and home-care patients is undeniable. But can we, or should we, turn the clock back? Whether most providers like it or not, chronic disease is now the central, not a peripheral, challenge in modern health care. And the preservation or restoration of functional ability is, or should be, the central goal of all such care (8,9), not a secondary consideration to be delegated to nonphysicians when the former have given up on the "interesting" aspects of a case, i.e., the diagnosis and treatment of reversible disease.

The potential significance of this new approach was suggested recently by Butler (10). Replying to the question of whether we may be entering a new era of hope for the elderly, he said:

> Definitely. We cannot prevent people from growing old and we cannot forestall death indefinitely. But we now have a chance to do something about the debilities of aging. We can intervene with treatments that relate to hormones, like estrogen; that relate to diet, such as calcium; and medications that control blood pressure, which is a high risk factor for strokes. And we have the new gerontology, which instead of focusing on disease, disability, and death, is beginning to get behind the underlying mechanisms of aging (10).

Indeed, most geriatricians think in terms of a comprehensive model that encompasses both curing (insofar as possible) and caring, the medical model and the social model, acute care and LTC. Among most third-party payers, however, the dichotomy remains as rigid as the Iron Curtain. Is this accidental, inevitable, or a consequence of present methods of financing?

My definition of LTC seeks to combine the two goals. The large caring component is recognized in the long-term coverage, the need for a multidisciplinary approach, and some additional managerial functions. But the basic goal of MFI preserves the activist, optimistic bias and related responsibilities characteristic of acute care medicine as opposed to "custodial care."

Undoubtedly, the definition could be improved, and the effort should be made, with inputs not only from all the relevant professions and interests in this country but from other countries with more, or different, experience. Such a definition of goal would then provide the base line for evaluation of programs, agencies, and institutions seeking recognition in the LTC field and for the design of appropriate financial incentives, including incentives for prevention and rehabilitation.

Relation to Other Health Care Programs: Mainstream Versus Separate?

This issue overlaps with the two previous points. The case for a separate LTC system is often supported by both those who believe it to be very important and those who do not. The former stress their fear of the "medical model," especially as embodied in Medicare, and the inadequacies of technological medicine in relation to chronic illness and disability. At the same time, some supporters of the acute-care system fear that extension of Medicare coverage to LTC could seriously dilute the funds now available for acute care.

Despite these understandable concerns the case for programmatic integration, or at least close coordination, seems compelling. In the first place, even a well-funded LTC program, if separate from the acute-care mainstream, will never achieve the same level of quality; it will remain a "stepchild," as Medicaid has been from the beginning. "Separate but equal" will not be equal in this area any more than it was in education. In the inevitable rationing of resources, it will be much easier to shortchange LTC if it is organizationally and financially separate from acute care.

Second, separation is not cost-effective. Despite the discrimination against LTC, the costs have grown astronomically. Nursing home and home care are now the fastest growing segments of the health care field. It may appear easier at the outset to limit Medicaid costs than to limit those of Medicare, but the final accounting has to consider the increased and often inappropriate demand on Medicare, increased demands on the VA, and other forms of cost-shifting.

One of the major causes of the current cost escalation is the duplication (along with remaining gaps) that inevitably results from a congeries of separate programs.

Primary Financial Responsibility: Public Versus Private?

Thus far, the private insurance industry has shown little interest in LTC, chiefly because the financial stakes seemed inconsequential and the potential market very poor (11,12). The first of these conditions is changing, especially with the rapid growth in nursing home expenditures, and this could change the prospects for marketing. There are some who now feel that new and "creative" financial instruments might enable private insurers to enter the market successfully (13). The best-known such proposal is the Social Health Maintenance Organization (S/HMO). Also mentioned is a possible Medical Retirement Account (MRA), modeled after the tax-subsidized Individual Retirement Account (IRA) (14).

The carriers are well advised to be cautious. It was their inability to successfully underwrite acute care for the elderly and disabled that led to Medicare in the first place; there is little reason to expect any better experience with LTC. There is a significant place for the private carriers and plans in the LTC field, but on a subsidiary basis.[2] A recent article challenges Blue Cross/Blue Shield to initiate innovation in this broad area, perhaps on a joint venture basis with some of the religious multihospital systems (15). As another example, the insurance industry could well decide to assume primary responsibility for promoting the exciting life-care or continuing-care retirement community concept, which could probably profit from some additional managerial and actuarial expertise (16–19).

A recent review of developments in the European health care systems, most of which have been experiencing the same financial problems as those in the United States, concludes that the future belongs to a public/private mix. The following refers specifically to The Netherlands but, by implication, to most of the Continent:

> It seems probable that the division of the population into two groups according to income level will be abolished, implying one uniform system for all people. At the same time it can be expected that market forces will be incorporated into the system. The most likely outcome will be a uniform public insurance scheme covering a minimum set of benefits, to be accompanied by regulated private insurance (20).

Some might say that such a formula could apply equally to the United States. If agreement could be reached on such a fundamental issue, research could then focus on the nature of the appropriate mix, especially in the LTC field, and on incentives relating thereto.

With respect to nursing homes and home health agencies, the private sector is dominant. Here, the division is between nonprofit and for-profit ownership. It appears, at least at the present time, that this is generally a healthy situation, conducive to innovation and constructive competition, provided that all conform to basic national and/or state standards respecting nondiscrimination in admissions and quality.

Public Responsibility: Federal Versus State/Local Governments

Within the public arena, however defined, there is the recurring issue of which level or levels of government should be responsible for administration. Medicare is or was, until very recently, a strictly Federal program. (Under new waiver authority, several states now have a large degree of control over financial arrangements and provider payments. How far this

---

[2] A decade ago, H. M. Somers and I suggested one such approach—an NHI model of "regulated competition" based at least partly on the Federal Employees Health Benefits Program. Under our plan, a limited number of approved public and private carriers would be permitted to compete for membership enrollment. But coverage of all Americans would be assured through a Social Security type of financing supplemented by general revenue funds. And all approved carriers would have to provide a basic package of defined benefits (14a). If my LTC proposal were accepted, the basic package would include LTC, as well as acute and preventive, services. Thus, the advantages of private enterprise could be combined with publicly assured universal coverage and an economical balanced package of basic benefits.

evolution of responsibility will be carried remains to be seen.) In Medicaid, the Federal role was much smaller to begin with, and even that is being rapidly eroded. Medicaid could end up simply as another block grant for states to use largely as they see fit.

Demands for the reconsideration of federal/state relations recur frequently but rarely result in significant action. The flurry of activity, and even excitement, that followed President Reagan's call for a "New Federalism" in his 1982 State of the Union message has almost completely disappeared. The possibility of federalizing Medicaid in return for state assumption of several welfare programs attracted considerable attention. However, with respect to LTC, it turned out that federalization was not being seriously considered. Medicaid was to be split into two or three segments, with the LTC segment remaining with the states, but with even less adequate federal funding than today. Given the recurrent fiscal plight of most states, the fate of LTC under such conditions would almost certainly deteriorate rather than improve (21).

The failure of the "New Federalism" proposal to generate any serious reforms, either in Medicaid or in LTC, is unfortunate. Certainly, there are no easy answers, but that should not discourage the effort to seek new approaches.

Public Programs: General Revenues Versus Special Taxes

Almost all public programs providing LTC in the United States are supported by funds derived from general revenues. This includes Medicaid, the VA, Titles III and XX, and state/local mental and chronic hospitals. The only exception is Medicare, whose relatively small contribution to LTC is financed in the same way as its acute care—primarily through the Part A (hospital insurance) payroll tax. About 75% of the funds for Part B, originally raised on a 50/50 basis between the premium tax paid by beneficiaries and general revenues, now come from the latter. Altogether, at least 90% of the public money spent for LTC comes from general revenues.

This contrasts sharply with the financing of acute care, where the proportions are roughly reversed. Does this dichotomy make sense? Is it a good way of "spreading the heat?" Or does it accentuate the Iron Curtain between acute-care coverage, with its near-universal and quasi-insurance entitlement, and LTC, with its highly limited welfare connotation? Or both? Assuming that it makes sense to tear down, or at least modify, this Iron Curtain and the Medicaid responsibility for LTC for the elderly and disabled is transfered to Medicare, a comingling of general and special revenues would result. If, at the same time, Medicare Parts A and B were merged, this would provide further opportunity for redesigning and strengthening the revenue structure.

A special federal excise tax on alcohol and tobacco products could also provide a source of additional funds. Such a tax, earmarked for the Medicare

Hospital Insurance Trust Fund, was recommended by the 1983 Advisory Council on Social Security "based on the demonstrated correlation between the use of these products and increased health care costs" (22).

Considering the huge sums involved in LTC in years to come, whether financed under Medicare or Medicaid, careful study should be given to the most equitable and effective distribution of the burden between different methods and levels of taxation.

Primary Setting: Institutional Versus Community/Home

The strong proinstitutional incentives in both Medicare and Medicaid and their expensive consequences have been recognized for a number of years. Some consider this the central issue in the entire LTC field. Why the failure to take corrective action? Most obviously, the strength of the vested interests that have grown up around the current arrangements makes it exceedingly difficult to effect any significant transfer of entitlements or funds, especially in a period of serious financial constraints. Indeed, there is fear on the part of many policymakers that effective transfer is impossible and that any addition of now-uncovered community- or home-based LTC benefits will inevitably end up not as substitutions but as "add-ons" to the existing benefit package. Moreover, they fear that any new benefits will result in many new beneficiaries. Many LTC patients who are now making do at home or in some residential facility with family or other informal supports would then end up on a public program. According to this view, even if the per capita costs of caring for individual patients could be cut by substituting more community/home care for institutional care, the total costs would rise substantially.

One result of these conflicting pressures—"Cut the costs of institutional care!" versus "Don't open the possibility of more beneficiaries!"—has been the series of extensive LTC demonstration projects sponsored by the Health Care Financing Administration and several private foundations (23). According to one review of 70 published studies relating to such projects, the most dramatic finding was the reduced mortality rate experienced by home health care patients (24). Other positive results included gains in contentment, mental functioning, and social activity.

With respect to cost savings, the results appear inconclusive (25,26). According to one interim report, average expenditures for 4,000 Medicaid patients under the New York State Long-Term Home Health Care Program, 1978–1982 were half the cost of an equivalent level of institutional care (27). A 1978 study by Weissert reported that adult day care offered the possibility of savings of 37 to 60% compared to the cost of nursing home care on a period-of-care basis (28). A Health Policy Alternatives study concluded, "Cost savings can be demonstrated in some, but not all, cases" (24).

Inconclusive or not, states are being pressured to move faster in this direction, strictly on the basis of economy. There is danger that the pendulum could now swing too far in the opposite direction, that we could repeat the earlier indiscriminate deinstitutionalization of the mentally ill, again with predictable results. Abuse and neglect are not limited to the institutional setting (29). Some experts on aging are already warning of this. Dr. Sidney Katz, Director of the Gerontology Center, Brown University, pointed out recently that "changing social demographics will force national policy away from the philosophy of reinforcing dependence upon family and friends for help, to greater support of the role of institutions in care for the elderly" (30).

Despite the idealistic motivation of many sponsors of the community- and home-based projects, there is some danger that this development will further exacerbate the acute care versus LTC dichotomy to the further detriment of the latter. What is badly needed at this time is recognition of the need and appropriateness of both institutional and noninstitutional modalities in given situations. Criteria should include the level and duration of care needed and the availability of family and other informal supports. Neither patients nor their care-givers should be locked into any one modality. Some way must be found, through objective functional assessment, case management, patient cost-sharing, appropriate reimbursement policies, tax incentives for family care, respite services, family education, etc., to facilitate access to the broad range of services that will make possible the most cost-effective and health-effective use of all our LTC resources. Clearly, research in this area is needed. One promising area for examination is the cross-cutting life-care retirement community.

Organization of Patient Care: Primary Physician Versus Case Manager

Long-term care generally involves a greater "management" function than acute care. First, the patient is likely to be older, poorer, to have fewer family supports, little or no health insurance and, of course, to be sick or disabled for a much longer period of time. Second, the length of time over which care has to be sustained usually involves changing physical and/or mental, economic, and familial conditions. Third, the frequent combination of physical/mental and socioeconomic dependence often calls for a finely tuned interdisciplinary approach that can rarely be achieved without an individual organizer or manager.

Recently, a new twist has been added, the "gatekeeper" concept. The gatekeeper is a generalist who has overall responsibility for the patient, without whose permission or referral specialist care will not be paid by a third party (31). The concept is by no means limited to LTC. It is common in HMOs, "primary care networks," and other forms of "alternative" care for younger populations. However, it is related to the case manager function and is an intrinsic part of the experimental S/HMO model.

If some form of case manager becomes increasingly common in LTC for the reasons noted above, the important question then arises: Who shall it be? At least three options are theoretically possible: (a) require all LTC patients to register with a primary practitioner or family doctor, who would then be responsible for all referrals, medical and social; (b) set up a separate system for LTC patients using a nurse practitioner, social worker, or other nonphysician as the case manager with full responsibility for referrals; or (c) compromise by assigning final professional, legal, and moral responsibility to a physician but delegate nonmedical referrals to an associated nonphysician. The financial incentives and implications of the different alternatives are important.

Cost Controls: Competition Versus Regulation

It is surely unnecessary to further document the need for cost controls in any viable LTC program. Nor is it necessary to review the multifaceted debate over competition versus regulation that has enlivened the health care scene during the past few years. It is significant, however, that the "procompetition" advocates rarely point to LTC as an area particularly well suited to the free market and price competition. On the contrary, the absence of private insurance from the LTC field emphasizes the generally poor fit between the LTC market and pure competition.

In the nursing home field the "for-profits" are dominant, but they now operate within a regulated environment that proved necessary as a result of extensive abuses in the early days of proprietary expansion. Efforts on the part of the current Administration to reduce Federal nursing home regulations, especially with respect to inspection and accreditation, have thus far been resisted by Congress and consumer groups. The recent creation of an independent commission under the National Academy of Sciences Institute of Medicine to reexamine the whole question of nursing home quality standards and controls is a more promising approach.

The for-profit home health agencies have shown considerable growth since the 1980 Congressional amendment permitting them to be reimbursed by Medicare. The fact that they are less regulated is a cause for some concern. Although there have never been the abuses, or even the allegations of abuses, that characterized the nursing home industry 15 years ago, the potential for such abuse is, unfortunately, even greater. It is hard to imagine a more vulnerable individual than an 85-year-old widow, aphasic and paralyzed from stroke, living alone in a rural area or high-crime inner city. It is inconceivable that any third party, public or private, would ever sanction, through reimbursement or otherwise, the entry of intravenous technicians, "homemakers," "home health aides," "chore workers," or any other paraprofessional category into such a home except on a regulated basis.

Neither regulation nor competition alone can solve all the problems of this complex industry (32, 33). What is needed is a flexible mixture, and this is another area for study.

Patient Cost-Sharing: Deterrence Versus Assistance

Recent confirmation of the common sense notion that substantial cost-sharing reduces the use and cost of health services by relatively healthy individuals under age 61 (34) is hardly a breathtaking discovery. The problem of cost-sharing by the elderly, especially for LTC, is as complex as it is important. The usual argument against cost-sharing—the danger of underutilization—has to be carefully balanced against the potential advantages of providing coverage to hitherto excluded individuals and/or of improving existing benefits.

For example, if reasonable cost-sharing for both acute and long-term benefits could make possible universal Medicare coverage of a substantial amount of LTC services as opposed to the current general exclusion, it would benefit many elderly. Moreover, since 43% of all nursing home costs are paid for directly by patients or their families (35), the substitution of a reasonable income-related cost-sharing schedule as the price of Medicare coverage could help to distribute this existing burden more equitably. To determine the viability and the terms of such a trade-off would require study of a number of issues including:

1. Effect of various cost-sharing formulas on the price of all affected services.
2. Effect on the use of such services.
3. Effect on patient health.
4. Potential for expanding coverage of LTC services.
5. Administrative feasibility and effect on costs of administration.

Two related approaches deserve consideration: (a) voluntary supplementation, now generally illegal under Medicaid, of LTC costs paid by a public program; (b) tax incentives to encourage and help families take care of patients at home (3). A score of Congressional bills authorizing the latter have been introduced in the current Congress but have been opposed by the Administration.

Payment of Institutional Providers: Prospective Versus Retrospective Rates

The absurdity of "reasonable cost" hospital reimbursement and its enormous inflationary impact on the costs of health insurance have been recognized by health care authorities for years. Nevertheless, it took nearly 18 years and the prospect of bankruptcy for the Medicare Hospital Insurance Trust Fund before Congress became willing to undertake serious corrective action. Now with the shift to DRGs—diagnosis related groups—incentives are being totally reversed, and concern shifts from the likelihood of overutilization to the possibility of underutilization (36). One can hope that the gradual phasing in of the new program and provision for complicated cases and other exceptional circumstances ("outliers") will permit this experiment to be more successful then the previous one.

At the moment, chronic hospitals and other LTC institutions are exempt from the DRG experiment. This was certainly wise. The feasibility of applying this methodology to LTC has yet to be demonstrated and at first glance seems unlikely. The very thought of using the payment mechanism to try to speed up patient discharge from a LTC facility or program appears a contradiction in terms. If a speedy cure had been possible, the patient would not require LTC at all. Moreover, many LTC patients defy being "pigeonholed" into a single diagnostic category. Multiple pathologies are the rule rather than the exception with the very old. Then, too, in the LTC field, unlike acute care, underutilization is already a widespread problem (32).

This is not to imply that retroactive cost-based reimbursement is any more appropriate for LTC than for acute care. But the alternative is not necessarily per-case reimbursement. Payment based on fixed prices or charges per diem, per week, or per month is also an alternative. The per-case system not only calls for fixed prices but also changes the unit or product that is being priced from a day to a case. This is a good way to confront alleged overutilization, but since this is not generally the problem in LTC, some other more relevant alternative will probably have to be sought. Among those suggested is a point system, perhaps based on an ADL (activities of daily living) index, which would reward admission to heavy-care patients. This system is already being tried out in a few states. An alternative could be an outcome-oriented system with payment based on whether the patient appears to improve or to decline as predicted by some neutral analyst (3,37,38). The current Congressional proposal, noted above, to establish an independent commission to review Federal nursing home standards could also provide an appropriate opportunity for simultaneous study of reimbursement.

Payment of Practitioners: Fee for Service Versus Capitation/Salary

Current interest in HMOs and related "alternative delivery systems" stems from much the same concern as the DRG movement. It is widely alleged that fee-for-service payment prompts overutilization of physician and other professional services whereas capitation or salary encourages more restrained and therefore more appropriate and less expensive use of services. As already noted in connection with institutional payment, testing this hypothesis is exceptionally difficult in the LTC field. It will be equally so for practitioners. Good geriatric doctors and nurses are very scarce regardless of how, or how much, they are paid.

It is possible that the S/HMO experiment will shed some light on this issue, although it is not clear how much use will be made of physicians in these projects. In any case, the crucial case-manager function, whether performed by a physician or nonphysician, obviously has to be paid for on a salary or capitation basis. If the entire array of home care personnel, including visiting nurses and therapists, could be maintained on a salaried basis, it would probably be much less expensive. But is this possible or equitable if most physicians continue to be on fee for service? These are not easily researchable issues, but they are crucial to the viable financing and success of any large-scale LTC program.

Perhaps even more urgent are the issues of (a) selective "assignment," which permits physicians to pick and choose among their patients those whom they will bill above Medicare rates, and (b) the strong protechnology bias in the existing Medicare and most private health insurance fee structures.

IMPLICATIONS FOR THE TEACHING NURSING HOME

The exciting concept of the teaching nursing home (TNH), which was launched by the National Institute on Aging under the leadership of Dr. Robert Butler some 3 years ago (39), is described and discussed in detail in this volume. At this point, we should focus on the financial issues as they apply to this particular type of LTC institution.

In his 1981 article in the *Journal of the American Medical Association*, Dr. Butler suggested that the concept could be launched for relatively modest sums. For 25 such programs at an annual cost of $100,000 to $300,000 each for "major teaching, logistical, and administrative arrangements," the overall cost would range from $2.5 to $7.5 million per year. Research and professional training in the TNH would, according to this view, be financed through conventional sources such as NIH and the Health Resources and Services Administration. Presumably, patient care would continue to be funded, as at present, through Medicaid, Medicare, and private funds.

Dr. Butler did not view this as a luxury or extravagance, even in these "austere times." On the contrary, he sees our present health care program for the elderly as "ineffective . . . and costing more than need be." He suggests that a strong effort of this type could actually save the nation billions of dollars. Just as vaccine replaced the iron lung in polio treatment, "today's nursing home—the 'iron lung' of geriatrics—will be transformed by a strong research effort."

Two years later, Dr. Edward Schneider, also of NIA, addressed the financial issue as follows:

> The introduction of research and training into teaching nursing homes may increase the costs of these institutions in the same manner that teaching and research in teaching hospitals may increase their costs. However, teaching nursing homes are not intended as a model to be applied to the 19,000 nursing homes in the country. Instead, they should serve as sites for research, training, and health services related to long-term care, just as the 450 teaching hospitals in the U.S. are sites for research and training related to acute disorders. The in-

creased costs of the teaching nursing home should therefore be considered in the context of their potential for helping to reduce the costs related to inappropriate institutionalization as well as in terms of their role in improving the health status and the quality of life of nursing-home residents (40).

Both of these points are appropriate in trying to defuse the almost automatic negative reaction to any proposal that implies additional costs for LTC today. At the same time, both points are more complex than may first appear.

Dr. Butler's analogy of the contemporary nursing home as the "iron lung of geriatrics"—a "half-way technology" that should be displaced as medical science gains more control over the prevention and treatment of chronic diseases—may or may not be accurate for the 21st century. Although his assessment may be correct, it is certainly premature to count on any such development as a basis for short-run economies in LTC financing.

Dr. Schneider's point—that the more expensive TNH should not be construed as a model to be applied to all nursing homes—is well taken but suffers by analogy to the teaching hospital. Although the logic of funding and maintaining both types of academic institutions as selected sites for research and training is very attractive, in practice the concept has not worked out this way in the hospital field, and there is no assurance that it will with respect to nursing homes. Far from recognizing the special status of a limited number of teaching hospitals, the majority of American community hospitals have attempted, with considerable success, to emulate the academic example in terms of tertiary care, training—at least at the graduate level—and even in some research.

None of this is to imply that the TNH is either undesirable or unaffordable as a matter of public policy. It does suggest that the conditions under which it is desirable and affordable are by no means automatically assured. Special provisions may be necessary.[3] For the TNH faces practically all the major issues raised in relation to LTC in general. For example:

1. What, and what size, population should it serve?
2. Should it relate primarily to Medicare, Medicaid, or both?
3. What is the basic patient-care goal of the TNH—cure or care? Or both?
4. Should the TNH be part of mainstream health care or of a separate LTC program?
5. Should the financial responsibility be primarily public or private?

---

[3] In one state, California, the legislature is considering a bill—AB 2614—authorizing grants up to $250,000 to each University of California medical school to establish a teaching nursing home program. Grants could not be used to buy or build a home but to operate training, patient care, research, and community service programs using the home as a base. A similar bill was passed by both houses in 1983 but vetoed by the Governor. In view of the state's improved fiscal condition, sponsors are optimistic of passage in 1984 (P.G. Weiler, M.D., Chair, American Public Health Association Gerontological Section).

6. To the extent that such financial responsibility is public, should the funding agency be primarily Federal or state/local government?
7. To the extent that it is public, should it be supported primarily from general revenues or special taxes?
8. Should it concentrate primarily on traditional institutional care or expand its role to be a hub for community outreach programs?
9. How does the TNH fit into a general scheme of managing or "channeling" LTC patients?
10. Is competition or regulation the better approach to controlling the costs of the TNH?
11. Should the TNH encourage or discourage patient cost-sharing?
12. What reimbursement methodologies are most appropriate for the TNH and for the professionals involved?

The originators of the TNH concept clearly favored "bringing geriatrics into the mainstream of American medicine where a thriving intellectual atmosphere exists" (39). It would appear to follow that the Medicare universal-access model is more appropriate than the Medicaid means-tested model and that effective rehabilitation and maximum functional independence are the most appropriate goals.

If this interpretation is correct, the implications are as great for mainstream medicine as they are for the TNH. If LTC is recognized as an essential aspect of mainstream health care, it follows that the latter will have to share its resources far more clearly and openly than has been true in the past, or would be true in the future, if LTC remained a separate "stepchild" type of program, as Medicaid has been from the outset. The only way that any such sharing can be equitably carried out is by tempering market forces with a significant degree of planning and regulation. Only thus can we insure even a chance that the lessons learned from the TNH will be translated into more cost-effective as well as more health-effective programs and facilities rather than simply more sophisticated and more expensive "iron lungs."

The exciting new concept of the TNH presents health care policymakers with a very important and urgent policy decision. Should chronic care be brought into the mainstream of health care policy and financing as logically dictated by its increasingly central role in the pattern of American morbidity, or should it be left to grow undirected by either public or professional leadership, devouring in the process enormous resources that were never intended for this purpose?

REFERENCES

1. National Center for Health Statistics: *Health—United States 1983*. Publication No. (PHS)81-1232. Washington, DC, Department of Health and Human Services, 1981, p 332.
2. Somers AR, Fabian DR (eds): *The Geriatric Imperative: An Introduction to Gerontology and Clinical Geriatrics*. New York, Appleton-Century-Crofts, 1981.

3. US Department of Commerce, Bureau of the Census: *Projections of the Population of the US: 1982–2050 (Advance Report) Ser. P-25, No. 922.* Washington, DC, US Government Printing Office 1982.
4. Department of Health and Human Services, Office of the Inspector General: Service Delivery Assessment. *Long Term Care.* Report to the Secretary, December 1981 (unpublished) 2 vols.
5. Neugarten BL (ed): *Age or Need? Public Policies for Older People.* Beverly Hills, CA, Sage Publications, 1982.
6. Somers AR: Long-term care for the elderly and disabled: A new health priority. *N Engl J Med* 1982;307:221–226.
7. Ruchlin HS, Morris JN, Eggert GM: Management and funding of long-term care services: A new approach to a chronic problems. *N Engl J Med* 1982;306:101–106.
8. Williams ME, Hadler HM: The illness is the focus of geriatric medicine. *N Engl J Med* 1983;308:1357–1359.
9. Kennie DC: Good health care for the aged. *JAMA* 1983;249:770–773.
10. Friggens P: Easing the problems of aging: An interview with Dr RN Butler. *Exxon USA Magazine* 1983 (first quarter), pp 12–15.
11. Murphy JF: The role of the insurance industry in long-term care, in Home Health Agency Assembly of New Jersey (eds): *Proceedings of an Invitational Conference: Broadening Access to Long-Term Care.* Piscataway, NJ, Home Health Agency Assembly, 1982, pp 27–30.
12. Slattery RM: Private insurance, in Home Health Agency Assembly of New Jersey (eds): *Proceedings of an Invitational Conference: Broadening Access to Long-Term Care.* Piscataway, NJ, Home Health Agency Assembly, 1982, pp 63–70.
13. Meiners MR: The case for long-term care insurance. *Health Affairs* 1983;2:55–79.
14. Minard DE: A role for insurance, in Home Health Agency Assembly of New Jersey (eds): *Proceedings of an Invitational Conference: Broadening Access to Long-Term Care.* Piscataway, NJ, Home Health Agency Assembly, 1982, pp 71–75.
14a. Somers HM, Somers AR: Major issues in national health insurance. *Milbank Mem Fund Q* 1972;50(1):177–210.
15. Griffith JR: The role of Blue Cross and Blue Shield in the future US health care system. *Inquiry* 1983;20:12–19.
16. Lanahan MB: Life care retirement communities. Pride Institute. *J Long-Term Home Health Care* 1983;2:41–42.
17. Fillenbaum GG: Portrait of a life-care community: An alternate living arrangement for the elderly. *Duke University Center for the Study of Aging and Human Development. Center Reports on Advances in Research* 1981, p 5.
18. Winklevoss HE, Powell AV: *Continuing Care Retirement Communities: An Empirical, Financial, and Legal Analysis.* Homewood, IL: Richard D. Irwin, 1983.
19. Rudnitsky H, Konrad W: Trouble in the elysian fields. *Forbes* August 29, 1983, pp 58–59.
20. Rutten FFH: Health care policy today: Making way for the libertarians? *Effective Health Care* 1983;1:35–43.
21. Somers AR: Long-term care for the elderly and disabled: An urgent challenge to the "New Federalism." Paper presented to Project Hope, Conference on the New Federalism and Long-Term Care of the Elderly. Millwood, VA, 1984.
22. Department of Health and Human Services: *Medicare Benefits and Financing: Report of the 1983 Advisory Council on Social Security.* Washington, DC, US Government Printing Office, 1983.
23. Department of Health and Human Services, HCFA, Division of Long-Term Care Experimentation: *Long-Term Care Demonstration Project Summaries.* Baltimore, Health Care Finance Administration, 1983.
24. Expansion of Cost-Effective Home Health Care. Testimony prepared by Health Policy Alternatives, Inc., for Home Health Services and Staffing Association. Presented to Senate Finance Subcommittee on Health. Hearings on Long-Term Care. Washington, DC, November 14, 1983. US Government Printing Office, 1984.
25. Hammond J: Home health care cost effectiveness: An overview of the literature. *Publ Health Rep* 1979;94:305–311.
26. Dunlop BD: Expanded home-based care for the impaired elderly: Solution or pipe dream? *Am J Publ Health* 1980;70:514–519.

27. Brickner PW: *Ten Years of Long Term Home Health Care, January 1973–December 1982.* New York, St. Vincent's Hospital and Medical Center, 1983.
28. Weissert WG: Costs of adult day care: A comparison to nursing homes. *Inquiry* 1978;15:10–19.
29. Hickey T, Douglass RL: Mistreatment of the elderly in the domestic setting—an exploratory study. *Am J Publ Health* 1981;71:500–507.
30. Stuart R: "Old-old" grow in number and impact. *New York Times*, June 20, 1983.
31. Somers AR: And who shall be the gatekeeper? The role of the primary physician and the health care delivery system. *Inquiry* 1983;20:301–313.
32. Rango N: Nursing home care in the US: prevailing conditions and policy implications. *N Engl J Med* 1982;307:883–889.
33. Speigel AD, Hyman HH, Gary LR: Issues and opportunities in the regulation of home health care. *Health Policy Educ* 1980;1:237–253.
34. Newhouse JP, Manning WG, Morris CN, et al: Some interim results from a controlled trail of cost-sharing in health insurance. *N Engl J Med* 1981;305:1501–1507.
35. Gibson RM, Waldo DR, Levit KR: National health expenditures, 1982. *Health Care Financ Rev* 1983;5:1–31.
36. Garber AM, Fuchs VR, Silverman JF: Case Mix, Costs, and Outcomes: Differences between Faculty and Community Services in a University Hospital. National Bureau of Economic Research Working Paper No. 1159. Stanford, CA, 1983.
37. Kane RL, Bell R, Riegler S, et al: Predicting the outcome of nursing home patients. *Gerontologist* 1983;23:200–206.
38. Weissert WG, Scanlon WJ, Wan TTH, et al: Encouraging appropriate care for the chronically ill: Design of the National Center for Health Services Research experiment in nursing home incentive payments. Paper presented to American Public Health Association, Detroit, 1980.
39. Butler RN: The teaching nursing home. *JAMA* 1981;245:1435–1437.
40. Schneider EL: Teaching nursing homes. *N Engl J Med* 1983;308:336–337.

The Teaching Nursing Home, edited by Edward
L. Schneider et al. © 1985 The Beverly
Foundation. Raven Press, New York.

Reimbursement Issues and Quality of Care

Linda Kaeser

Oregon Teaching Nursing Home Program, Oregon Health Sciences University School of Nursing, Portland, Oregon 97201

Encouragement of quality care within restricted dollars is today's major long-term care (LTC) issue. Within this broad framework, reimbursement may be the most critical issue, since it provides incentives and disincentives that drive decisions about the population to be served, the services, and the providers of services. Teaching nursing homes (TNHs) are interested in educating health care professionals and developing new knowledge to improve the care for LTC clients and/or reduce the numbers needing such care. Since reimbursement decisions will profoundly affect the character and amount of LTC that can be given, it behooves TNHs to expend some of their energies on these important matters.

REIMBURSEMENT AND POPULATION

Reimbursement policies, to a large extent, determine the numbers and characteristics of the population that can be provided health services under a particular program. Persons may be deemed eligible to become program participants by virtue of a variety of characteristics (e.g., age, sex, relationship to another, ability to pay, place in line, health status, mental health status). Medicare, the major insurance source for the elderly in need of acute-care services, uses an age criterion (over 65) or a health criterion (permanently disabled and unable to work) for inclusion purposes. Medicaid, the major insurance source for the elderly in need of LTC services, uses an ability-to-pay criterion set by each state for eligibility determination. In addition, states often add to the Medicaid eligibility requirements: a residency requirement (e.g., in the state, in a nursing home in the state), a relationship requirement (e.g., children, who can, shall pay for care), a health status requirement (e.g., must be dependent in at least one activity of daily living), and/or a mental status requirement (e.g., must not be mentally ill).

As the proportion of physically and financially dependent persons is increasing, the proportion of persons who can physically and financially care for others is decreasing. This is driving decisionmakers to examine their criteria for potential Medicare and Medicaid beneficiaries. The size of this poor, chronically ill, dependent, largely female elderly population may be perceived by policymakers as too large a burden for the public to carry. This could lead to a severe tightening of eligibility requirements or to an abandonment of the programs. Since this population is unable to lobby for itself, it must rely on others. Teaching nursing home staff, with their multiple political access points and their high level of expertise, have a responsibility for providing leadership relative to Medicare and Medicaid eligibility requirements for this vulnerable population.

REIMBURSEMENT AND SERVICES

There are two major categories of services needed by any LTC client: health services (e.g., nursing services, medical services) and hotel services (e.g., dietary services, housekeeping services, laundry services). Medicare and Medicaid do not restrict the payment for most health services to hospitals or nursing homes. However, both Medicare and Medicaid restrict, without a waiver, the payment for hotel services to hospitals and nursing homes. Since LTC clients need a basic level of hotel services concurrent with the necessary health services, they may be unable to find a way to pay for these services outside of the nursing home setting. The current policy of coupling health and hotel services in hospitals and nursing homes and uncoupling them in congregate care facilities or private homes has led to a disporportionate use of the more restrictive and, in some cases, more expensive settings. It has also restricted our ability to compare the quality and cost of specific health and/or hotel services across sites. The uncoupling of health services from hotel services would enable public policymakers to set different reimbursement standards for health services and hotel services, thereby gaining greater control over both costs and quality. To accomplish such a task, Federal and/or state governments might need to transfer some funds into or out of Medicaid, Medicare, Social Security, Old Age Assistance, Title XX, food stamps, and Housing and Urban Development. Planners of TNHs should examine this issue and develop research and demonstration projects to test the viability of such a strategy.

Within the health services category, LTC clients need large, frequent doses of high-touch services (e.g., nursing) and small, infrequent doses of more technical services (e.g., surgery). Medicare and Medicaid policy makers have never valued, as evidenced by reimbursement policies, high-touch services as much as they value the technical (medical) services. In addition, they have valued almost any service provided in a hospital above that same service provided in a nursing home. Furthermore, professional groups with a high proportion of physicians have been given preferential treatment over groups with a high proportion of high-touch practitioners (e.g., social workers). Teaching nursing home staff who understand the importance of high-touch services need to lobby for a raising of the priority of this set of services.

Medicare and Medicaid have looked more favorably on reimbursement for LTC health services for some sets of conditions than for others. In general, health services related to injuries receive a higher priority than those related to disease; services related to physical disability (e.g., physical therapy) receive a higher priority than services related to emotional disturbance (e.g., counseling) or cognition or communication difficulties (e.g., speech therapy); and services related to organic disease (e.g., heart disease) receive a higher priority than services related to deficits related to brain malfunction (e.g., Alzheimer's disease). In addition, services are usually valued above durable medical supplies (e.g., eyeglasses, hearing aids). Clients and providers are often frustrated and angered by this piecemeal rather than holistic approach to services. For example, what good does it do to teach a man to walk if he needs a hearing aid and speech therapy in order to communicate with other human beings? Teaching nursing home personnel who can relate to these problems should examine ways to solve them.

Medicare and Medicaid have largely ignored issues surrounding hotel services with the possible exception of dietary services. We know that hotel services must be packaged and delivered to client's homes in order for them to be in a position where they can utilize health services. Some multilevel complexes (e.g., apartments, congregate living facilities, and nursing homes) have been developed throughout the country to solve this problem. However, these complexes are primarily for persons with money and/or persons of a particular racial or religious subgroup. Some TNHs might experiment with developing similar arrangements between government-subsidized units for the elderly and existing nursing homes. Others might experiment with offering hotel services to the catchment area surrounding the nursing home.

REIMBURSEMENT AND PROVIDERS

Physicians, as a class, have traditionally received the highest priority rating for reimbursement as health care providers, and nurses the lowest. Other classes of health care providers (e.g., dentists, pharmacists, physical therapists, social workers) have been ranked between these two. In general, the professions with a large proportion of high-touch practitioners (e.g., nursing, social work, physical therapy) have a lower priority rating than professions such as medicine.

Most state reimbursement systems do not adequately address the need for more and better LTC staff even though the client mix is becoming more difficult to serve. Nursing home personnel are under ever-increasing pressure to care for a growing proportion of clients needing complex and extensive health care services. Hospitals, including mental hospitals, are reducing lengths of stay in response to regulations and reimbursement policies (e.g., Medicare, DRGs). Community noninstitutional programs are being used more frequently for clients needing less complex care. Advances in medical technology are increasing the numbers of persons surviving with severe illness and/or disability, and the total number of aging persons is increasing. As a result of forces such as these, nursing home staff are being asked to provide care for an increasing number of very sick and/or disabled clients.

The very phrase "nursing home" implies nursing services within a residential setting. Registered nurses, licensed practical nurses, and nursing assistants supply the overwhelming majority of the care to clients. Indeed, the registered nurse may be the only health professional in a LTC facility. In fact, because of current reimbursement policies and institutional practices, the "highest ranking" of the service personnel during evenings, weekends, and nighttime hours may be a nursing assistant or a licensed practical nurse.

Most current reimbursement systems do not adequately address the need for greater competency requirements for nursing services personnel. The plethora of titles, degrees, and certifications for persons providing nursing care to patients is often confusing and bewildering. The general public, and sometimes even nursing home administrators, do not have a clear idea about what is an appropriate role and level of responsibility for each category of nursing preparation. For example, the term licensed personnel may refer to a practical nurse with one year of training or to a clinical nurse specialist with a Master of Science degree in nursing. Clearly, these persons have different levels of competence and should have different roles and responsibilities. The lack of interest in making meaningful distinctions between nursing service personnel is often attributed to reimbursement policies. Reimbursement policies need to encourage LTC institutions to hire and retain nursing staff that have the qualifications necessary for their roles and responsibilities. In addition to providing educational opportunities for current and future nursing service personnel, TNH leaders can help formulate and implement the reimbursement policies that encourage the recruitment and retention of nursing service personnel who can assure clients of receiving safe, therapeutic nursing care.

Other health personnel are also adversely affected by unfavorable reimbursement policies. Social workers, occupational therapists, recreational therapists, and pharmacists have been traditionally underfunded in LTC facilities, although the value of their services to a dependent population and their families cannot be overrated. The physical therapy profession has fared somewhat better, although, like many others, physical therapists face the cost and "red tape" requirements of required physician referral. Traditionally, most professional groups have attempted to align themselves with physicians who, within reimbursement guidelines, determine access to clients for individual providers. This pattern may not serve LTC clients as well as it has served acute-care clients. The TNH staff have the opportunity to examine the different reimbursement patterns for different health care providers for the purpose of designing and testing new models that provide higher quality and more complete health services for every dollar spent. These efforts, concurrent with education efforts, are necessary to insure the recruitment and retention of quality staff.

Teaching nursing homes also have the opportunity to develop education and training relationships with schools that educate (or can educate) persons to manage hotel services and business services. For example, schools of home economics and hotel management could become participants in TNHs, thereby educating persons to administer the hotel service aspects of LTC, providing faculty expertise for consultation and research, and providing a broader base of support for LTC reimbursement issues. Schools of public administration and business administration as well as health professions (e.g., nursing, social work, public health) that have graduate programs in administration could also be asked to participate in the TNH program for the same general reasons.

SUMMARY

What services are provided—in what settings, by which kinds of providers, to which groups of clients—is largely determined by reimbursement policies. Current Medicare and Medicaid reimbursement policies are not favorable for providing LTC clients with quality health and hotel services in the least restrictive environment suited to their needs. The TNH personnel have the professional expertise and political clout necessary to address the many complex reimbursement issues that have an impact on quality of care. A variety of areas have been suggested as reimbursement issues worthy of examination. Among the suggestions are to uncouple health services and hotel services, raise the status of high-touch services, eliminate restriction of services for specific conditions, develop a non-setting specific system of LTC services, develop meaningful reimbursement distinctions for various levels of nursing service personnel, standardize reimbursement methodologies across health profession groups, and develop TNH relationships with schools of home economics, hotel administration, public administration, and business administration.

PART II
Teaching Nursing Home Models

The Teaching Nursing Home, edited by Edward
L. Schneider et al. © 1985 The Beverly
Foundation. Raven Press, New York.

Introduction

Ewald W. Busse

Duke University Medical Center, Durham, North Carolina 27710

A model teaching nursing home (TNH) must be an excellent service unit and, in addition, a high-quality learning facility. Learning includes the retention and the application of knowledge. Learning is influenced by previous and current events as well as social and physical environmental factors. For a student, it is particularly important that early learning experiences be positive. The successful learner has the ability to solve problems and to develop skills that are energy efficient and beneficial.

A TNH must provide a favorable milieu that includes excellent role models at all levels of personnel including those responsible for direct and indirect patient care and administration. Role models are excellent teachers, capable of conveying to the learner the principles of problem solving, the satisfactions inherent in acquiring new knowledge, and the capacity to demonstrate successful techniques and maintain positive attitudes. The student who learns in an environment that is less than excellent develops bad habits and low expectations. A good learning environment must include diversified experiences with an underlying system of humanistic values. Criteria need to be developed to identify those factors that are basic for a model TNH and include a mechanism of correcting deficiencies and making improvements. These basic assumptions and principles can be met in many ways.

The present oversupply of physicians, which will likely continue for years to come, will provide a major resource for geriatrics.

At present there is no identifiable system of long-term care (LTC). Chronic-care facilities and levels of professional skills are poorly coordinated. The nursing home is a major component in LTC, and the establishment of TNHs is very likely to make a major contribution in the development of a LTC system.

It is repeatedly stated that medical students learn exclusively in hospitals. It is preferable to state that the nurse or medical student is enrolled in an academic health center. An academic health center includes hospitals, diagnostic facilities, clinics, and extensive programs that deal with ambulatory patients. In establishing a TNH, another needed resource is added for the education of health service personnel.

The chapters in this section present several TNH models. They discuss the complexity of affiliation arrangements. Liaison among affiliated institutions must take place at all levels, not only at the administrative levels. In fact, most affiliations that are unsuccessful fail because of defects of communication between personnel responsible for the care of patients. If those responsible for a service and for teaching work in harmony, administration is likely to be flexible.

The Teaching Nursing Home, edited by Edward
L. Schneider et al. © 1985 The Beverly
Foundation. Raven Press, New York.

The Beverly Enterprises Teaching Nursing Home Program

Larry J. Pipes

Beverly Enterprises, Pasadena, California 91109

In the fall of 1982, Beverly Enterprises issued a corporate policy statement and guidelines supporting the teaching nursing home (TNH) concept because of its potential to improve patient care and the training of health professions in geriatrics. In taking this action, Beverly Enterprises responded to shared interests of schools of nursing and medicine throughout the country to generate affiliations with company nursing homes.

Teaching nursing homes can play an important part in the training of health professionals and provide much-needed opportunities for geriatric research. They may also serve as a focal point for developing innovations and improvements in the delivery, financing, and quality of long-term care (LTC).

The Beverly Enterprises approach is to develop replicable and successful models for the TNH. Although there are many examples of affiliations between academic research and training centers and health care facilities, the suitability of many of these for TNHs is questionable. Suitability is questioned, in part, because of financing and reimbursement limitations faced by nursing homes, the regulatory environment within which nursing homes must operate, the proprietary operating structure of the majority of nursing homes, and the lack of a prior association or experience between nursing homes and higher education. If TNHs are to serve as a model for the LTC industry, these issues of suitability must be addressed. The alternative would be for TNHs to represent only ideal situations and not serve as role models for the industry. Beverly Enterprises supports the TNH as a role model for addressing issues of critical importance in LTC.

By developing more effective relationships with the academic and research communities, both the nursing home industry and LTC patients will be drawn into the mainstream of American medical care. Success in developing these relationships will depend on several factors: mutually agreed-on goals for the affiliation, the commitment of necessary and sufficient resources to accomplish those goals, and flexibility in identifying joint roles and responsibilities.

71

SCOPE AND FRAMEWORK OF THE BEVERLY PROGRAM

Beverly Enterprises recommends that at least three operational elements be considered as fundamentals to the TNH concept. First, the nursing home can be seen as midway between the acute-care hospital and the wide range of deinstitutional alternatives. For example, in a teaching or research affiliation, the nursing home could be used as the "hub" or management point for a wide array of LTC services, which could include home health care, adult day care, rehabilitation, social services, nutritional counseling, and family and bereavement counseling. Second, since nursing home patients demonstrate a range of functional and psychosocial disabilities that are best managed by a variety of medical, health, and social science disciplines, an interdisciplinary approach to patient management is needed. Third, a liaison between the nursing home and the academic center should include an affiliation agreement.

In taking into consideration these operational elements and various management issues and perspectives, Beverly Enterprises developed the following corporate TNH policy:

> Beverly Enterprises encourages the affiliation of Beverly nursing homes with a teaching institution or research center provided such affiliation is feasible and contributes to:
>
> - The improved care and quality of life of nursing home patients.
> - The education and training of health professionals and allied personnel for LTC.
> - Better nursing home administration, operation, and staffing.
> - Innovations in the financing, management, and delivery of LTC services to the elderly.
> - Increased community, public, and professional relations.

Although there are important benefits to be gained through the successful establishment of TNHs, not every facility is suited to become a TNH. Also, not every affiliate relationship between Beverly Enterprises and a university training or research center must be nursing home based.

Beverly Enterprises encourages the pursuit of discussions with teaching institutions and research centers involved in the training of health professionals of all disciplines who will pursue careers as clinicians and/or researchers in LTC. Such discussions potentially lead to the establishment of mutually beneficial affiliate relationships between operational settings (nursing homes) and the training institution or research center.

An affiliation agreement should be drafted to clarify responsibilities and future courses of action regarding patient care, operational administration and management, professional and support staff training and education, the conduct of research, financial feasibility and responsibility, and programs of community, public, and professional relations.

The following guidelines direct teaching institutions and research centers in discussion, negotiation, and, ultimately, affiliation:

1. Throughout the affiliate relationship, control of the daily administration, operation, and patient care functions of the nursing home must remain with Beverly Enterprises management.
2. The relationship must not interfere with the nursing home's ability to comply with applicable local, state, and Federal laws and regulations.
3. Special attention should be given to proposed activities affecting patient's rights, confidentiality of patient information, legal liability, and financial reimbursement. No teaching or research action or activity involving patients should be undertaken without an express participation agreement of individual patients or guardians.
4. High priority will be given to proposed affiliate relations that emphasize the development of methods to improve overall patient care, nursing home operations, and support staff training.
5. Costs and sources of revenue for the development, teaching, and/or research phases should be projected and identified. In particular, the extent of increased cost and overhead for the nursing home and the likelihood of increased revenue and/or improvements to patient care must be investigated.
6. The use of interdisciplinary and interinstitutional liaisons and arrangements should be identified and encouraged.
7. A system of internal project review, development, and management and impact evaluation should be developed.
8. Acceptance of the TNH by appropriate community elements should be demonstrated.
9. An arrangement should be included for the exchange of relevant information between the nursing home and teaching institution or research center.

CHARACTERISTICS OF THE BEVERLY PROGRAM

Beverly Enterprises maintains that the quality of care and life of patients in nursing homes, as well as aspects of nursing home operations, should be improved through affiliations with academic training and research centers. As a result, a corporate program has been developed to explore and provide opportunities for establishing clinical and nonclinical affiliations. Some of these affiliation models are inappropriate for TNHs. Certain structural elements in other models may be useful, but the preferred model will likely result from a blending of both existing and new elements. Therefore, Beverly's approach allows the TNH model to evolve dynamically through developing and testing of alternative affiliations and evaluation of results.

Beverly Enterprises has provided financial and other support to developing projects located in different parts of the country. Financial support is attempted on a joint-venture or shared basis. Through working directly with the different projects and assessing their progress, Beverly Enterprises hopes to learn the necessary and sufficient conditions and requirements for successful affiliations and research projects.

Not all affiliations necessarily require corporate financial support to a university. In cases in which student training in the nursing home is the focal point of the affiliation, the potential benefits to both sides would appear to justify each handling its own expenses and committing sufficient effort and resources to make the affiliation successful. In such cases, the role of Beverly Enterprises is to provide a well-managed, quality facility, and the university is responsible for providing a quality educational and training program.

For projects to be successful, it is very important that they be goal oriented. To help insure success, projects must identify realistic and mutually agreed-on goals, provide a management structure that monitors and reports on progress toward those goals, and take necessary corrective action. When modifications are warranted, all parties to the affiliation or project should collaborate in an effort to insure appropriate input toward a consensus.

Our approach to TNHs accommodates both secondary and primary affiliations. There is support for affiliations that focus on student training rotations through the nursing home. Primary affiliations go beyond student training to include such elements as joint appointments, joint operational planning, and joint development and implementation of research projects. This approach does not require joint appointments as a mandatory element, nor does it require the use of a nursing home in all cases. The TNHs should serve as role models to be followed by other homes. There are likely to be more benefits to nursing homes and their patients if the TNH concept encompasses "typical" nursing homes and addresses their problems.

Beverly Enterprises' approach supports the involvement of community colleges in the TNH concept. Since many aides in nursing homes have received their training in community colleges, interaction is symbiotic. A major objective of the Beverly TNH is to contribute to the function and effectiveness of nursing aides. Thus, the community college is felt to be an important element in the TNH concept.

As of December, 1983, a number of different affiliations were in various stages of development and implementation. The following selective summary highlights the variety of ongoing activities.

Duke University

Through the Geriatric Division of the Duke Center for the Study of Aging and Human Development, Beverly Enterprises sponsors a postdoctoral Geriatric Fellowship Program that enables a physician who is board eligible in internal medicine, family medicine, or psychiatry and who has an excellent academic–research background and training to complete a year of postgraduate study and research. The Beverly Fellow pursues scholarly research and works with Beverly Enterprises' Durham Care Center Nursing Home on methods for improving geriatric care. An advisory committee composed of Beverly Enterprises and Duke personnel assists in the Fellow's selection in addition to recommending other types of collaborative arrangements.

East Carolina University

The Schools of Medicine and Nursing are working with Beverly Enterprises' Greenville Villa Nursing Home in implementing an interdisciplinary approach to physician and nurse training in geriatrics. Physicians in the Department of Family Medicine are on the staff of Greenville Villa and provide direct care to the patients. Arrangements for student nurses to undertake part of their training at Greenville Villa have been made. In addition, faculty members from both schools assist in developing improved methods of care and management for the nursing home. Research projects in geriatrics are being considered.

Medical College of Virginia

The Department of Health Administration and Beverly Enterprises' Eastern Division are developing a three-part training and research program that focuses on administrative internships and residency training for students majoring in LTC administration, continuing education and training for executives, managers, and administrators in LTC, and graduate student/faculty research in LTC administration.

Santa Monica Hospital Medical Center Family Practice Residency Program

The program provides physician care to patients admitted to the Beverly Manor facility in Santa Monica who are otherwise lacking a physician. Program faculty and residents conduct teaching rounds on attended patients and will participate in the nursing home's case conferences and staff meetings. For discharged patients, some rounds are made at patient's private homes. In addition, the program provides physician backup on after-hours urgent calls for program-attended patients.

University of Arkansas for Medical Sciences

The University's Department of Medicine and Division of Geriatrics have an arrangement with Beverly's Central Division to use the Little Rock Nursing Center in a program involving patient care, staff education, and research. The Division of Geriatrics will assume responsibility for the management of patients and for developing a multidisciplinary care team. The College of Pharmacy has developed a student rotation program. The inclusion of other Beverly Enterprises' homes and development of an innovative delivery system aimed at optimizing the management of care of elderly residing in rural areas is currently being explored.

University of California, Los Angeles

A research project to improve the assessment and management of urinary incontinence in nursing homes has been initiated with faculty in the School of Medicine. The project should result in a system of assessment and monitoring procedures which, after refinement, should contribute to patient-care management and control cost. Arrangements to disseminate results of this research are being made, and plans for clinical trials are being considered.

University of Maryland

An experimental design and research evaluation project is being developed with faculty in the School of Nursing to determine the impact of a "short-stay training program" proposed by the staff of the Sligo Gardens Nursing Home in Takoma Park. Family members of nursing home patients requiring stays of 90 days or less will be trained at the nursing home in certain aspects of patient care to prevent the need for readmissions and to reduce costs. The School of Nursing's role is to aid in the design of a pilot project, to collect and analyze resulting data, and to provide general consultation on the project. Plans include the submission of a research proposal to the Health Care Financing Administration to demonstrate this approach in multiple sites.

University of Southern California

Projects involving alternative LTC delivery methods have been initiated with the Department of Nursing and a Family Practice Residency Program in the School of Medicine. The roles and effects of geriatric nurse practitioners and physician's assistants within the typical nursing home are being addressed. Resident physicians in the Family Practice Program provide care to nursing home patients. In-service educational programs for the nursing home staff are included. Future plans include internship arrangements for student nurses, nursing faculty–management personnel exchanges, submission of a joint research project to the Health Care Financing Administration, and other collaborative research. A project to develop a career ladder program for nursing service employees is also under way.

In addition to these specific arrangements, discussions regarding joint projects and affiliations are currently ongoing with faculty at other universities including the Florida University System at Pensacola and Tampa, Georgetown University, Oregon Health Sciences University, Stanford University, and the University of Texas. At Pensacola, a newly constructed

Beverly Enterprises' nursing home, built next to the college campus, includes classrooms for student training and office space for faculty members' use. Other training arrangements have been made with community and state colleges across the country.

RESEARCH OPPORTUNITIES

With respect to research, many past investigations of nursing homes and patient conditions have been criticized because of limited scope and size. However, Beverly Enterprises' network of approximately 900 nursing homes and retirement centers spread throughout 43 states and the District of Columbia provides a potentially vast and powerful research resource. In certain parts of the country, the complement of services includes home health agencies and pharmacy operations. There is a good distribution of facilities in terms of the geographic location, economic status, type of facilities, and patient characteristics. This overall resource could be utilized for large clinical trials. Commitments have already been made for some homes to participate in multisite research projects.

Beverly Enterprises' management is currently moving toward the development and implementation of information systems to record, analyze, and merge nursing home operational and medical care data. The uses for the resulting information include patient assessments, care plan development and analysis, and the prediction of patient needs and resource utilization. The information could also be used to directly measure the quality of patient care. Beverly's quality assurance process has recently been revised to allow computerized analysis of facility review data based on a standard review instrument. These efforts to automate certain aspects of the quality assurance processes should enhance patient care and contribute to LTC and geriatric research.

Consideration is also being given to ways of increasing the presence of health professionals trained in geriatrics in the nursing homes. Although this is only in the initial stages, increased patient care benefits could result from this increased presence and should be demonstrated in an objective manner. The TNH may provide a vehicle for collaboration in each of these research areas.

SUMMARY

Long-term care delivery systems in general and private enterprises in particular can play important roles in the development of TNHs. Ideal affiliations and collaborations include those in which well-managed and good-quality nursing homes are matched with excellent training and research programs. Since it is doubtful that there will be a significant increase in funding for nursing homes, it is essential that training institutions and research centers become familiar with the requirement for operating on low reimbursement and consider incorporating this financial necessity into TNH models. The nursing home industry and the residents served can certainly benefit through academic and research affiliations. Working together, the private and public sectors can help insure that the TNH becomes an effective partnership expanding education, research, service, and training.

The Teaching Nursing Home, edited by Edward L. Schneider et al. © 1985 The Beverly Foundation. Raven Press, New York.

The Robert Wood Johnson Foundation

Mathy D. Mezey,★ Joan E. Lynaugh,★ and Linda H. Aiken†

★*Teaching Nursing Home Program, University of Pennsylvania School of Nursing, Philadelphia, Pennsylvania 19104*
†*The Robert Wood Johnson Foundation, Princeton, New Jersey 08540*

The Robert Wood Johnson Foundation, with the cosponsorship of the American Academy of Nursing, is supporting a five-year initiative that links 11 university schools of nursing and other health disciplines in affiliations with 12 nursing homes for the purpose of pooling personnel and physical and financial resources for the mutual benefit of both institutions and society. The project is being administered by the School of Nursing at the University of Pennsylvania.

CONTEXT FOR THE TEACHING NURSING HOME PROGRAM

The context for this teaching nursing home initiative can be traced to simultaneous changes occurring in the care of the elderly and in nursing education. There is every reason to believe that nursing homes will increasingly be called on to care for a significantly more impaired and diverse patient population. Some of the changes in the case mix of nursing home patients have already occurred (1–6). The rapidly growing numbers of very old people and their increasing need for and use of health services and nursing home beds have been discussed in depth by Brody and Foley (*this volume*).

There is little doubt that these changes pose a serious challenge to a sector of our health care system that is having great difficulties meeting current obligations without taking on new responsibilities. With implementation of prospective reimbursement for acute hospital care, the diversity of nursing home patients will become further apparent. Without any deliberate planning in that direction, acute-care hospitals have become institutions serving the needs of the elderly. As hospitals seek to facilitate earlier discharge of their elderly patients, nursing homes will be called on to care for people with increasingly complex health problems requiring application of sophisticated compensatory technologies to monitor, sustain, and improve outcomes. Although many homes currently have neither the personnel nor the environmental capacity to absorb such patients, continued inability to care for sicker short- and long-stay patients will place homes in severe financial jeopardy.

Changes are also occurring in nursing education and practice. For both altruistic and financial reasons, professional schools, especially those in the health fields, are seeking ways to bridge the gap between education and practice. A small but significant number of university nursing schools have, for many years, been centrally involved in the delivery of nursing services in their affiliated teaching hospitals (7–9). Increasingly, leading university nursing schools have organizationally merged with nursing services in their teaching hospitals, creating unified models of nursing education and practice. Nursing schools have also assumed management responsibility for other clinical services, including ambulatory clinics and visiting nurse programs (10,11). As a result of these initiatives and other faculty training projects such as the Robert Wood Johnson Foundation Primary Care Fellows (12) and the Clinical Nurse Scholars Program, clinically sophisticated nurse educators and seasoned nurse administrators are now assembled and prepared to contribute to advances in nursing practice, education, and research. University nursing schools are therefore well positioned to forge effective clinical affiliations with nursing homes.

The interest of nursing education in clinical practice initiatives is augmented by a small but growing interest on the part of clinician practitioners in working with the elderly. Experience with primary care practice during the 1970s clearly showed that nurses can and do manage a broad spectrum of medical/nursing/social problems when certain organizational, financial, and professional barriers are lowered (13,14). Since 1973, over 41 masters level nursing programs have graduated a cadre of gerontologic nurse practitioners and gerontologic nurse clinical specialists prepared to meet the acute and chronic care needs of older people in a variety of settings. These nurses are already assuming many formal responsibilities in long-term care (LTC). They modify diet and medication, develop diagnostic treatment and monitoring schedules, execute bowel and bladder regimens, and deliver supportive rehabilitative and personal care services for LTC patients (15,16).

The above formulation serves to highlight the special interest of nursing in the Teaching Nursing Home Program (TNHP). Nurses are eager to respond to the needs of the institutionalized elderly. Nursing homes offer a productive environment in which nurses can assume autonomous and collaborative roles in clinical management and leadership, and they offer an arena in which to further demonstrate the competency of nurse practitioner/clinicians in the delivery of health care services. Moreover, the TNHP affords a mechanism to demonstrate to as yet unconvinced or reluctant practitioners, researchers, and nurse administrators the potential benefits of involvement in LTC. Nursing homes, therefore, are a unique service arena in which professional nurses' skills and interests are particularly well matched with patient needs.

THE TEACHING NURSING HOME PROGRAM CONCEPT

The affiliations forged under the sponsorship of the Robert Wood Johnson Foundation Teaching Nursing Home Program capitalize on the congruency of interests between nursing homes and schools of nursing on issues of patient care, education, and research.

Many of the problems of nursing homes are attributable to their relative isolation from mainstream medical care. Most nursing homes are small in scale, having an average bed capacity of 75. Most are freestanding without formal organizational links to other health providers, and most are physically isolated from community hospitals, physicians' offices, and other community health care resources. Affiliation contracts with major mainstream medical institutions provide a mechanism that has been used in the past to assist isolated health care institutions to attract professional staff and improve quality of care (17–20).

Affiliations with medical schools have been proposed for some years as a strategy for improving nursing homes (21). Indeed, where nursing homes have been large enough to support full-time medical staff, or where long-term beds were physically or organizationally part of a hospital system, as with some VA homes, medical school affiliations have been successfully implemented (22), and model demonstration grants intended to stimulate research on LTC problems have now been funded by the National Institute on Aging (23,24).

Critics of medically affiliated nursing homes point to the hazards and costs of "medicalizing" and overtreating the normal processes of aging and death, and the inappropriateness of limiting geriatric training to institutionalized patients (25). Moreover, nursing homes have traditionally been the purview of nurses. The emphasis on nursing in the description of LTC institutions and definitions of levels of care, i.e., "skilled nursing care," implies that nursing care is the core service required and provided in nursing homes. Physicians operate as consultants in an institution where nursing care is central and constitutes nearly all direct patient contact. Although physicians can assume a more valuable role in diagnosis and treatment, some medical educators advise against a more dominant medical presence, which could undermine the central role of nurses (26,27).

An affiliation model linking nursing homes and university nursing schools, however, holds promise not only for improving education and research opportunities for all health professions but also for restructuring and enhancing the clinical care capacity of nursing homes. The Robert Wood Johnson Teaching Nursing Home Program affiliations are initiatives in which two (or more) agencies or institutions collaborate in the development of a new activity or service. This collaboration involves fundamental reshaping or innovation that exceeds that which each partner could do alone. Such joint ventures are shaped from the beginning not only by interorganizational linkages but to a great extent by intraorganizational factors (28,29). Successful affiliations, therefore, require that both partners in the venture undergo internal and mutual recalibrations. These affiliations are not simple mergers in which schools of nursing carry out education and research while nursing homes continue clinical care of older people. The 11 projects in the program are developing areas of shared activities and responsibility: innovations in patient/resident health care, more and better education for health professionals, and new understanding of care needs through clinical research.

INSTITUTIONAL CHARACTERISTICS OF THE ROBERT WOOD JOHNSON TEACHING NURSING HOME PROGRAM

In 1981, applications to the Robert Wood Johnson Teaching Nursing Home Program were generated from a pool of approximately 130 eligible universities with baccalaureate and higher degree programs in nursing. The 11 participating sites were selected from among 53 applicants. These sites include six public and six private education institutions located in nine states and the District of Columbia (30).

Certain characteristics of the program's schools of nursing are of particular interest. As of 1982, participating schools tended to be larger, both in terms of faculty size and undergraduate nursing students, than schools of nursing nationally. Of the participating schools, the average faculty size was 53 FTEs, and 50% of the participating schools had 400 or more undergraduate students compared to 20% of all schools of nursing nationally (31).

Funded schools demonstrated a strong interest in and prior commitment to gerontological nursing. Three-fourths (75%) of the participating schools had 10 or more school of nursing faculty publications in gerontological nursing. Of the 27 schools that had received Division of Nursing funding for masters level preparation in gerontology, 14 submitted applications for the TNHP, of which seven were funded.

The degree of experience with affiliations may have been a factor in the choices made by schools of nursing in their selection of nursing homes. Five of the funded sites had a strong history of prior affiliation activities, defined for this purpose as (a) responsibility for administration of nursing service and (b) a mechanism for joint appointments of faculty that involves joint funding. Six sites had little or no experience with this type of activity. Schools with strong experience with clinical affiliations tended to select homes that had a past history of having one or more masters-prepared nurses and/or strong physician backup or potential for such backup and/or strong preexisting linkages with acute-care facilities (30).

The 12 nursing homes originally participating in this project included two county facilities, two proprietary facilities, including one facility that was a member of a large corporate chain of nursing homes, and eight voluntary nonprofit homes including six church-related homes. One site has affiliation agreements with two different nursing homes. Five homes had a close corporate relationship with acute-care facilities. Two were part of organizational structures that encompassed a continuum of care, including independent living units, and/or had linkages with a home health agency.

In general, the participating nursing homes tended to be larger and better staffed than the national average. All of the participating homes had more than 100 beds. Whereas 73% of the nursing homes in this country do not have 24-hr RN coverage (6), the level of nurse staffing in the TNHP homes appeared to be higher than in nursing homes nationally. The figures for beds per nurse (RN plus LPN) in the TNHP homes ranged from 3.5 to 8.2, whereas nationally the data ranged from 7.5 to 13.4 beds per nurse when averaged by type of facility (e.g., SNF/ICF, SNF, ICF) (SysteMetrics, Division of Data Resources, Bethesda, *unpublished data*).

OUTCOMES

Although the primary objectives of the Robert Wood Johnson TNHP are to improve quality of life and care for nursing home patients, it is anticipated that the program will have a significant impact on preparation of geriatric nurses and on the advancement of clinical research. To achieve quality of care outcomes, sites are concentrating their efforts on implementing programs for the prevention, identification, and management of common health problems encountered in nursing homes. Problems of concern include infection, incontinence, ambulation impairments, iatrogenic responses, and altered sleep patterns. In order to successfully achieve the primary clinical objectives of this project, health professionals in general and physicians and nurses in particular are working to arrive at a new mechanism for collaboration and shared decision making. As indicated previously, physicians are relatively absent from the nursing home (32,33). Only 17% of physicians who would normally be expected to serve the elderly (general practitioners, family physicians, internists) actually make nursing home visits. Primary care physicians spend, on the average, less than $1\frac{1}{2}$ hr per month caring for their patients in nursing homes (34).

Since nurses are the health professionals on the scene, their capacity to act must be assured. Current customs of delayed response, *de facto* delegation, or absentee health care management need to give way to a more rational and realistic reappointment of decision-making responsibility. To successfully develop nurse–physician collaboration, a skilled, well-prepared nurse and a responsive, knowledgeable physician are required. Considerable mutual benefit to the two health professionals is possible in a shared model, and care for the elderly or chronically ill client is likely to be more individualized, prompt, and cost-effective.

The increased level of acuity of people now admitted to nursing homes raises questions about the utility of the current measures of the intensity of care, and what constitutes appropriate staffing patterns for patients with differing nursing care needs. There is a general agreement, however, that recruitment and retention of qualified nursing staff is essential.

Unfortunately, although the nursing profession is responding to the care needs of the elderly, there continues to be a lag in the recruitment of sufficient numbers of nurses into LTC. Currently, 101,000 nurses, 8% of the RN work force, and only 400 of the 20,000 nurse practitioners are involved in LTC (35,36). The reluctance of nurses to pursue careers in nursing homes is understandable given the regulatory statutes and reimbursement schedules, which serve to limit numbers of personnel and salaries. For example, only 15% of nursing home staff are registered nurses. This translates into one RN per 49 patients. In acute-care hospitals, there is one RN per four to five patients, and professionals make up about 46% of the total hospital staff. Nursing home residents receive on the average 12.5 min of RN care per 24 hr (37). In 1979, the average nurse working in LTC was 45.8 years old. The average salary was $13,000 (range $11,000–$17,000), with an average hourly reimbursement rate of $5.93/hr. These figures are quite striking when contrasted with those of nurses working in acute-care settings who received $6.86/hr. Nursing home nurses receive few employee benefits as compared to nurses in general. As of 1977, only 7.2% had paid vacations or sick leave, only 11% had retirement programs, and very few had tuition reimbursement (38). Given these statistics, it comes as no surprise that geriatric patients and facilities are consistently cited as the least desirable specialty by nursing students. Fewer than 5% of students identify a commitment to work with the elderly despite the need for a fourfold increase in gerontological nurses (39).

Nursing school affiliations should bring a new source of potential recruits to the nursing home setting. Nurses will be more willing to work in homes affiliated with university nursing schools just as they have preferred teaching hospitals because of increased visibility, greater colleagueship, and opportunities for continuing education and career advancement. Affiliations are also likely to result in more competitive salary and benefit packages for nursing home nurses, which will enhance recruitment efforts. Moreover, in recent years the job market for nurses has tightened and is expected to remain this way for the rest of the decade (40,41). Many more nurses can be expected to consider nursing home employment than in years past, making this an ideal time to recruit nurses. Furthermore, the program should expand the pool of nursing faculty specialized in geriatrics by incorporating the pool of qualified nursing home personnel into faculty positions and affording easily accessible practice and research opportunities.

EVALUATION

The evaluation of the TNHP, which is cofunded by the Robert Wood Johnson Foundation and the Health Care Financing Administration, is being conducted at the University of Colorado Health Sciences Center by the Center for Health Services Research. The major focus of the evaluation is to determine measurable evidence of the project's impact on selected quality-of-care indicators. The evaluation should help to identify potential areas of cost saving that could serve to offset anticipated increased expenses of incorporating more and higher-paid nurses and other professional staff into the nursing home.

In addition to assessing the general quality of care for patients in the TNHP homes in comparison to patients in matched control homes, the evaluation will pay specific attention to the "hidden expenses" of nursing home care, use of emergency rooms for diagnostic evaluations, prevalence and reasons for hospital admissions, transfer of patients from the nursing home immediately prior to death, and impact of the project on discharge of "hard-to-care-for" patients awaiting nursing home placement.

SUMMARY

At present, far too few health professionals, nurses, and physicians devote their careers to the care of the elderly. In each of the three settings where nurses and the aged ordinarily encounter one another, the home, the hospital, and the nursing home, different factors currently operate to inhibit the full practice of excellent nursing. The Robert Wood Johnson Teaching Nursing Home Program affords an opportunity to demonstrate the benefits of pooling service and educational resources to create centers for excellence in practice, education, and research in the care of the elderly.

REFERENCES

1. Brody S, Magel J: DRG, The second revolution in health care in the elderly. Paper presented at the APHA annual meeting, Dallas, TX, November 1983.
2. Brody S, Persily N: *Hospitals and the Aged—The New Old Market.* Rockville, MD, Aspen Publications, 1984.
3. Fox P: Long-term care: background and future directions. Office of Policy Analysis, Office of Legislation & Policy, HCFA, unpublished document, 1981.
4. Liu K, Paksh Y: The nursing home population: Different perspectives and implications for health policy. *Health Care Financ Rev* 1981;3:2.
5. Mezey M, Lynaugh J: Facts and issues for nursing in long-term care. Paper prepared for the American Hospital Association National Commission on Long-Term Care, 1983.
6. DHEW: *The National Nursing Home Survey: 1977, Summary of the United States,* #43, DHEW Pub. No. 79–1794. Washington DC, US Government Printing Office, 1979.
7. Christman L, Grace H: Unification, reunification: Reconciliation or collaboration, in *Modes for Collaboration, Fall Conference Proceedings, Midwest Alliance in Nursing,* September, 1980–1. Unpublished document.
8. Ford LC: Creating a center of excellence in nursing, in Aiken L (ed): *Health Policy and Nursing Practice.* New York, McGraw-Hill, 1981, pp 242–255.

9. MacPhail J: *An Experiment in Nursing: Planning, Implementing, and Assessing in Planned Change.* Cleveland, Case Western Reserve University, 1972.
10. Lundeen S: Erie Family Health Center, Inc: An interdisciplinary nurse-managed center, in Mezey M, McGivern D (eds): *Nurses, Nurse Practitioners: The Evolution of Primary Care.* New York, Little Brown, 1984 (in press).
11. Herman C, Krall K: University Sponsored Home Care Agency. Paper presented at Clinical Experience Today & Tomorrow. College of St. Catherine, St. Paul, ME, July 22–24, 1983.
12. Nurse Faculty Fellowships in Primary Care, A National Program of the Robert Wood Johnson Foundation, September, 1976. Unpublished document.
13. LeRoy L, Solkowitz S: *The Implications of Cost-Effectiveness of Medical Technology: Case Study #16: The Costs and Effectiveness of Nurse Practitioners.* Washington, Office of Technology Assessment, 1981.
14. Fagin C: Nursing's pivotal role in achieving competition in health care. Address given to the American Academy of Nursing, Washington, 1981.
15. Ebersole PA, Smith EW, Dickey L, et al: Roles and functions of geriatric nurse practitioners in long term care as viewed by physician GNP and administrator. *Am Health Care Assoc J* 1982;3:2–7.
16. Henderson M: A GNP in a retirement community. *Geriatr Nursing* 1984;5:109–112.
17. Aiken L: Nursing priorities for the 1980's: Hospitals and nursing homes. *Am J Nursing* 1981;81(2):324–330.
18. Mechanic L, Aiken L: A cooperative agenda for medicine and nursing. *N Engl J Med* 1982;307(12):747–750.
19. Ginsberg E, Columbia University Conservation of Human Resources Staff: *Urban Health Services: The Case of New York.* New York, Columbia University Press, 1971.
20. State Study Commission for New York City: *Health Care Needs and the New York City Health and Hospitals Corporation.* New York, The Commission, 1973.
21. Pawlson LG: Education in the nursing home: Practical considerations. *J Am Geriatr Soc* 1982;30(9):600–602.
22. Farber SJ: The future role of the VA hospital system: A national health policy dilemma. *N Engl J Med* 1978;298:625–628.
23. Schneider E: Teaching nursing homes. *N Engl J Med* 1983;308(6):336–337.
24. Butler RN: The teaching nursing home. *JAMA* 1981;245:1435–1437.
25. Ahronheim J: Pitfalls of the teaching nursing home, a case for balanced geriatric education. *N Engl J Med* 1983;308(6):335–336.
26. Gillick MR: To the care of the chronically ill a medical prerogative? *N Engl J Med* 1984;310:190–193.
27. Kane RL, Hammer D, Byrnes N: Getting care to nursing-home patients: A problem and a proposal. *Med Care* 1977;15:174–180.
28. Hirschorn L: *Joint Ventures and the Reshaping of Relationships Within Organizations. Retrenchment/Redevelopment Series Working Paper.* Philadelphia, Management and Behavioral Science Center, Wharton School, University of Pennsylvania, Winter 1983.
29. Charns MP, Laurence P, Weisbord M: *TIMS Studies in the Management Sciences,* vol 5: *Organizing Multiple-Function Professionals in Academic Medical Center.* Amsterdam, North-Holland, 1977, pp 71–88.
30. Mezey MD, Lynaugh JE, Cherry JE: The teaching nursing home program: A report on joint ventures between schools of nursing and nursing homes. *Nursing Outlook* 1984;32(3):146–150.
31. National League of Nursing: *Nursing Data Book, 1981.* New York, National League of Nursing, 1981.
32. US Senate Special Committee on Aging: *Nursing Home Care in the United States: Failure in Public Policy, Supporting Paper No. 3, Doctors in Nursing Homes: The Shunned Responsibility.* Washington DC, US Government Printing Office, 1975.
33. Kane R, et al.: The future need for geriatric manpower in the United States. *N Engl J Med* 1980;302:24.
34. Center for Health Policy Studies, Georgetown University: National Physician Study conducted by Robert Mendenhall, University of Southern California School of Medicine (ICPSR 7782) (unpublished report).
35. American Nurses Association: *Fact Sheet on Registered Nurses.* Washington DC, ANA, Government Relations Division, 1980.

36. Health Resources Administration: *Health Personnel Issues in the Context of Long Term Care in Nursing Homes.* Washington DC, Public Health Service, HRA, 1980.
37. Shields E, Kick E: Nursing care in nursing homes, in Aiken L (ed): *Nursing in the 1980's Crisis, Opportunities, Challenges.* Philadelphia, JB Lippincott, 1982, pp 195–210.
38. DHEW: *The National Nursing Home Survey: 1977, Summary of the United States,* #43, DHEW Pub. No. (PHS) 79–1794. Hyattsville, MD, US Government Printing Office, 1979.
39. Strumpf N, Mezey M: A developmental approach to the teaching of aging. *Nursing Outlook* 1980;20:12.
40. Aiken L: The nurse labor market. *Health Affairs* 1982;1:30–40.
41. Institute of Medicine, Health Care Services Division, Nursing and Nursing Education Committee: *Nursing and Nursing Education: Public Policies and Private Actions* (Pub. No. ISEN 0-309-03346-2). Washington, DC, National Academy Press, 1983.

The Teaching Nursing Home, edited by Edward L. Schneider et al. © 1985 The Beverly Foundation. Raven Press, New York.

The NIA Teaching Nursing Home Award Program: A National Program of Research on Geriatrics and Long-Term Care

Noel D. List, Marcia G. Ory, and Evan C. Hadley

National Institute on Aging, National Institutes of Health, Bethesda, Maryland 20205

Despite the burgeoning of the elderly population in the 1980s, the academic community has devoted little attention to research on medical or social aspects of geriatric care. The National Institute on Aging (NIA) initiated its Teaching Nursing Home (TNH) Program in 1982 to stimulate high-quality research on the development, course, and treatment of diseases and disabilities prevalent in old age that have often been neglected in the past. Jointly sponsored by the two extramural programs at the NIA, this program encourages both biomedical and behavioral sciences research on clinical or functional problems of the elderly. The NIA concept is not limited to research on health problems of the nursing home population but also considers biomedical, behavioral, and social factors influencing the health and functioning of older people and their need for long-term care (LTC) services. The purpose of this chapter is to provide a brief description of the goals of the NIA TNH program, the scope of the solicited research, the eligibility criteria and award structure, currently funded projects, and recommendations for future research directions.

GOALS AND OBJECTIVES

The National Institute on Aging's legislative mandate is to conduct and support biomedical, social, and behavioral research and training related to the aging process and the diseases and other special problems and needs of the aged. To date, research on chronic diseases and disabilities prevalent in old age is not being aggressively addressed by the academic research community and is not keeping pace with the rapid growth of the elderly population and their escalating needs for health care (1–4). The Teaching Nursing Home Award of the NIA is a special grant mechanism designed to support investigator-initiated research by academic centers and nursing homes on health problems, therapies, and health maintenance strategies for older people in nursing homes as well as other institutional and community settings.

Some confusion exists concerning the definition and implementation of TNH concepts. This is in part because different TNH models place different emphases on geriatric research, training, and care. The program's title is intended to emphasize the analogy between the teaching hospital as a setting for research in acute-care settings and the "teaching nursing home" as a site to develop research in LTC settings (5–7). Despite the title, however, teaching, training, or service activities per se are not directly supported by this mechanism.

The TNH program of the NIA supports research in a variety of LTC settings, with the nursing home as just one of the sites. The NIA has selected this multisite approach for several reasons. If the health problems responsible for placement in nursing homes are to be successfully prevented, they must be studied in their early stages, prior to institutionalization. Furthermore, the conduct of LTC research in multiple clinical settings allows comparisons of alternative therapeutic strategies.

Similarly, the emphasis of the NIA program is multidisciplinary. Recognizing that the health of older people is determined by complex and interacting biological, social, and psychological processes that occur over the life course, the NIA program is sponsored jointly between NIA extramural research programs, the Biomedical Research and Clinical Medicine Program, and the Behavioral Sciences Research Program. Thus, multidisciplinary research is encouraged on the roles that biomedical, behavioral, and social factors play in the etiology and course of chronic diseases and disabilities in the middle and later years. A goal of the TNH program is to generate information on strategies to maintain health and prevent or postpone disease in a variety of LTC settings.

The TNH award focuses on such clinical issues as understanding and treating chronic diseases that result in significant morbidity, institutionalization, or mortality of the elderly. Chronic diseases and disabilities associated with aging can seriously affect patients who are "geographically and intellectually removed from traditional academic medicine interests and concerns" (7). Senile dementia, urinary incontinence, osteoporosis, osteoarthritis, depression, falls, and a number of other medical conditions in the elderly have been the subject of only limited research despite the fact that they are major causes of disability and demand costly health and social services.

The lack of knowledge about the causes and consequences of such diseases may result in inappropriate, indifferent, or inadequate care. In some cases this lack of information can lead to the failure to recognize and properly treat reversible conditions, a situation that can have untold medical and social consequences for patients and their families. To make matters worse, health care professionals in the United States are not consistently trained to care for the special problems and concerns of older people. This situation is changing, but there is still a severe shortage of geriatricians in this country (8).

Congress has recognized the need for more research and training in geriatric medicine and has provided special funding for NIA's TNH Awards. As the present time, the NIA TNH Program is designed (a) to encourage investigators to turn their attention to the field of aging and to the health problems of the elderly; and (b) to increase understanding of ways to prevent and treat chronic diseases and disabilities that contribute heavily to the need for institutionalization and other LTC services. Although the NIA program does not support training or service, the underlying expectation is that the research stimulated by model TNH programs will lead to improvements in geriatric training and care.

SCOPE OF PROPOSED RESEARCH

The NIA's broad definition of the TNH Program acknowledges the need for a greater understanding of the biomedical, behavioral, psychosocial, and environmental problems associated with health problems, treatments, and health maintenance strategies of older people. Therefore, research is solicited in four broadly defined areas:

- Epidemiology, pathophysiology, diagnosis, and therapy of specific disorders causing significant morbidity and mortality in the elderly, such as dementia, incontinence, sleep apnea, musculoskeletal disorders, and infections.
- Behavioral, psychological, social, environmental, and organizational influences on health and health care of the elderly, such as effects of social supports, stress, and coping patterns on health and well-being and the impact of alternative LTC strategies on functioning of aged patients and their families.
- The roles of nutrition, exercise, and other factors in the prevention of diseases and functional disability in the elderly.
- Rehabilitative and prosthetic techniques for ameliorating chronic musculoskeletal, neurologic, and other health problems of the elderly.

ELIGIBILITY CRITERIA

The TNH award is only one of several NIA funding mechanisms that provide support for geriatric research. The TNH award is based on the program project mechanism and is appropriate in one or more of the following situations.

1. Unlike most program project grants, which often involve only one discipline and are required to have a central theme or approach, the

TNH program projects encourage multidisciplinary investigations. Further, since biomedical, clinical, and behavioral science aspects of geriatric research have long been neglected, research depth may not be available in any one area. Therefore, to achieve research goals requires exchange of data or services among several research projects from one or more disciplines.

2. Several discrete research projects depend on a core resource for the research activity. Core functions appropriate for this mechanism might include: (a) recruiting, clinical screening, and/or follow-up of subjects for the TNH research projects; (b) providing biostatistical support in design and analysis of individual research projects and in the overall evaluation of the project; (c) developing a central data file on individuals participating in the TNH clinical studies and/or incorporating test results and other data from the base data set and research activities from these studies into a standardized accessible format for analysis; and (d) planning for program review and development of existing and new pilot studies and research projects.

3. Several detailed projects are beyond the capacity of any single investigator. Frequently, interlocking questions must be addressed simultaneously in order for the researchers to attain a desired goal. For example, understanding the etiology, course, and treatment of the dementias may involve projects in epidemiology, neurobiology, neuropathology, neuropsychology, and psychiatry as well as the behavioral sciences. In these cases, the principal investigator must be a senior scientist who is able to organize, supervise, and produce a research outcome from diverse elements that will contribute to our knowledge base in geriatrics and gerontology.

4. A TNH provides the best mechanism for several schools or institutions to collaborate in a research program. It permits investigators to share resources and facilities to pursue research goals that might otherwise be impossible.

The rules and regulations for the TNH program are described in detail in the guidelines for prospective applicants (6). Two basic components must be present in any TNH program and are therefore mentioned here. First, each TNH must include at least three individual research projects that are coordinated under the supervision of an experienced research investigator. The TNHs may either address multiple health problems or different aspects of a single health problem. Second, each TNH project should include plans for a central core that will provide research support, data management, and the development of supplemental projects that may be added to the TNH base.

The applicant may request up to $500,000 for direct costs during the first year of the overall TNH program project with appropriate annual incremental increases in future years. The initial award may run for 5 years and may not exceed $3 million in direct costs. The maximum duration of new awards, and of competitive renewals of awards, is 5 years. Projects may be extended, through competitive renewal applications, up to a maximum total project period of 10 years.

There are several unique requirements that prospective applicants must meet to be eligible for the TNH Award. These prerequisites reflect the NIA's desire to promote an increased interaction between academic and nursing home personnel as a means of furthering clinical research on aging. To be considered for the Award, prospective applicants must document the participation of one or more nursing homes, a school of medicine, and a school, division, or department of nursing. Additional participation of other institutions (a school of public health or department of behavioral sciences) is desirable. Any participating institution may serve as the grantee, subject to NIH policy. Components need not represent a single academic center.

Individuals from each of the three essential components should have significant responsibilities in TNH projects. These responsibilities may involve the operation of the TNH center core and/or the conduct of one or more research projects. The proposed research projects need not include a project from each component.

Although the primary research goal of the NIA TNH program is to further knowledge relevant to geriatric medicine, a secondary goal is to bring the resources and personnel of academic centers into LTC settings. The best parallel to the expected outcome would be the changes that resulted from the integration of Veterans Administration hospitals and academic teaching medical centers. In this latter program, the medical school faculty receive support from the Veterans Administration hospitals of which they become staff, and monies are made available through separate Veterans Administration sources for research. It is hoped that changes and improvements in research and practice will result from the collaboration of the medical and nursing schools with the nursing home and other LTC settings.

CURRENT NIA TNH PROGRAMS

Since NIA's initial announcement of the TNH program in 1981, over 45 applications have been submitted for review. As of April 1984, NIA has funded teaching nursing homes at six sites: (a) Albert Einstein College of Medicine and Montefiore Medical Center and associated chronic care facilities; (b) Philadelphia Gerontology Research Consortium, consisting of The Philadelphia Geriatric Center, the Medical College of Pennsylvania, and the University of Pennsylvania; (c) Case Western Reserve University School of Medicine in collaboration with the School of Nursing, affiliated teaching hospitals, and nursing homes; (d) the Hebrew Rehabilitation Center for Aged in conjunction with the Beth Israel Hospital, Massachusetts General Hospital, the Harvard Medical School, and the Boston University

School of Nursing; (e) The Johns Hopkins Medical Institutions in affiliation with Baltimore City Hospitals and the Mason F. Lord Chronic Care Hospital; and (f) The University of California, San Diego School of Medicine, San Diego State School of Nursing and affiliated nursing homes and geriatric-service-based programs. These consortia of academic nursing homes have received approximately $3 million for their first year of operation with a cumulative 5-year commitment for $17.5 million.

The individual projects supported by the first five TNH awards are listed in Table 1. This listing indicates that the majority of projects focus on distinguishing between normal aging and disease processes and on increasing our understanding of the major chronic diseases and conditions associated with aging. For example, there are five research projects on Alzheimer's disease and other causes of dementia, three projects on sleep disorders, two projects each on the relationship of exercise and nutritional factors to the health of the elderly, two projects each on falls, infections, pulmonary function, and functional assessment, and one project each on arthritis, rehabilitation, incontinence, and osteoporosis. In addition, there are socioepidemiological/behavioral sciences studies focusing on factors associated with functioning in community and nursing home settings and on risk factors for institutional placement. Detailed information on any one of these programs can be obtained from the individual principal investigators.

DISCUSSION AND FUTURE DIRECTION

We are pleased that the NIA TNH award has brought increased research attention to chronic diseases and conditions of the elderly population. In addition, several interdisciplinary collaborative research efforts have been stimulated by this award mechanism. The TNH mechanism has also stimulated affiliations and mutually productive arrangements between academia and LTC institutions. Medical and nursing directors at these institutions have been given faculty appointments, and agreements have been made for medical and nursing students, house staff, and fellows to rotate through the nursing homes.

Although NIA's TNH program is intended to stimulate both biomedical and behavioral sciences studies relevant to geriatric research, there are few funded behavioral sciences projects in the currently funded TNH programs. Thus, there is a need for more social and psychological research. Also, a greater emphasis should be placed on the development and testing of both biomedical and behavioral interventions for helping older people maintain maximal functioning whether at home or in institutions.

Behavioral sciences research in the TNH program can contribute to our knowledge in two major ways. First, separate projects can focus on understanding how social, psychological, or environmental factors influence older people's morbidity, risk of institutionalization, or mortality. For example, little is known about how organizational characteristics of the nursing home

TABLE 1. *Teaching nursing home projects, 1982–1983*

Albert Einstein College of Medicine (1982)[a]	Case Western Reserve University (1983)[a]	Hebrew Rehabilitation Center (1983)[a]	Johns Hopkins University (1983)[a]	Medical College of Pennsylvania (1982)[a]
Dementia studies in context of TNH	Cleveland GAO study of elderly: a follow-up	Syncope and blood pressure homeostasis in the elderly	Cardiopulmonary effects of training in an aging population	Urinary tract infections in a geriatric population
Osteoarthritis: synovial cell–cartilage interactions	Performance and control of the respiratory muscles	Bladder function and incontinence in frail elderly	Aging, adiposity, physical fitness, and endocrine metabolic function	Cognitive rehabilitation of stroke
Falls in the elderly	Autonomic and airway reactivity in the aged	Vitamin D nutrition in the institutionalized elderly	Aging, adiposity, and sleep-disordered breathing	Regional metabolism and flow in aging and dementia
Cognitive and genetic aspects of Alzheimer's dementia		Identification of persons at risk of institutional placement	Neurobehavioral performance in aging and the role of sleep-disordered breathing	Modification of exercise capacity in the elderly
		Clinical and neuroendocrine measures of depression in SDAT		Sleep apnea syndrome in the elderly
		Vasopressin release in dementia		
Robert Katzman, M.D.[b]	Amasa B. Ford, M.D.[b]	John W. Rowe, M.D.[b]	William Hazzard, M.D.[b]	Donald Kaye, M.D.[b]

[a] Year of grant award.
[b] Principal investigator.

affect patient survival and well-being. Second, the TNH concept can help integrate behavioral sciences research questions into other, more traditional biomedical or clinical studies. This might involve the examination of social factors as determinants or consequences of medical treatments. Behavioral scientists can also provide valuable expertise on questions of methodology, research design, or analysis of longitudinal data for individual study projects.

Although the primary focus of the NIA TNH research projects should be on clinical or functional endpoints, there could be more research on economic or health services aspects of chronic diseases and disabilities prevalent in old age. Few studies have systematically addressed how the structure and delivery of health care services affect or are affected by the physiological changes people experience as they grow older. There has been little interdisciplinary research aimed at understanding social and behavioral factors as they affect patients' or providers' health attitudes and behaviors and the delivery and utilization of health care services for older people.

Significant scientific and public policy issues and questions surround the TNH concept (9–12). Some people fear that the academic centers' incursion into LTC settings will introduce high-cost, high-technology methodologies into the nursing home. This is not an inevitable conclusion. The information gained from research conducted in TNHs will facilitate the choice of appropriate levels of technology for optimal care. The need for this knowledge is increasingly urgent because of the growth of the very old population and the escalating costs of nursing home care, which are projected to quadruple by 1990 to more than $90 billion. There is a need to develop improved diagnostic and therapeutic methods, encourage preventive self-care strategies, increase support of existing family and informal caregivers, and stimulate other LTC alternatives. Additionally, it is not anticipated that every nursing home will be a teaching nursing home. Rather, NIA envisions a small number of model teaching nursing homes that should contribute to our understanding of significant biomedical, social, and policy questions about the health and health care of a rapidly aging population.

REFERENCES

1. Brody JA, Brock DB: Epidemiologic and statistical characteristics of the U.S. elderly population. Draft 1982, in Finch CE, Schneider EL (eds): *Handbook of the Biology of Aging*, ed 2. New York, Van Nostrand Reinhold (in press).
2. Federal Council on the Aging, US Department of Health and Human Services: *The Need for Long-term Care: Information and Issues*. Washington, Government Printing Office, 1981.
3. Rice D, Feldman J: Living longer in the United States: Demographic changes and health needs of the elderly. Milbank Mem Fund Q 1983;61:362–396.
4. US Department of Commerce, Bureau of the Census: *America in Transition: An Aging Society. Current Population Reports*, Series P-23, No. 128. Washington, Government Printing Office, 1983.
5. Butler RN: The teaching nursing home. *JAMA* 1981;245:1435–1437.
6. Department of Health and Human Services, National Institute on Aging: Guidelines for Prospective Applicants: NIA Teaching Nursing Home (TNH) Awards for Geriatric Research, November, 1982.

7. Schneider EL: The teaching nursing home. *N Engl J Med* 1983;308:336–337.
8. Kane RL, Soloman DH, Beck JC, et al: *Geriatrics in the United States*. Santa Monica, Rand Corporation, 1981.
9. Ahronheim JC: The teaching nursing home. *N Engl J Med* 1983;308:335–336.
10. Kapp MB: Nursing homes as teaching institutions: Legal issues. *Gerontologist* 1984;24:55–60.
11. Libow LS: Geriatric medicine and the nursing home: A mechanism for mutual excellence. *Gerontologist* 1982;22:134–141.
12. Weiner AS, Lichtman M: The nursing home as a teaching and research center. *J Long-Term Care Admin* Fall 1982, pp 2–8.

The Teaching Nursing Home, edited by Edward
L. Schneider et al. © 1985 The Beverly
Foundation. Raven Press, New York.

Mount Sinai School of Medicine

Robert N. Butler

Ritter Department of Geriatrics, Mount Sinai Medical Center, New York, New York
10029

It has been clear for some time that revolutionary reforms are necessary in medical education, services, and research if our society is to meet effectively the challenge posed by an unprecedented increase in absolute numbers as well as the relative proportion of older persons. The rapid increase in longevity, especially among the oldest segment of the population, requires creative innovations in service, alterations of the biomedical and behavioral research agenda, reconsideration of dollar allocations, establishment of innovative health and social policies, and the systematic integration of gerontology into professional education. There must be an aggressive pursuit of the study of aging from the biological, psychological, and social perspectives with the application of this knowledge to prevention, diagnosis, care, and treatment of the elderly. Geriatrics must be integrated throughout contemporary medical undergraduate and postgraduate education. The modest incremental change in activity in geriatrics that is occurring today is inadequate considering the impressive growth of the elderly population.

The creation of the National Institute on Aging provided multiple opportunities to develop a research program that could support and/or conduct studies that would examine the rates of aging of various systems, distinguish the changes of aging from those of disease, identify biomarkers of aging, abate or delay aging and its consequences, and, where possible, provide the means for social and personal adjustment. The problem, then, has been to develop a mechanism that could accomplish this and be positively integrated into the care system.

It was felt that the Teaching Nursing Home Award could alter the traditionalism of the medical schools which continued to act as though the population was not aging and as though the typical patient was the young or middle-aged individual suffering from a single identifiable and perhaps even "exciting" medical illness. The basic concept of the teaching nursing home (TNH) to many agencies is the creation of a mechanism capable of precipitating major reforms in areas including the reimbursement systems, with renegotiations of the fee schedules of Medicare, Blue Cross–Blue Shield, and commercial carrier insurance systems to ensure success beyond a scope limited to research. Such reimbursement changes would have to be brought into conformity with the changing demography of the nation and, therefore, with the changing incidence and prevalence of disease. These changes might occur even within constant dollars by evolving alterations in benefit structure, including greater attention to preventive care (check-ups), outpatient care (e.g. outpatient coverage of medication), home care, and long-term care (LTC). There is an obvious need for expanded nursing home insurance as well. Comprehensive assessment, which is so vital and cost-effective and "human effective," must be more appropriately reimbursed.

Many practitioners of LTC felt that efforts should be made to bring together acute care and chronic care. The Commission on Chronic Illness, as early as 1952, urged that separation of acute and chronic care be avoided. The advice of this distinguished blue-ribbon commission was not followed. With the passage of Medicare and Medicaid as amendments to the Social Security Act in 1965 came an explosion of a separate nursing home industry. Much of nursing home care is currently outside of the mainstream of medicine and nursing; in fact, the nursing home remains outside of academia.

It seems reasonable that just as teaching hospitals are the standards against which community hospitals can compare themselves, the development of their counterpart, the TNHs, could become the standard for all homes for the aging and the measure against which evaluation can occur. Is it too much to ask that each of our 127 medical schools have affiliations with at least one TNH just as they do with the teaching hospital? All together there are 416 teaching hospitals in the United States.

In retrospect, it might have been better to speak of an academic nursing home to make clear the fact that the concept would have to fulfill the classic academic goals not only of teaching but of the creation and implementation of innovative services and the ability to conduct research. The need is for the "teaching medical school" with reforms made in the methodology of teaching and the material content of our medical schools, not only in relationship to geriatrics but to capitalize on the extraordinary advances in knowledge and the changing needs of society. The realities of advances such as recombinant DNA and hybridoma technologies parallel the need to advance our abilities to deal more directly and effectively with the "stuff of life," nutrition, bereavement, death. The TNH is a device to improve nursing homes and to advance our fundamental knowledge base. There is a dire need to build and flesh out those laboratories. Many efforts have been made to alter the behavior and therefore the attitudes and activities of nursing homes through regulation. Regulations and the enforcement of regulations have not been altogether successful. It is unlikely that education will do the total job either, but it could create important standards and provide preservice and in-service training for those who work within nursing homes by introducing the kinds of disturbing and penetrating questions that students always ask and by stimulating the intellectual curiosity, even passion, that dedicated physicians, nurses, social workers, and other health professionals are able to provide in the nursing home setting.

There are other important elements including a need for imaginative studies of operating in the "real world." The Department of Health and Human Services and other regulators and suppliers must understand the multifactorial needs and realities of both private and nonprofit nursing homes, the importance of introducing prosthetic environmental design in old and new nursing home environments, and the necessity of pioneering efforts toward meeting the mobility, sensory, communicative, and psycho-social deficits of older patients and of meshing these with teaching and research within a reasonable economic construct. Nursing home architects and suppliers can respond through their capacities to design an environment to meet the need of the patient yet be compatible with the goals of the TNH. There is the need to build or renovate hospitals and nursing homes phys-ically and conceptually to better fit with the 21st century, when geriatrics will truly dominate the health care system.

The nation's first Department of Geriatrics and Adult Development at the Mount Sinai School of Medicine, in concert with the Jewish Home and Hospital for Aged (JHHA), which functions as a traditional medical school affiliate, has formed a partnership that is leading toward the integration of acute and long-term care. The JHHA was an academic and teaching nursing home which, in its 114th year of history, has moved toward a goal of be-coming a TNH. In 1925, Frederick Zeman, one of the pioneers in geriatrics, instituted a complete physical examination and history at the JHHA. In 1927, a social service program for the aged was established for the first time in any nursing home. In 1948, home care began. In 1950, a psychiatric program led by Alvin Goldfarb and Eli Savitsky was pioneered. Dr. Manuel Rodstein did important clinical studies in cardiology and on falls at the JHHA. The JHHA cares for 1,200 individuals at two complexes, one across New York's Central Park from The Mount Sinai School of Medicine and the second directly across from the Bronx Veterans Administration Hospital.

A major thrust of the Department of Geriatrics and Adult Development is the creation of a consultation service available to the nursing home in-dustry. We believe that such a geriatric consultation service would increase the effectiveness and efficiency of client institutions or agencies by providing the methodology for the most up-to-date care of patients and families. Its objective is to be implemented by field training workshops, seminars for facility staffs, career development of staff leaders through a program re-quiring attendance at Mount Sinai Medical Center, creation of clear, up-to-date guidebooks for caregivers dealing with practical care problems, rapid dissemination of patient care information in the form of newsletters and hotlines, and access and consultation services provided on site or tailored to specific client needs. In addition, the service will conduct research to improve techniques of care and aid in the organization of the delivery of services and the development of policies of reimbursement coupled with quality assurance. It would help to administer program reviews. The consultation service will also be involved at the interface between long-term and acute care, for example, the hospital response to the needs of nursing home residents. Finally, it would offer assistance to nursing homes desiring to develop a teaching or academic nursing home. The consultation service is a conceptualization of an additional way to extend the concept of the TNH without walls.

Under Dr. Leslie S. Libow, the Director of Medical Services of the JHHA and the Vice Chairman of the Department of Geriatrics and Adult Development, the present medical student teaching program at JHHA was created. All 132 Mount Sinai fourth-year students are required to take a 4-week rotation full-time in geriatric training, which started with the academic year beginning in the fall of 1983. A block of 11 students was scheduled for each rotation in the TNH setting at JHHA. A department faculty member supervises the rotation. Programs include didactic lectures, readings, home visits, weekly subspecialty rounds, weekly teaching rounds, and monthly patient staff conferences at JHHA. There are also routinely scheduled rounds in ethics.

Attitudinal surveys are taken before and after each rotation. The program staff realizes that the pressures of heavy programs coupled with the relative absence of much geriatric content in medical education are not conducive to a strong interest in geriatrics among the senior medical students. Through the implementation of this complex curriculum in the first year, and given the reality of the learning process for this department (which is striving to create a desire for changes and improvements against an attitude of passive disinterest), there has been surprising success for the staff. There now is the reward of discovering major changes in attitude and a new recognition of the validity and importance of geriatrics by many of these students on completion of their rotation. The objective of this experience is not to develop geriatricians but to sensitize students to the special needs and problems of the elderly, build their knowledge about geriatrics, and expose them to the many sites in which geriatric care is delivered: an acute-care hospital, home, clinic, and LTC facility.

The JHHA rotation in particular has become popular with medical students. There is a very different set of activities and, in fact, purpose in a LTC institution, which, for these residents, is their home. The nursing home is different from a high-technology acute-care medicine environment. The students learn about the elderly and about LTC issues by participating in the "nursing home without walls" program through home site visits. Such "house calls" were the first in the medical school experience of Mount Sinai medical students. It was their opportunity to become acquainted with the life conditions of older persons. In addition, there are several fellows in geriatrics who also participate through rotation at the JHHA and act as models for the medical students. The fellows have passed their boards or are board eligible in medicine. It is a 2-year fellowship, the second year of which includes half of the time spent in research. Several social workers and nurses in training are participating in the program.

With support from the Federation of Jewish Philantropies, a 25-bed geriatric rehabilitation unit was opened at the Jewish Home and Hospital for Aged in July, 1983. With the collaboration of the Department of Geriatrics and JHHA, this program offers a comprehensive rehabilitation program for elderly patients in the convalescent phase of medical or surgical illness. The program is directed at those patients who require a 2- to 3-month period of rehabilitation in order to achieve a level of independence that can allow discharge to home. Patients recovering from stroke, hip fracture, and limb amputation (prosthesis training) are prime candidates; general debilitation and respite care are also appropriate within this program. Only patients who have adequate cognitive function are eligible; this is a prerequisite for entry into the rehabilitation program because of the need to be able to understand and follow directions.

A nursing-home-based rehabilitation unit whose objective is the discharge of patients to their homes when possible is an expensive concept but one that has been shown to be cost effective. However, the standard nursing home bed reimbursements by third-party payers do not cover the cost of such programs, special therapies or therapists, prostheses, or other aids. A proportion of the costs have been covered by the JHHA through other sources. This Department plans to address the various reimbursement obstacles in providing geriatric care through its policy research component and perhaps ultimately through direct negotiations with third-party payers to obtain waivers.

Geriatric medicine lacks adequate resources and manpower. There is a desperate need for a Federal geriatric manpower bill and, most significantly, for incorporation of rehabilitation into all geriatric centers in the United States. Rehabilitation in Great Britain has helped tie together the continuum of acute and long-term care. Rehabilitation symbolizes effective intervention in geriatrics. This is augmented by the team approach, which is used both for admission screening and during the process of rehabilitation. It includes geriatric and other appropriate physicians, occupational and physical therapists, geriatric and rehabilitation nurses, social workers, activity therapists, dieticians, and others as appropriate. The staff psychiatrist evaluates each patient on admission and plans an individualized program. When appropriate, the services of a speech therapist and audiologist are utilized. Auxiliary services including podiatry, ophthalmology, and other subspecialty clinics are made available.

Because educational and clinical programs had to be operational almost instantly, planning and implementing them formed a major task for the Department. Funding, as well as time for research, was and continues to be limited. The research arm of the Department's activities is the least developed. However, through the generosity of the Robert Wood Johnson, Jr. Charitable Trust and the Willard T. C. Johnson Foundation, there is a developing program in Alzheimer's disease. There is active development of a special research experience for fellows and electives for medical students involving several concepts and techniques of aging research. There is active development of laboratory space and a vivarium.

The Department has major funding to create excellent laboratories. This TNH will concentrate on the neurobiology of aging as well as on problems found mainly in nursing home populations such as bed sores, functional assessment, urinary incontinence, infectious disease. Within all of the above activities, special care is taken to protect the rights of human subjects, especially the frail elderly in the nursing home setting, for whom there is need for special sensitivity. This is especially true in light of the need for eventual autopsies on these patients.

Relationships must continually be developed with the new nursing home for the Mount Sinai Medical School at the Bronx Veterans Administration Hospital affiliate. The Veterans Administration Nursing Home residents will be predominantly male, which should provide a very different population than that of JHHA.

The unique features of the JHHA are its organizational strengths, its funding sources, and its location in the city of New York. Government as well as private funding resources are important; private sector philanthropy, individuals, and foundations as well as cooperation with the existent (for-profit and nonprofit) nursing home enterprise must all be interrelated in a manner that will yield the creation of the TNH.

The partnership of JHHA and Mount Sinai is the beginning of the bridge that allows the Department of Geriatrics to have the ultimate laboratory, a TNH, which must be part of any genuine program in geriatrics building toward a model of coordinated services, teaching of medical students, and research.

PART III
Crosscutting Issues in the Teaching Nursing Home

The Teaching Nursing Home, edited by Edward
L. Schneider et al. © 1985 The Beverly
Foundation. Raven Press, New York.

Introduction

Anne Wilder Zimmer

*Biomedical Research and Clinical Medical Program, National Institutes of Health, Bethesda,
Maryland 20205*

Planning for a teaching nursing home requires more than simply transplanting researchers, teachers, and clinicians from the teaching hospital into a long-term care facility. There are existing patterns of behavior that require adaptation, and there are familiar issues that take on new meaning in this new environment.

The average nursing home is vastly different from a teaching hospital. Nursing home administrators are unfamiliar with research and training and are generally budget oriented and isolated from service staff. The composition, roles, and relationships within and between the professional team and support staff are different in the nursing home than in academia. Nursing home residents with chronic diseases require long-term care with the goal of maximum function instead of an emphasis on diagnosis and cure of acute diseases. Issues such as ethics, administration, assessment, and the quality of life of the resident are of concern in all clinical care. They take on new dimensions and importance, however, in long-term care because of the unique characteristics of the older population, the environment, and the nature of chronic diseases. Team management and participation skills must be learned; the physician may need to function either as a team member or team leader as required. Extra time must be allowed for clinical procedures on research subjects with multiple chronic conditions. Careful attention must be paid to the obtaining of consent for research on residents in long-term care facilities. Assessment can be used in new ways to facilitate care and research and to benefit the resident. Administrators must be involved and understood, and throughout, the welfare of nursing home residents must be a priority. Awareness of and joint planning for these challenges are critical.

The Teaching Nursing Home, edited by Edward
L. Schneider et al. © 1985 The Beverly
Foundation. Raven Press, New York.

The Teaching Nursing Home: Ethical Concerns

Christine K. Cassel

Department of Geriatics, Mt Sinai Medical Center, New York, New York 10029

Although there are many different models of what a teaching nursing home (TNH) could be and of what kinds of activities may be conducted within its boundaries, this chapter addresses a general model in which both research and teaching of students and trainees occurs. This approach seems most realistic, since it does in fact reflect the model of the teaching hospital, which is a kind of paradigm for what we might look at in the TNH.

TEACHING

It is entirely possible to have a good educational program in which students, residents, and fellows are taught about the care of institutionalized elderly persons without including a research component. Given the moral hazards inherent in using institutionalized persons as research subjects, one might be tempted to limit the research component and concentrate on the educational aspects. There will be little argument in any professional group that health professionals in training need a better understanding of the organizational and clinical realities of long-term care. In order to achieve this better understanding and to develop the skills necessary to improve the quality of care in nursing homes, it seems necessary that we place students and trainees in an actual setting.

We have not found a way to teach effectively by proxy: hands-on care is a *sine qua non* of education in any of the helping professions and especially those most clinically oriented. And yet, educating students through clinical exposure is the first step in the existential reality of "objectifying" human beings—using people as a means toward an end rather than treating them as having meaning inherent in their very being. This is the initial Kantian transgression (1), and we see examples of it everywhere in teaching hospitals, regardless of whether there is research actively being conducted or not. The 90-year-old man with aortic insufficiency may not mind, or may even enjoy, the interaction with eager stethescopes numbering in the hundreds over the years. Our obligation is to make sure he does not object, and also, to add to the interaction a conscious component of humanism, e.g., to engage the students in learning other aspects of the gentleman's story in addition to auscultation of the heart murmur.

RESEARCH

Human experimentation carries an even greater risk of objectifying (and therefore dehumanizing) persons. It can put them at greater risk than most clinical care and often is directed at a distant accretion of scientific knowledge not likely to directly benefit the subject himself or herself. But research is also an important aspect of the TNH concept.

The factors favoring the inclusion of research have to do with the image of the nursing home as an important place where learning goes on not only by the trainees but also by the graduate physicians and faculty. Unanswered questions are explored, and new knowledge is discovered—this kind of learning is called research. It creates an atmosphere of striving for excellence that could promote not only better care for the institutionalized elderly but also, by extension, improve the negative stereotypes of aging in our culture. It is additionally clear that much research needs to be done on the common and debilitating disorders of the institutionalized elderly population (2), and, therefore, there is probably greater moral pressure toward achieving better practical clinical knowledge in these areas.

THE HISTORY

In 1966, Henry K. Beecher published "Ethics and clinical research" in the *New England Journal of Medicine* (3). In this article, he called into question the ethics of clinical research, citing a number of examples of research projects that, either by lack of protection of subjects or by inadequate research design, were unquestionably unethical. This classic article marks a new period in our understanding of ethics as an important discipline and as a part of the endeavor of research. It gave birth to scandals and also to scholarly and institutional approaches to the problem of protecting human research subjects (4). Many of the exposes of unethical practices were of research projects that were being conducted in nursing homes. At that time, nursing homes were a common site for clinical research. It was a very convenient place to find research subjects: they were all in one place; the researcher did not have to travel around to find them; they were usually of a homogeneous population; and if findings might be confounded by chronic disease, at least the chronic disease was widely prevalent. These reasons are not unethical in and of themselves and provided enough incentive for researchers to quickly look to institutionalized populations for subjects. Care to rule out risky ethical practices was often inadequate or based on justifications not always strictly value neutral. For example, there was a devaluing of the remaining lifetimes of severely impaired persons. Should harm ensue, presumably it was felt it would be less damaging if it occurred to people whose life horizons were so sorely constricted and for whom the end of life appeared much closer than for "normal people.

One of the most well-known of these incidents occurred when two highly respected researchers from the Sloan-Kettering Institute conducted a project to test immune reaction to foreign cancer cells, based on the hypothesis that cancer cells may cause less of a non-self response because of some altered immune characteristics of those cells (5). Thus, live cancer cells were injected into many nursing home patients at the Jewish Chronic Diseases Hospital of Brooklyn, New York. Many of the patients who were subjects in this project were either extremely demented, aphasic, or non-English speaking. When asked at the court hearing whether or not patients really understood what was happening when they gave informed consent, one of the researchers replied, "Of course they didn't understand that these were cancer cells. If they did, they never would have agreed to it" (6).

Ethical problems with institutionalized populations were not limited to nursing home residents but also included prisoners, who comprised the other group commonly used as subjects in research projects (7). The third institutionalized group at risk were children who required institutionalization because of mental retardation, emotional disturbance, or both. The Willowbrook School experiments caused much notoriety—in this group, experimental hepatitis vaccine was given to institutionalized retarded children with parental consent obtained under significant coercion; i.e., the children would not be admitted unless the parents gave consent for the research (8,9).

These three distinct institutionalized groups share certain characteristics that put them at higher risk for unethical exploitation as research subjects. The National Commission for the Protection of Human Subjects in Biomedical and Behavioral Research therefore focused a major part of its work on the problem of research with mentally infirm institutionalized populations (10). Although not all nursing home residents are mentally infirm, there are many who are, and thus the case for consideration by the Commission was the protection of the most vulnerable.

There was a difference of opinion as to whether institutionalized persons should participate in research when suitable noninstitutionalized subjects are available and whether institutionalized persons should participate in research that is not relevant to their own clinical conditions(s). Some commissioners felt strongly that an individual who is institutionalized as mentally infirm should not participate in research in which other persons would be suitable subjects because (a) institutionalized persons are especially vulnerable to exploitation and (b) because they already carry burdens from their disability and their institutionalization, and it is therefore unjust to ask them to assume any additional burdens for the benefit of society. This reflects the fear that institutionalized persons will be used disproportionately and unfairly in research because they are convenient—the research might therefore be more efficiently conducted and perhaps even less costly. People with similar disabilities outside of institutions are more likely to have caring persons who could act as their advocates. These considerations argue that whenever possible, it is more just for research subjects to be sought outside of the institutional setting.

On the other hand, some commissioners argued that it is wrong to assume that research must always be a burden, that it in fact may have beneficial effects including increased social interaction and relief from boredom. There may even be positive meaning in an altruistic act. Although these points are well taken, and respect for persons argues in favor of treating nursing home residents as much as possible like other people rather than as a special class, the scandals revealed by Beecher and others alert us to the need for some safeguards beyond simply trusting the moral fiber of the research community.

The resolution reached by the Commission in their 1978 report, when considering only those institutionalized as mentally infirm, was (a) to place the burden on the investigator to justify the need to involve the nursing home population and (b) to permit institutionalized individuals to particpate in research that is not specifically relevant to their condition only if they are capable of giving informed consent and the research presents no more than minimal risk. Thus, even those who are not mentally infirm are thought to be more vulnerable to exploitation, however subtle, so that non-therapeutic research of greater than minimal risk was proscribed by the Commission even in those persons able to give informed consent. As the risk of the research increases, justification of the use of institutionalized subjects must include an increasing relevance to the subjects' own clinical conditions and a likelihood of benefit directly to them.

THE ISSUES

Consent, Freedom, and Respect

The main characteristic distinguishing institutionalized populations from other people is that they are not free. This factor is one that prisoners share with residents of nursing homes (11). Although residents of nursing homes are not restrained by law in most cases, it is, in reality, their chronic illnesses and their dependence that strictly limits their freedom, whereas in the prisons, walls, bars, and legal proscriptions act as limits to freedom. In both cases, however, there is an inherent limit to the degree of autonomy the person excercises in responding to a request to participate in research. There may be a sense that participation is "expected" by the "administration" or by the physician. There may be peer pressure from roommates and others to agree or to disagree, and people who are not accustomed to making decisions of any kind on their own behalf may find such a situation terribly anxiety provoking.

However, not all these limits to freedom are immutable. Studies have shown improvement in mood and cognitive function in nursing home residents who are allowed and encouraged to make even minor decisions about the character of their environment and the structure of their days (12). In establishing conditions to correct for limited autonomy, one could look to aspects of the general situation and to the specific interaction with the researcher in which personal choices can be made and be respected. It is possible to actually enhance autonomy if health professionals are aware that in full respect for persons more than kindness and compassion are required: one must support autonomous choice on all possible levels.

In the conduct of educational programs, basic tenets of respectful treatment include (a) identification of students to the residents as students, and thus allowing the resident a free and informed choice about participation in the educational program, (b) careful supervision of trainees by qualified faculty, and (c) careful maintenance of confidentiality. Legal liability can be minimized by attention to and documentation of these considerations (14).

Competence and Consent

Although not all patients in nursing homes have cognitive impairment, it is the one place in our society where one finds the highest density of persons with these kinds of disorders. Cognitive impairment, especially that caused by chronic dementing illness that is irreversible, calls into question the first component of free and informed consent, that the patient be competent. This is an area in which there is a great deal of room for more study and more research (15). The question of competence is addressed by the courts, but its relevance to a person's consent to participate in research is severely limited. "Competence" as a legal concept refers to standards of a person's ability to care for himself or herself, which might lead to guardianships or conservatorships being imposed in order to fulfill the state's responsibility to care for those who cannot care for themselves. Inability to handle finances, get dressed, or cook a meal, however, does not necessarily imply inability to make judgements for oneself about medical care interventions or (even) participation in research. Even disorientation to time, place, and persons does not automatically prove a person incapable of giving meaningful consent.

Another limitation of the notion of competence is that it has been established by courts in an adversarial context. It is therefore not designed to protect the patient's rights as vigorously as we would like or to enhance what autonomy the patient may have left by allowing him or her to choose to participate in research. Our understanding of the moral role of the mental competence determination is limited by the lack of a clear concept of what kind of understanding is necessary for a valid consent to participate in research. Many studies (10,16) have shown that even among a normal population very few people actually understand fully what is told to them in the informed consent process, which calls into question whether a test of comprehension is, in fact, discriminatory against the cognitively impaired elderly in this regard.

Memory is also problematic: when persons can understand something but not remember it, should we invalidate all of their strongly held preferences and desires? The Commission in 1978 felt that full consent may not be possible in some patients but did not want to impede the possibility of certain kinds of beneficial therapeutic research, and therefore developed a category of "assent" in which a patient may not fully understand all of the medical aspects of what is being done, but it is to the satisfaction of the researcher and other primary people involved that the patient does not object, and in fact there is a tacit, if not verbal, assent to the procedure (17). Obviously, this limited form of consent can be sufficient only in a relatively nonrisky, noninvasive procedure in which therapeutic benefit is likely.

The President's Commission for the Study of Ethical Problems in Medicine was directed to look toward ethical dilemmas in clinical practice as well as further issues in research and produced a careful analysis of this issue (18). In order to clarify the confusion inherent in using the word "competence" with its legal connotations (which vary from state to state), the Commission used the concept of "capacity." In the Commission's view, decision-making capacity is specific to a particular decision and depends not on a person's "status" (such as age or diagnosis, e.g., SDAT) or on the decision reached (e.g., a decision that differs from that which might have been made by the physician or other caregiver is not necessarily evidence of incapacity), but on the person's actual function in situations in which a decision about health care is to be made. This is another kind of "functional assessment" in geriatrics, in which the patient's functional capacity to make a health care decision on his or her own behalf must be judged in relation to all the specific factors in that particular situation and not on some unitary examination yielding a diagnosis of capacity or incapacity.

Thus, a conclusion about a patient's decision-making capacity necessarily reflects a balancing of two important objectives: to enhance the patient's well-being and to respect the person as a self-determining individual. Capacity (or "competence") must thus reflect the balance of these possibly competing interests.

The elements of capacity are (a) the possession of a set of values and goals, (b) the ability to communicate and to understand information, and (c) the ability to reason and to deliberate about one's choices. Notice that nothing has been said about memory per se, or about the "rationality" or "reasonableness" of the choice, which are criteria often used by the courts in evaluating "competence" (19). This is, in contrast, a rather minimalist and process-oriented set of criteria for capacity. In the name of balancing the best interests of the patient with full respect for individual autonomy, it also requires the caregiver to exercise a truly benevolent analysis of the risks involved. There is a relativism based on level of risk. When the consequences for well-being are substantial, there is a greater need to be certain that the patient possesses the necessary level of capacity. When less turns on the decision, the level of capacity required may be reduced, even though the constituent elements remain the same.

To Do No Harm

We have a responsibility to all of our patients to protect them from harm (20). This principle of "beneficence" is one of the most basic to the professions of medicine (21) and nursing (22). It stems from the early Hippocratic writings in which very little or nothing is said about respect or autonomy or informed consent, but the emphasis is on doing what is best for the patient and not doing harm.

The inherent conflict of interest between the roles of physician/caregiver and physician/investigator has been described in depth by philosophers (23), social scientists (24), and clinical researchers (25). Briefly, it is that the attitude of a physician acting on behalf of his or her patient, with only that particular patient's well-being in mind, cannot be sustained by a physician whose goals include the completion of a successful research project. The patient may feel pressured to consent, however subconsciously, by a fear of "disappointing" the physician and perhaps spoiling the relationship. Physician investigators may be influenced to make decisions in the interest of the research project rather than the individual patient, e.g., if a patient near the end of life requests no aggressive life-prolonging therapy, that request may conflict not only with the physician's discomfort in confronting death but also with his or her discomfort in a seemingly premature end to a clinical trial.

Some writers recommend that the two functions of primary care and research never be joined in the same person, thus avoiding the risk of conflict of interest. Others regard the intrusion of a "stranger" in the form of a researcher as more potentially damaging to the world view of the patient and thus would depend on procedural safeguards and an emphasis on the ethics of clinician researchers to ensure the moral integrity of the clinical research enterprise (26).

To take the injunction, "Do no harm," seriously in the TNH is to be extremely careful not to devalue the people who are the objects of research in favor of some future benefit to other persons. This trade-off, a risk in the present for the sake of future knowledge and for the benefit of future human beings, is an important aspect of research that deserves close attention. One of the problems with the National Commission's 1978 exclusion of institutionalized populations from most research is the disqualification of nursing home residents from participation in altruism. Although we may forget in more cynical moments that the human spirit has many positive aspects toward fellow human beings, it is important not to limit the nursing home residents to a too strictly narrow definition of self-interest. For many people, altruism and altruistic activity provide one way of giving meaning to life. Certainly, a sense of purpose is something that could benefit many nursing home residents. The limitations of life in an institutional setting, added to the limitations of advanced age and chronic disability, may obscure the meaning of life and lead to depression, apathy, and a feeling of being disconnected from the rest of the human community (27). The philsopher Hawerwas asserts that the challenge of suffering that cannot be erased is to invest it with meaning—thus, suffering can be channeled to include, not to exclude, the victim from a meaningful human context (28). To participate in a research project that might bring understanding of the cause of disability and suffering in future generations can sometimes give meaning to that disability and suffering that cannot be cured. Thus, we must be careful not to cut these patients off from a very important source of contribution to the human community.

Some theories extend the "privilege" of participating in research to a duty, claiming that:

> all persons, insofar as they are members of a social community, have a duty to help others in that community. Because reciprocal duties of beneficence apply to all persons, an enhancement of benefits for society as a whole will result. Thus, persons who are mentally infirm share to an equal degree with other persons this duty of beneficence; and it might even be argued that it would be a violation of their right to pursue their moral obligations is if this class of individuals were categorically excluded from participation (29).

Nontherapeutic research of minimal risk could, according to this theory, even involve mentally infirm nursing home residents as long as the method for selection of subjects was equitable, i.e., included equally other categories of subjects.

Equity

Other issues of equity apply. We generally view health care and supportive systems for the vulnerable or disabled as rights of a liberal and compassionate society (30). The stated values are not always reflected directly in policy; distributive justice and its manifestation in the world of health care change distinctly from one administration to another, suggesting that the value of just distribution is in fact more controversial than most philosophers would admit. Let us assume that we would like to distribute the goods of care, in this case long-term care, most fairly to those who need it. This always seems the most rational principle for distribution and is supported by a utilitarian demand to use resources perspicaciously as well as by a more formalist demand to care for one's fellow human beings in need (31). In fact, a great deal of modern health services research attempts to define, discover, identify the "needs" that are more likely to respond and to benefit from the application of health care resources or institutions. Ideally, we would not want to waste resources, nor would we want real needs to go unmet.

In long-term care, inequities of great magnitude are longstanding (32). The efforts of the TNH and the broad field of gerontologic research and education are a response to needs that are perceived and, in many cases, fairly carefully described. In short, there is a great deal of room for improvement in our institutions of long-term care. Justice is confounded on many fronts: people who do not receive the level of care they need, people who are inappropriately or unnecessarily institutionalized. If it is true that the resources added to a nursing home by a TNH grant will upgrade the care received by the residents (in an immediate, not a future sense), and if it is true that being a resident in an active, busy TNH is overall a positive experience, then we are faced with a problem of distributive justice which can be posed as follows: Should the resources of the TNH be allocated to only the highest quality nursing homes, where the residents are more likely to be treated with more respect so that the moral risks of objectification are less? Or should those resources be applied to institutions that need the upgrading (notice the need criterion arising here), where the residents are likely to benefit to a much greater degree from the improved quality of care and level of attention because they are starting with lower standards and therefore have more room for improvement? Would research studies from such institutions, which we believe to be more typical, thus provide more useful knowledge overall because they apply to the more common situation? A third option would be to distribute the available resources more widely, thus making smaller grants to more institutions and using selection criteria related to the likelihood that the particular research and educational program proposed would directly benefit the residents of the home.

Some of these points are drawn as extreme in order to illustrate the principles that conflict in the ethical dilemma raised by the question of justice in the notion of the TNH. All of the options painted thus far are evaluated in terms of their benefit to existing persons who are nursing home residents. In the current programs, the major consideration is often that of benefit to future nursing home residents. Consideration of present benefit exists, but almost as a fortunate side effect of the increased knowledge to be gained by research and the improved competence and better attitudes of providers to be gained by the educational programs.

Serious concern for justice would require us to take seriously the resources of the TNH as social goods and to carefully weigh these different and sometimes competing benefits in decisions of allocation. Science is not value-free even when there is no direct risk to subjects.

The Priorities of Research

Any discussion of the value base of science, must consider the moral aspects of the selection of specific research for funding (33). Similar considerations of present versus future or near future versus far distant future are at play here. For example, clinical research into the treatment or prevention of pressure sores, depression, or urinary incontinence are likely to have a benefit sooner, perhaps even to the residents who are participating in the trials. This kind of research is aimed generally at improving quality of life in the most proximate time frame. On the other hand, we want to support more basic research which asks questions about the etiology and genetics of Alzheimer's Disease. In this latter case, benefit to future patients is likely although not certain. Benefit to current residents who participate in the studies can only be counted in terms of the general improvement in care that comes from being in a TNH, perhaps greater levels of social interaction, and perhaps the knowledge that one is helping to increase the fund of knowledge of medical science.

These two extremes are presented to make the point that we have other values than the benefit to current patients and residents. We value knowledge, sometimes even for its own sake. It is this phenomenon that sometimes leads to the claim that science is value-free.

The funding for today's projects is in some way or another public—even if it is not directly federally or state supported, foundation philanthropy entails public responsibility as well. It seems logical then that the distribution of such resources ought to reflect some social values. If all projects cannot be funded, what should be the principles by which to choose between them? Scientific quality is the current baseline, the value underlying the peer review process, but it is only a baseline. Social utility and probable benefit to the residents of nursing homes or to the aging population in general should weigh heavily in the determination of funding.

TOWARDS METHODS OF RESOLUTION
Ethics Research

The moral risks involved in using extremely vulnerable, already devalued, institutionalized persons as research subjects are major. Those moral transgressions of researchers before the establishment of institutional review boards were mostly simple ethical "oversights." These physicians and scientists were not scurrilous, malevolent geniuses. On the contrary, many of them were driven in a search for knowledge that would relieve suffering in future generations. But in so doing, they used research subjects only as a means to an end and thus committed the principal Kantian sin. In order to proceed ethically in TNHs—both with education and research—we must insist that what is returned is as valuable as what is given. To calculate a cost or risk–benefit analysis based on numbers of future lives saved, productivity increased, days of hospitalization and disability decreased is far easier, especially in a more reductionist scientific context, than to calculate the much more inchoate but no less significant qualities of the respect of a society for its people, particularly those most vulnerable (33). We do not know exactly how to value progress in the humanization of society at least partly because we do not have quantitative terms for measurement. Nonetheless, progress is possible on this front. A qualitative methodology (34) will enable the questions of values and standards to be investigated alongside the questions of pharmacology and pathogenesis.

We need to do research in ethics in these settings. We need philosophical and clinical investigation into the thorny questions that lie in the tension between beneficence and respect for autonomy. We need data about the effectiveness of ethics committees and how they might be improved. We need data about elderly persons who are research subjects—their attitudes toward research, their problem-solving abilities using research protocols, their interpretation of risk, intrusiveness, and autonomy, their idea of proportional participation versus the burden of institutionalization. We need data about the effectiveness of care delivery structures and innovative experiments in improving environments and practices in nursing homes. We need to find a way to include autonomy and the meaning of life in our outcome measures.

Ethics Teaching

Identifying, analyzing, and resolving ethical issues are important aspects of the body of knowledge and the skills we should be teaching in TNHs. These should be done not only by role modeling (35), an acceptance of the importance and willingness of teachers to discuss, but also by structural events: law and ethics seminars, ethics rounds or case conferences, assignment of relevant readings, and inclusion of capable philosophers in the faculty.

Ethics Committees

It is because of these moral risks that care must be taken in bringing education and research activities into the long-term care setting. But the risks of not doing so are equally great, if not greater. We owe it to the present and future persons who will need nursing home care to find better ways of caring. We want to avoid exploitation and also avoid unjustifiable paternalism (an overprotectiveness that can be just as dehumanizing as exploitation). The fundamental golden mean in this regard should be to treat nursing home residents as much as possible simply as persons, using special considerations and cautions, as conceived by philosopher John Rawls (36), only when necessary to maximize the autonomy of the disadvantaged.

The challenge is to build a process consistent with this principle. The model of a consultative "Ethics Committee" or "Care Committee" can be recommended for several reasons. Ideally, it is interdisciplinary and thus reflects varied perspectives and value orientations. A competent ethicist can clarify that nature of the ethical problem and frame the issues to allow for a meaningful interchange. A representative group would include a philosopher/ethicist, physician, nurse, attorney, clergy member, administrator, social worker, investigator, and nursing home resident and/or family member. Such a committee can be viewed either as arbiter or facilitator of communication, depending on the specific situation. Its very existence and the process it enables to occur raise the awareness of everyone concerned about the issues of values and ethics that frequently will arise in a TNH and will acknowledge that a broad expertise does exist to deal effectively with such issues. If it meets on a regular basis, staff may be relieved of the discomfort of carrying unacknowledged doubts and questions indefinitely. With the multiplicity of ethical issues raised by the TNH, it may be wise to consider making a structural requirement for such a committee.

One of the major complaints research scientists have with the institutional review board system for the protection of human subjects is that it is too cumbersome, too time-consuming, and excessively complicated. There is no reason to expect that the conduct of ethical research should be simple. Quite to the contrary, it is an undertaking of great complexity, requiring insight, intelligence, and information not only about science and clinical medicine but also about interactional psychology, professional sociology, philosophical ethics, and the content and structure of the meaning of human life. The TNH thus poses a unique opportunity for the humanization of institutions. We should not let this opportunity pass.

REFERENCES

1. Kant I: *Foundations of the Metaphysics of Morals*. Indianapolis, Bobbs–Merrill, 1959.
2. McCally M, Greenlick M, Beck JC: Research in geriatrics: Needs and priorities, in Cassel CK, Walsh JR (eds): *Geriatric Medicine*, vol II. New York, Srpinger-Verlag, 1984, pp 451–462.
3. Beecher HK: Ethics and clinical research, *N Engl J Med* 1966;271:1354–1366.
4. Freund PA (ed): *Experimentation with Human Subjects*. New York, George Braziller, 1970.
5. Editorial. *Science* 1964;143:551.
6. Guttentag OE: Human experimentation. *Science* 1964;145:768.
7. Hodges RE, Bean WB: The use of prisoners for medical research. *JAMA* 1967;202:513–515.
8. Krugman S: Experiments at the Willowbrook State School. *Lancet* 1971;1:966–967.
9. Goldby, S: Experiments at the Willowbrook State School. *Lancet* 1971;1:749.
10. The National Commission for the Protection of Human Subjects of Biomedical and Behavioral Research: *Report and Recommendations: Research Involving Those Institutionalized as Mentally Infirm*. Washington, DC, DHEW Publication No. (OS) 78-0006, 1978, pp 113–121.
11. Beanchamps TL, Childress JF: *Principles of Biomedical Ethics*. New York, Oxford University Press, 1979, pp 163–164.
12. Schulz R, Hanusa BH: Long-term effects of control and predictability—enhancing interventions: Findings and ethical issues. *J Pers Soc Psychol* 1978;36:1194–1201.
13. Lipp M: *Respectful Treatment: The Human Side of Medical Care*. Hagerstown, MD, Harper & Row, 1977.
14. Kapp MB: Nursing homes as teaching institutions: Legal issues *Gerontologist* 1984;24:55–60.

15. Cassileth BR, Zupkis RV, Sutton-Smith K, et al: Informed consent—why are its goals imperfectly realized? *N Engl J Med* 1980;302:896–900.
16. Lidz CW, Meisel A, Osterweis M, et al: Barriers to informed consent. *Ann Intern Med* 1983;99:539–543.
17. President's Commission for the Study of Ethical Problems in Medicine and Biomedical and Behavioral Research: *Making Health Care Decisions*, vol I: *Report*. Washington, DC, US Government Printing Office, 1982, pp 55–62.
18. Abernathy V, Lundin K: Competency and the right to refuse medical treatment, in Abernathy V (ed): *Frontiers in Medical Ethics*. Cambridge, MA, Ballinger, 1979, pp 79–98.
19. Jonsen AR: Do no harm. *Ann Intern Med* 1978;88:827–832.
20. Veatch R: *A Theory of Medical Ethics*. New York, Basic Books, 1981, pp 15–24.
21. Jameton A: *Nursing Practice: The Ethical Issues* Englewood Cliffs, Prentice-Hall, 1984, pp 89–98.
22. Jonas H: Philsophical reflections on experimentation with human subjects, in Reiser SJ, Dych AJ, Curran WJ (eds): *Ethics in Medicine: Historical Perspectives and Contemporary Concerns*. MIT Press, Cambridge, 1977, pp 304–315.
23. Barber B: The ethics of experimentation with human subjects. *Sci Am* 1976;234:25–31.
24. Spiro HM: Constraint and consent—on being a patient and a subject. *N Engl J Med* 1975;293:1134–1135.
25. Cassel CK: Senile dementia of the Alzheimer's type: ethical issues involving informed consent. In Dubler N, Melnick V (eds): *Alzheimer's Dementia*. Clifton, NJ, Humana Press, 1984.
26. Cassel CK, Jameton AL: Dementia in the elderly. An analysis of medical responsibility. *Ann Intern Med* 1981;94:802–807.
27. Hawerwas S: Reflections on suffering, death, and medicine. *Ethics Sci Med* 1979;6:229–237.
28. Capron AM: Human experimentation: Basic issues, in Reich WT (ed): *Encyclopedia of Bioethics*, vol 2. New York, Macmillan, 1978, pp 692–697, 700–701.
29. Menzel PT: *Medical Costs, Moral Choices*. New Haven, Yale University Press, 1983, pp 1–23.
30. Outka G: Social justice and equal access to health care. *J Religious Ethics* 1974;2(1):11–32.
31. United States Senate Subcommittee on Long-Term Care, The Special Committee on Aging: *Introductory Report: Nursing Home Care in the United States: Failure of Public Policy*. Washington, DC, US Government Printing Office, 1975.
32. McKee PL (ed): *Philsophical Foundations of Gerontology*. New York, Human Sciences Press, 1982.
33. Van Maanen J, Dabbs JM, Faulkner RR: *Varieties of Qualitative Research*. Beverly Hills, Sage Publications, 1982.
34. Seigler M: A legacy of Osler: Teaching clinical ethics at the beside. *JAMA* 1978;239:957–966.
35. Rawls J: *A theory of Justice*. Cambridge, Harvard University Press, 1971, pp 108–113.

The Teaching Nursing Home, edited by Edward
L. Schneider et al. © 1985 The Beverly
Foundation. Raven Press, New York.

Management and Administration

Mitchell M. Waife

The Jewish Home and Hospital for Aged, New York, New York 10025

Health care professionals have predominantly hospital-based educations and
bring practices . . . to nursing homes that are often counterproductive to the
care of residents. On the other side, many nursing home administrators and
owners have never been associated with hospitals, so they are unable to clearly
explicate the desired differences (1).

Long-term care has evolved its own model of behavior over a long period,
and yet it still faces frequent rejection by the hospital fraternity. Some of
the differences between nursing home and hospital care have to be delineated and faced objectively before the teaching nursing home (TNH) can
reach its true potential. These differences include the social basis of care
versus the scientific model, emphasis on the best possible functional improvement in life versus the treatment and discharge of patients, and dis-
similarities in expectations of patients versus staff.

Overshadowing these differences is the basic reason for the nursing home:
to provide an atmosphere that encourages self-direction for the patient. This
requires compromises in the daily routine that acute care hospitals can not
tolerate. Thus, the nursing home must be able to accommodate appointments missed, physicians kept waiting, or family involvement in minor matters—all of which seem to prevent application of the "scientific method."
Such compromises can mean the expenditure of needless energy and time
by the professional. And time is money in hospital–university settings as
everywhere else.

Final decision making in hospitals rests with the physician, although staff
from the other disciplines play a supportive role. The nursing home setting
is more diffuse, and patient management includes input from social workers,
nurses, families, and others. Staff coming from the monolithic environment
of a unversity hospital to the seemingly chaotic world of the nursing home
can suffer culture shock. "Nothing ever gets done" is descriptive of the
nursing home, whereas "This must get done" is the cry of the hospital.

Introducing the TNH into the traditional mold of the long-term care
facility represents a challenge amid change. The challenge comes from the
involved relationship between hospitals and nursing homes. Very often, the
nursing home self-image is the result of interaction between these two care

providers. The hospital represents the historical basis for much of the nursing home's history and work procedures, and the hospital is the source of most of the nursing home's professional personnel, who often come to the new facility with built-in prejudices and preconceived notions. Those professionals who have worked in both settings are best adapted for change, since they can relate both acute- and long-term levels of care to the specific needs of patients.

It is the hospital-based or hospital-trained personnel without nursing home experience who require orientation and briefing in moving from an acute-care to a long-term care setting. We must know each other before we can be co-workers. From the very beginning, administrative matters of concern to both parties should be delineated and shared. Frequently, the nursing home staff will identify areas of possible conflict. The hospital and the related nursing or medical schools, often encapsulated in a large university setting, loom huge beside the self-contained, limited-sized nursing home. So the nursing home staff will begin expressing their concerns and desires at the first mention of the potential opening of a TNH.

The first step in the process of introducing a TNH is to open up communications between the principals at the hospital and nursing home. The nursing home administrator should take the initiative for this. Often, a series of simple sessions between the policymakers at both facilities will clear the air for the moment and at least show equality of purpose and effort. The administrator should establish clear-cut avenues of communication early on, so that the principals all have a single source of information and communication. In addition, the nursing home director should delineate the operative guidelines, set up regular conferences of the policymakers, and establish an exchange of correspondence among them. These may appear to be very elementary considerations, yet they are often forgotten in the rush toward progress.

TNH directors must be aware of and understand the differences in professional training and experience between personnel at the hospital and the nursing home and the resultant threat of the new relationship between them. They must anticipate resistance to change and deal with it effectively.

The limited resources of the nursing home should be considered in all ongoing arrangements, and the status of the administrator—often a jack-of-all-trades—must be respected. Hospital staff must realize that their usual habits of doing business may not be appropriate in the TNH. In fact, the hospital's usual staffing, particularly at the administrative level, is totally out of synchrony with that of the nursing home. The administrator or lone eagle at the nursing home, who must be a planner and doer, often brings a pragmatic approach to concepts and plans that may be alien to the teaching center.

Clearly defining job titles and reporting responsibilities—and then explaining them to personnel—is a standard procedure in the beginning of any new project. But nowhere is it more important than in the implementation of a TNH, since the greatest sensitivities are required to overcome the initial resistance to major change. The introduction of highly qualified peers who have a totally new relationship with the nursing home can cause disruption if the administrator feels threatened by them. This one aspect of staff integration is a closely kept secret to avoid embarrassment and the consequent questioning of the chief executive, which creates an obstacle to progress. Lack of frankness among decision-making principals, however, can cause good projects to fail.

Critical to the success of the project is the existing senior medical officer, the medical director of the nursing home, whose worth to the facility may exceed that of his/her equivalent in the TNH program. Concerned nursing home medical officers have years of experience in direct patient care, although they may have overlooked the many newer approaches to geriatrics. This type of physician can be invaluable to the facility and its patients and yet be a negative force with the arrival of the TNH. But this need not work against the program. The contribution of staff can mean different things to different people. The so-called obstructionist may very well be the best doctor in the world when it comes to treatment of the dying. Or he/she can be that rarest of all breeds, the physician who loves paper work and enables the facility to sail through state surveys because of his/her devotion to rules and regulations. Is it truly necessary to convert such valuable medical colleagues to conventional TNH home physicians? Not necessarily. But executive tact and skill are required to keep the rest of the staff happy and productive when this doctor views the arrival of the TNH as an intrusion and a nuisance.

A most important executive act needed as the facility appears on the scene is to establish the administrator's role so that he/she can participate in every aspect of the initial planning. Why every aspect? The early days, when resistance may run high, are critical to the program's success. Once roles and expectations are determined, it becomes relatively easy to proceed to delegating tasks.

The usual array of administrative devices such as staff meetings, brainstorming sessions, conferences, and organization charts are put into play at the outset. Then, the chief administrative goal, besides integrating the program, is to allow the TNH staff to implement new modalities and concepts without massive dislocation of existing operations. A smooth transition can be achieved by an educational process that requires the new personnel to tour the home and learn about its operation, needs, goals, and accomplishments. The new staff can be shown the positive in what they see and be encouraged to indicate, tactfully, how they can work together with the nursing home's permanent staff. But even under the best of circumstances, a key member of the nursing home staff may be unable or unwilling to cooperate with the new program and thus will be a continual handicap. A very valuable staff member, usually of department head rank, may fall by the wayside, a victim of sudden change. The choice of whether to retain this individual or to force him/her out for the ultimate benefit of the TNH program is an administrative problem of the first rank. Its solution will depend on the executive's ability to handle the situation with sensitivity. It is happy for all concerned when the rare staff member who leaves the facility under such circumstances does so on his/her own initiative.

It is the implied goal of the TNH program to effect change within the facility. The skills, knowledge, and experience of the new staff members must be accepted where appropriate and put into effect without significant dislocation in the life of the institution. This can occur within the guidelines of the administrative organization and personnel changes mentioned previously and with good leadership that anticipates dislocation and views the entire institution before authorizing any changes.

TNH programs bring two new personnel types to the facility. One is the faculty person accomplished in his/her field who can serve as role model for the analogous professional at the nursing home. If the individual is a member of a nursing faculty, then the nursing staff can take pride in the leadership recognition accorded their profession and benefit from the proximity of the role model. An on-the-job consultant is available, as well as an advocate who will enhance their own position within the organization.

If the faculty person is from the medical school, then a new closeness between physician and staff should result, since the first realization about the program is that accomplishment occurs only with the assistance of nurses and other personnel. Physician to physician is not the nursing home chain of authority, rather, it is physician to nurse. The positive result, then, is the seldom-realized goal of intensive medical input for the nursing home patient that is on a par with the hospital case.

The administrator should take advantage of the part- or full-time injection of faculty in accomplishing the quality program goals of his/her long-range planning efforts. Medical faculty, even with a limited agenda, can contribute to other areas of the home's endeavors, for example, by introducing advanced medical techniques or scheduling visiting lecturers. Bringing such knowledge and observations that are beyond the nursing home's training and experience can have lasting effects. What the nursing home staff learns can be applied in ways not necessarily apparent at first.

This is particularly true in the area of medical ethics. The choices made by a medical faculty in a large teaching facility with a wide variety of case management problems mean that they are in a position to influence those medical ethics decisions that constantly arise in the nursing home but are seldom addressed.

The first new person at the teaching nursing home, then, is the faculty person—either medical or nursing. The second new type is the professional student—again, either nursing or medical. Here the importation of attractive, alert, young people sets them apart in the age-dominated nursing home. One can sense the appreciation elderly patients feel for the attention of people in their grandchildren's generation. The infectious good humor and dedication of many of the new generation of students is a decided plus for the staff. Good administration has the clear responsibility for fostering staff morale that translates into efficiency, economy, and, of course, good patient care. New ideas, new treatments, and ever-questioning students give the administrator a rare opportunity to offset the rigid regulatory atmosphere often created in the home.

Effective programs frequently involve a rapid turnover of students in an otherwise stable atmosphere. This can be a positive experience when the student is an enthusiastic and rapid learner. But with staff turnover, episodic care and concern can develop as differences in attitude and motivation begin to show up. The informal communications system prevalent in all academic institutions is particularly active in medical school settings. Thus, a poor experience with one group of students can have a chilling effect on future groups. The patients themselves may sense this loss of interest and feel abandonment as they see a constant flow of students entering and leaving. Positive results can occur, however, when the patients are informed about changes and are made to understand that greater good will result in the long run if students have broader educational opportunities.

Effective liaison with the hospital facility and the TNH eliminates operational problems resulting from expenditures of effort and talent that may be beyond the capacity of the nursing home to make. The physical plant of the TNH is often one of the first concerns of the faculty and students. It is the rare facility that has spare space to give new personnel, especially the part-timers who seem to occupy space in name only.

Thus, integrating students from either the nursing or medical school requires arranging meetings and allocating specific areas that may seldom be used yet are coveted by others. Available space must be allocated with normal functioning of the facility as first priority. Dislocation from one's turf often results in emotional upheaval and should not occur without clear acceptance of the purpose. A tactful TNH leader will soften the demands for nonexistent space and will avoid at all costs comparing the functions of the new and regular staffs. Only the administrator of the facility can do this. TNHs will come and go, but the regular staff remain, so the total experience should promote the continuing functioning of the nursing home.

The economics of long-term care has no record of providing operating funds for the TNH, so the financing must come from grants and other fund-raising efforts. Often, the requirement of continual funding after the grant ends is a condition of the original disbursement. The administrator then faces a problem. Although the use of grant money and the expansion of staff enhance the operations of the home, the future looms just over the horizon. Almost as much effort is expended in seeking future funds as in maintaining current operations. This may require integrating some of the teaching functions provided by the grant into current operations, adding them to the budget, and then attempting to get a government agency to pick up the tab. Very often this will mean a state-wide lobbying role that seeks to expand the state's reimbursement policies in order to continue the new programs.

The most effective TNH program may bring on change that alters future reimbursement negatively. At best, state reimbursement is complicated and responsive in ways that are obscure and strange. An institution may find that progress in improving patient care means a change in patient mix, which in turn brings on a less desirable reimbursement. This can often occur as the balance changes among Medicare, Medicaid, and private-paying patients.

In summary, the following questions should be asked before we, as administrators, begin formulating the policies for a TNH:

1. Is the purpose of the TNH clearly defined as one that will be of benefit to the entire institution and not restricted primarily to the professional growth of faculty or students?

2. Has the proposed program been clearly integrated into the operation of the facility with regard to service and personnel practices?

3. Is it clearly understood that patient needs and rights come before any program requirements?

4. Do both parties realize that the patient remains the responsibility of the institution and that the teaching program can advise but cannot take authority without responsibility?

5. Are all financial implications clearly understood and payment mechanisms in place?

The TNH can be a positive, energizing force leading toward desirable change. It only requires the cooperation and understanding of all the parties.

REFERENCE

1.   Gordon KG, Stryker R: *Creative Long-Term Care Administration*. Springfield, IL, Charles C Thomas, 1983, p. 14.

The Teaching Nursing Home, edited by Edward
L. Schneider et al. © 1985 The Beverly
Foundation. Raven Press, New York.

Functional Assessment: Its Use in the Teaching Nursing Home

Marsha D. Fretwell and Sidney Katz

Southeastern New England Long Term Care Gerontology Center, Brown University, Providence, Rhode Island 02912

The concept of the teaching nursing home (TNH) has developed as part of an effort to bring a major site of health care for the elderly into the mainstream of medical care in the United States. Paralleling the model of the teaching hospital, TNHs add teaching and research activities to those of patient care or clinical service, and this is expected to improve the quality of those services. In this chapter, the broad application of functional assessment as the "common language" of teaching, research, and clinical services is proposed to improve the quality of care for older individuals in the nursing home.

FUNCTIONAL ASSESSMENT

Functional assessment is a systematic approach to the collection of patient data that allows evaluation of the patient's health status and disabilities in multiple areas or domains. Not only are the elderly subject to multiple diseases, but their physical, mental, and social health and well-being are also closely interrelated. Thus, measures of functional status that examine the ability of the individual to function independently in a variety of areas are more useful than a list of diagnoses in identifying health problems and planning services.

Significant advances have been made in the area of functional assessment (1,2). The beginnings of contemporary systematic approaches to measuring levels of functioning appeared in health interview surveys of the late 1800s and early 1900s and were intended to describe entire populations of people. Such survey information was often reported in terms of days of sickness per person or rates per 1,000 persons. Between 1940 and 1980, more specific and reliable measures of function were developed. These measures began to describe function on an individual task-oriented basis such as the ability to walk, dress, or use the toilet. As different investigators worked toward refining this type of measurement of function, it became apparent that there were ways of grouping different functional measures to achieve a single score or level representing the sum of function in a particular area. These indicators of functioning (walking, dressing, using the toilet) were grouped and referred to as activities of daily living (ADL). More complex self-maintenance skills (cooking, shopping, banking) were clustered to form a measure referred to as instrumental activities of daily living.

This reduction of a series of complex functions into a single composite level set the stage for expanding descriptions of an individual function beyond the functioning of separate parts (upper and lower extremity, for example) to a more complete description of the whole individual. This method of clustering different descriptions of function into a single profile of function in a given area was used as assessment technology expanded into other domains of function such as physical health, psychological function, social function, and cognitive function.

Between 1960 and 1980, systems of comprehensive functional assessment emerged. These were multidimensional scales of function used to provide a broad overview of patient status. The elderly, especially those residing in a nursing home, most often present with a complex mixture of physical, mental, and social dysfunction. To optimize their overall functional ability, consideration had to be given to the physical and social environment in which they lived as well as to each aspect of their "function" itself. The use of multidimensional functional assessment was especially valuable for providing more systematic descriptions of individuals in the long-term care system.

The final phase in the historical development of functional assessment occurred as a result of the collaboration of leading researchers with users of this long-term care information base. This collaboration resulted in the introduction of two systems of patient classification by function: *Patient Classification for Long-Term Care: User's Manual* and *The Long-Term Health Care: Minimum Data Set* (3,4). These classification systems were developed for broad use to accumulate national information in objective and commonly understood terms. These data-based systems revealed an increasing consensus concerning the type of information that should be included in multidimensional functional assessments. The range of available measures of physical, mental, and social function can be found in numerous reviews (5–10).

APPLICATIONS OF FUNCTIONAL ASSESSMENT

Uses and Users

These systems of functional assessment have valuable application in the TNH for direct care of the residents, training of health professionals and staff, and the conducting of research in the home. In each of these three activities, there are various functional assessment uses:

1. Description of the individual or the entire population in the TNH. This establishes a body of information about the population along multiple parameters such as physical, emotional, and social functioning. It is important to be able to describe the TNH population as a whole in order to assess service needs and staffing. At the level of the individual client, one needs to record the outcomes associated with care (improved mobility, for instance). In research efforts, one must test hypotheses about the effectiveness of various interventions.

2. Screening or identification of need for further clinical investigation. In this use, assessment is not expected to give an in-depth description of an individual or population. Rather, it is expected to identify specific problems (incontinence, etc.) in order to target further evaluation.

3. Identifying problems or making diagnoses. This is, by definition, the basic multidimensional assessment leading to diagnostic conclusions and assignment of specific therapeutic interventions. As previously noted, all domains (mental, social, and physical) must be considered to allow for the frequent interaction of problems within the elderly nursing home patient.

4. Predicting probable outcomes. As more information about changes in function in the elderly is gathered over time, with or without professional intervention, the ability to predict the outcome or result of our intervention is increased. Again, prediction in one domain, such as physical function, must take into account the influence of other domains, such as mental status and environmental barriers.

5. Planning for care. This aspect represents the most concrete application of this systematic data collection. Functional assessments are used to develop interdisciplinary care plans for an individual and assign tasks to the care staff.

6. Monitoring is the use of the assessment information to measure changes over time in relevant parameters (5).

In the TNH, there will be users of functional assessment who are either uniquely involved in one area of activity or involved in overlapping areas of activity. For example, the licensed practical nurse is primarily identified with the delivery of direct care to the patients. In this role, the nurse may be exposed to assessment as a means of identifying problems, planning for care, and monitoring changes in function over time. The Director of Nursing, on the other hand, has administrative responsibilities and may use assessment technology to monitor the efficacy of the nursing care, to make decisions concerning staff and resident assignments, and to develop institutionally relevant educational programs that are based on patient needs.

Clinical faculty involved in training programs will be involved in both direct care and teaching. For them, assessment provides a means of assisting students and staff in identifying problems, planning care, and monitoring results of care over time. For one to be an effective teacher and clinician, the ability to predict outcomes is crucial, and assessment provides the systematic data collection that supports more accurate predictions.

Full-time academic faculty may be active in all spheres of activities but have primary responsibility for introduction of research into the TNH. For them, assessment may be used as a descriptive device to evaluate the effectiveness of various interventions and as a screening device to determine the prevalence of certain disabilities in the TNH that bear further evaluation.

There can be a tremendous overlap in the uses and the users of assessment technology in the TNH. The same overlap traditionally exists whenever one examines an academic institution dedicated to the care of patients (i.e., a teaching hospital). As a way of systematically evaluating and describing patients, functional assessment has the ability to capitalize on that similarity of involvement. By introducing "a common language" of description to all interested participants in the TNH, it provides a means of facilitating communication and cooperation in the home.

Despite the mutual interest, there are potential barriers to the broad application of systems of assessment in all activities of a TNH. A major question is whose system should be used? The administrator's? The clinician's? The teacher's? Or the researcher's? In addition to identical questions or items found in the systems preferred by each interest group, there are unique questions of each system that might appear unimportant to all other interested groups. For example, the number and detail of questions that the researcher or administrator may desire could lengthen the assessment process to a degree that would seem unreasonable to the direct care providers or teachers.

In practice, for clinical care and teaching, the assessment process has two phases that may be used to facilitate a solution to this problem. At admission, there could be a comprehensive assessment including questions covering most domains (i.e., demographic, medical problems, drugs, physical functioning, social resources and functioning, cognitive and emotional functioning, and economic and environmental issues) in order to generate a complete care plan for the patients and predict needed services and staff. Over time, selected domains such as ADLs, instrumental ADLs, cognitive function, mobility, medical problems and drugs, or merely selected questions from these domains are sufficient for monitoring changes in function that might occur. Researchers will find this basic set of data useful but may need to add questions depending on the particular research topic under study.

Potential conflicts between the users and uses of assessment can be solved in the following manner. The home would have a comprehensive assessment data form for admission and from that would select certain questions for ongoing clinical care and teaching. If additional questions are needed for research, they could be added, but the researchers, not the providers of direct care, would have the responsibility for the collection of those data.

Examples of Application in Clinical Services and Education

Comprehensive functional assessment on admission to the TNH allows a baseline description of the resident that can be used to generate an individualized care plan, place the individual in a unit with appropriate and/or special services, and generate a monthly summary of function, which is useful for monitoring changes over time. Discharge planning is facilitated by providing a broad base of information about the resident and the environment to which he or she might return.

For care and training purposes, this comprehensive assessment aids the staff and practitioner in organizing a vast array of information about an individual for clinical decisions (11). By leading the staff and students through a systematic search of patient information to identify problems, it emphasizes the multicausal basis of disease and dysfunction in the elderly (12). More complete diagnoses, descriptions of functional disability, psychological health, and social well-being will be obtained through the organization of this large amount of data. Reversible and interacting problems are more likely to be identified and appropriate care plans generated. By systematically introducing psychosocial health concepts into every patient evaluation, this approach can balance the dominance of physical disease and its cure through traditional medical care. Therapeutic goals can be broadened beyond the cure of medical diseases to include maintenance and improvement of function in both physical and psychological domains. Residents and their families are, in fact, more sensitive to the loss of physical and mental function than to the presence of certain diseases and are gratified when care plans are focused on reversing functional disabilities.

Over time, it will be a change in functional status that most often heralds the progress of chronic conditions or the onset of acute illness. Baseline and monthly assessments of function increase the sensitivity of staff and students to these changes and are of great importance to the early detection and initiation of specific therapy. Because of the elderly resident's diminished capacity to withstand the stress of serious illnesses, prevention and early detection of illness are major contributors to improving the quality of care for this group of individuals.

By providing a systematic framework for collecting and displaying patient information over time, functional assessment can be used in staff or student educational programs to promote a clear understanding of the relationship among patient functions, clinical interventions, and patient-oriented outcomes. For example, functional data that might be routinely recorded on monthly summary sheets for each patient can be organized as suggested in Fig. 1 and reviewed with clinical staff.

		ADL dependencies at admission							Totals
		0	1	2	3	4	5	6	
ADL dependencies 6 months after admission	0			Mrs. J.					
	1			Mrs. M.					
	2			Mr. L.					
	3				Mrs. P.				
	4								
	5				Mr. K.				
	6					Mrs. N.	Mrs. O.		
	Deceased								
	Total								

FIG. 1. Comparison of ADL dependencies at admission to the nursing home and 6 months later. Activities of daily living (ADL) include bathing, dressing, use of toilet, transfer, continence, and feeding.

This display allows the portrayal of the changing well-being of patients over time as well as the description of possible determinants of such changes. In the example cited (Fig. 1), Mrs. J. was dependent at a level of 2 at the time of admission and improved to a level of 0 by 6 months. Mr. K. deteriorated from 3 to 5 during the 6 months. With regard to determinants, it can be observed that patients who functioned at higher levels at admission were the ones who improved, whereas those who were more dependent at admission did not. A noteworthy feature of this type of display is the fact that any person whose name appears in one of the diagonal blocks is a person who has neither improved nor deteriorated (i.e., remained the same in ADL). Moreover, anyone to the right of the diagonal is a person showing improvement, and anyone to the left has shown deterioration. The display, therefore, makes possible the consideration of individuals or the summarization of the experiences of groups of individuals. When relationships are associated with other characteristics of the individuals (e.g., age, diagnosis, mental status) or of the environment, potential risk factors can be discovered.

Example of Application in Research

This type of clinical and educational exercise using functional assessment allows the introduction of research into the TNH in a practical and acceptable manner. Although there are a broad range of research questions that could be asked in the TNH setting, it seems appropriate that an initial focus of research be clinical in nature, e.g., research aimed at providing information for improved clinical care and improved managerial decisions. Because functional assessment routinely gathers information about multiple domains (physical, social, emotional, and cognitive function), its use as a clinical data-collecting method would greatly facilitate implementation of health care trials in the TNH. Variables needed in this type of research include "sociopersonal" information such as a patient's physical, social, and emotional function, his/her attitude toward illness, and features of daily life including interactions with nursing staff and family. Because the nursing home is a unique setting that is both a treatment and living situation, this type of patient information is pertinent in evaluating the impact of any intervention, whether it be a conventional therapy or a change in the way services are organized and delivered.

In summary, the broad application of functional assessment in the clinical, educational, and research activities of the TNH will allow the development of a common language in the TNH. By structuring both clinical service and education within the framework of functional assessment and by using these functional clinical data as a core element in the information of research, the language of function develops credibility among all professionals. Since the language of function is also meaningful to the nursing home residents and their families, it generates a circle of communication among staff, clinicians, administrators, residents, and their families. Use of a common language promotes integration of goals and the achievement of coordinated care. This cooperative involvement is basic to the success of any clinical research or educational program that might be proposed for the nursing home setting, thereby making possible their optimal contribution to the quality of care and quality of life of their residents.

REFERENCES

1. Katz S, Akpom CA, Papsidero JA, et al: Measuring the health status of populations, in Berg RL (ed): *Health Status Indexes.* Chicago, Hospital Research and Educational Trust, 1973, pp 39–58.
2. Katz S: Assessing self-maintenance activities of daily living, mobility, and instrumental activities of daily living. *J Am Geriatr Soc* 1983;31:721–727.
3. Jones EW: *Patient Classification for Long Term Care: User's Manual.* Washington DC, Bureau of Health Services Research & Evaluation, DHEW Publication No(HRA) 74-3107, 1973.
4. US National Committee on Vital and Health Statistics: *Long-Term Health Care: Minimum Data Set.* Hyattsville, MD, NCHS/DHHS Publication No(PHS)80-1158, 1979.
5. Kane RA, Kane RL: *Assessing the Elderly.* Lexington, MA, DC Heath, 1981, pp 25–67.
6. Skinner DE, Charpentier PR, Wissman KG, et al: *Major Experimental Design Considerations of a Prospective Study of Clients Served by Alternatives to Institutional Care: Interim Report No 4 Prepared by Applied Management Sciences.* Washington DC, DHEW(OS) 74-294, 1976.
7. Stewart AL, Ware JE, Brook RH, et al: *Conceptualization and Measurement of Health for Adults in the Health Insurance Study, vol II. Physical Health in Terms of Functioning.* Santa Monica, The Rand Corporation, 1979.
8. Ware JE, Johnson SA, Davies-Avery A, et al: *Conceptualization and Measurement of Health for Adults in the Health Insurance Study, vol III. Social Health.* Santa Monica, The Rand Corporation, 1979.
9. Donald CA, Ware JE, Brook RH, et al: *Conceptualization and Measurement of Health for Adults in the Health Insurance Study, vol IV. Social Health.* Santa Monica, The Rand Corporation, 1978.
10. Brorsson B: *ADL-Index: Sammanfattande Matt pa Individens Fromage att Klara det Dagliga Livets Aktiviter.* Gotab, Sweden, Medicinska Forskningsradet, 1980.
11. Besdine RW: The educational utility of comprehensive functional assessment in the elderly. *J Am Geriatr Soc* 1983;31:651–656.
12. Rubenstein L: The clinical effectiveness of multidimensional geriatric assessment. *J Am Geriatr Soc* 1983;31:758–762.

The Teaching Nursing Home, edited by Edward
L. Schneider et al. © 1985 The Beverly
Foundation. Raven Press, New York.

And *This* Is Home?

Carter Williams

Jewish Home and Infirmary Day Services, Rochester, New York 14621

In *Webster's New World Dictionary*, a home is defined as "a place where one likes to be; [the] place thought of as the center of one's affections; [a] restful or congenial place." In contrast, an institution is defined as "an organization having a social, educational or religious purpose, [such] as a school, church, hospital, reformatory, etc." (1). The dictionary does not confuse home and institution, nor should we, but we are dealing with an environment where the essential qualities of the two must meet for the benefit of the people living in it.

It has been my privilege over the past 10 years to work with many persons in their eighth, ninth, and tenth decades of life for extended periods of time both before and after they entered long-term care institutions. Because of this experience and my knowledge of nursing homes through consulting work, I have accepted the challenge of speaking for others—that is, for the people living in institutions.

Recognizing that one can only figuratively walk in another's shoes or sit in a restraint in another's wheelchair, we shall enter into the lives of some people I have known and worked with. In this way, we can perhaps gain a common basis of understanding about the problems with which these individuals are trying to cope. We can then proceed to some questions about how teaching and research activities in long-term care facilities may affect them and, in turn, the job of the health care professional.

The transition from home to institution is a time of crisis for all involved, but most especially for the person making the move, so a look at this period serves as a good starting point for understanding the experience of institutional living. We now meet a woman who was my neighbor for many years, whom we shall call Mrs. Eckland, just as she is experiencing this transition.

Mrs. Eckland was 90, divorced following a brief marriage in her 30s, and was living alone in her small third-floor apartment, which she had occupied for 25 years. A licensed practical nurse, she had worked part-time into her early 80s. She had never had children, and her only close relatives were

---

* *Present address*: 5202 West Cedar Lane, Bethesda, Maryland 20814.

two sisters almost as old as she, both in institutions and both largely alienated from her and from each other. She was tremendously proud of her career as a nurse in a period when most women were not financially independent. And she was proud that her earnings had been substantial enough to result in Social Security payments that allowed her to meet her monthly expenses and pay for a personal care aide for a half day each week. She was also proud of her family background, which included early settlers in the city, and of her past relationships with a number of influential people. She was an avid reader, keenly interested in politics, vehement in her political opinions, and a warm supporter of the women's movement.

Along with this pride in family and in her own accomplishment ran a prickly, at times tempestuous, personality. This temperament, accompanied by increasing immobility, meant that she had few relationships: one or two by telephone and a few in the neighborhood. Her world had shrunk into the three rooms of her apartment. Always, she told me, she was complimented by others on the transformation she had wrought there. She recounted in detail her choice of the deep blue rug, her delight in her beautiful pink bathroom, her dressing table with the fabric ordered from a certain store, and the set of gold-plated toilet articles carefully arranged on top. There were her books, too, four shelves of them, and her family pictures, the clothes she cared so much about, and the mementos from her trips to India. She sat in her fanback chair and controlled her world, with spirited comments about the failure of the politicians in Washington to manage their world as well.

This home, special and beautiful to her, was to others an attic apartment, poorly lighted and inconveniently arranged. The blue rug was usually covered with lint, and the odor of urine was strong. There were many piles of books and papers about her room.

However, she persevered in her full determination to remain at home where she was content to be, selecting resources she wanted to use from those I told her about, and she brushed aside with anger attempts to discuss future planning and consideration of entering a long-term care facility.

Then, as had happened four or five times previously within the year, she fell. But this time she lay on the floor many hours, unable to reach either of her telephones, which had been appropriately lowered according to instructions from a consulting occupational therapist. Her *Daily Hello* caller alerted a neighbor when she received no answer, and Mrs. Eckland was admitted to the hospital for the second time in several months in severe congestive heart failure.

With this background, we may now picture her after a period in the hospital on the way to a nursing home, which her doctor has told her can no longer be avoided. She is out of the hospital gown for the first time in many weeks and is wearing her familiar raincoat and her fur hat. She is expressing conflicting feelings of hope and apprehension as we make the trip in the chairmobile.

There is no one to greet us at the door. Mrs. Eckland is wheeled upstairs by the chairmobile attendant and helped to sit in a chair beside a bed in a double room. The nurse in charge on the floor introduces herself and welcomes Mrs. Eckland to her new home. She is thinking and responding slowly and does not do very well with the questions addressed to her. She tries to focus as others come in to see her: the social worker, the dietitian, and an aide in fairly rapid succession. Some address her by her first name or call her "honey" though they do not know her, and most speak in loud voices though she is only slightly hard of hearing. All speak kindly, but rapidly, and she does not quickly apprehend what is expected of her in the discussion of food preferences, nor does she seem to comprehend some of the routines they describe. Some try to take time to listen to her, but they are obviously under pressure of time; their responses tend to be stereotyped.

From controlling her own small domain at home, Mrs. Eckland has been thrust into a 24-hr-a-day situation in which she is to live by a schedule decided by others in a setting where she cannot even maintain control over the position of the items on her bedside table, or for that matter what she wishes to have on top of the table and what is to be in the drawer, a detail that throughout her year and a half in the nursing home particularly annoyed her.

To observers this loss of control seemed appropriate to her condition, which included lack of urinary control, inability to walk, and some lack of judgment. To her this experience meant loss of identity. All material clues as to who she was and what her life had been were absent—no royal blue carpet to reflect her taste, no books, no family pictures, no closets of clothes, no mementos of her travels. Wiped away also were the freedoms of living at home: sitting up reading into the early morning hours, perhaps never going to bed, or sleeping until 11 a.m., and eating when and what she wanted. And, finally, the loss of freedom was literally and figuratively signified by the experience of being placed in a vest-like garment with long belts attached by which she was tied into her chair because of her tendency to slip out of it.

Psychologically, environmentally, and socially, Mrs. Eckland's familiar world had disappeared. She had lost control of most aspects of daily living. She felt vulnerable, acted upon by others. Her personal living space was greatly reduced and was often invaded by other people. There was little privacy and no solitude. From the limited social contacts she had at home at times of her own choosing, she was thrust into constant contact with others, beginning with a roommate who was a complete stranger. And she was visibly imprisoned in her wheelchair. Small wonder then that I would find her in her first days sitting in her chair almost bent double, her eyes closed. She handed me on my visit to her the day after her admission this message written on the back of the card I had left her the previous day with a message of love on it from me and my husband. This is what she wrote:

> Dear Carter——You know this was not the place I wanted to come. Please come to see me and really prove that you love me. Also please get Mr. B. (my lawyer) to come here. I must talk to him. I loved you more than you loved me and trusted you. How can I trust you now?

A long period of grieving and depression followed in which Mrs. Eckland questioned the value of living. She was accusatory toward staff and her few visitors, including her lawyer. The staff social worker and I did what we could to ameliorate the situation, with varying degrees of success: cherished items of her selection were brought from home as soon as possible—her chair, family pictures, and clothing both precipitated more grieving and very gradually helped her to begin to reestablish her sense of identity and self-respect. She decided which pictures she wanted hung and where they were to be placed. Aides were encouraged to ask her to select what she wanted to wear each day, but this was only minimally successful because aides were constantly rotated. Her hair style also changed with the aide of the day, varying from loose and free-flowing to tight knots and coy ornaments and bows. Sometimes spots of rouge and very bright lipstick were applied, though she had never used cosmetics previously. Mealtime was often difficult; she had to sit at table for a half hour or more while others gathered, and she longed for a really hot cup of coffee and real china and metal cutlery rather than the array of plastic with which she had to cope.

Gradually, several distinctly positive developments occurred: she formed good trusting relationships with the social worker and two aides. She began to discover that she could help some other residents through her conversational ability and the encouragement she offered them. And through the chaplain, she was reunited with her church from which she had long been estranged.

Mrs. Eckland's story has elements common to the experience of the many older people in our communities who are precipitously transferred from home to institution via the hospital because of major health crises. But as hard as the move to an institution was for her, it was probably not as great a change as some people experience. She also had greater coping abilities than many who have led more protected and circumscribed lives. She did not have to be separated from a spouse or other family members, nor did she leave behind a treasured pet. She also had no language problems. One must try to imagine what it must be like for the aged immigrant who has learned little or no English to enter an institution, or for a black person or others of another racial cultural minority to enter our overwhelmingly white institutions. What must it be like for people who have lost much of their hearing to enter the nursing home environment, experiencing all the loss of identity and control that Mrs. Eckland did and in addition hardly being able to communicate with others?

What lies ahead for people who make their homes in long-term care institutions if teaching and research functions are added? Even without the advent of research and teaching, the medical and nursing routines of long-term care facilities tend to medicalize the smallest details of life. For example, Miss Cohen cannot enjoy her Sabbath Eve challah when it is reduced from the warm fragrant chunk she has enjoyed Friday evenings all her life to a thin cold slice because of her restrictive diet. So great is her indignation, that her response is to refuse all food. And how can Mr. Denby, the courtly, dignified former executive, be saved from embarrassment and identity loss when he is unable to rise to greet or bid farewell to his guest because he is tied to his chair out of fear of his falling? He tries at times to work up a little levity about the restraint by calling it his "male brassiere," but another day he says quietly, "It's a terrible thing to lose your freedom." Indeed, his sense of imprisonment is so great that I found him in tears on another occasion because he was certain the doors were locked and his wife, who was soon to return from a trip, would not be allowed in by the jailor to see him. And where is there privacy for him and his wife when he shares a double room, and not only is the roommate present but at unexpected moments a loud voice comes over the intercom demanding to know where this or that aide is? These are hardly the circumstances and setting in which two people can share intimate moments, whether they be times of quiet conversation or longed-for sexual intimacy.

For anyone who has been in an acute hospital bed, these experiences, and many more, often strange and dehumanizing, are familiar. But we must remember, the long-term care facility is usually the person's permanent home, and the problems are chronic and have to be dealt with not for a limited number of days but, for most, for the rest of their lives.

Will the meaningful events of every-day life, already so greatly reduced, be further medicalized by teaching and research activities? When planning and carrying out these functions, will health professionals take time to plan their interventions into the lives of residents so that their contacts enrich them and lighten their loads rather than add to their burdens? If the health professional recognizes Mrs. Eckland as the proud woman who struggled for a means of supporting herself after what was at the time the disgrace of divorce and rejection by her family, he/she will contribute to the regaining and affirming of individual identity. One also hopes that he/she will take the time to look for her strengths and not only for her frailties and weaknesses. If one goes further to discover how life feels to Mrs. Eckland now, a new relationship will result. If this relationship can be of enough duration to provide some enrichment and dependability in her life, he/she will avoid becoming a part of another bewildering parade of faces. For, unfortunately, some homes deliberately rotate aides every week. The rationale offered for this policy is that they do not want individual residents to become attached to any one aide. Yet this practice runs exactly counter to what the sick, older person needs in terms of familiar faces, procedures, and continuing dependable relationships. There is a slight possibility of unhealthy relationships developing. But with monitoring for signs of destructive behaviors, this practice of cutting off people living in institutions from attachments to staff can be avoided. Grief is always involved when a relationship ends, but with appropriate support both to the older person and to staff, this grief can be worked through. The risk of loss, after all, is one we take throughout our lives. If we deny ourselves and others all attachments because of the potential of pain, we deny something essential to us as human beings.

When one has given up much that was formerly meaningful and has lost a large measure of personal freedom, one is particularly sensitive to an attitude of being used—used as an object of teaching or research. So to every resident of a nursing home who may participate in any project, careful explanation and feedback about what has been learned by such research are needed. And time is needed as well to avoid mistaking diminished hearing, sight, and voice strength for lack of response capabilities.

One research nurse wrote me of her experience in this regard as follows:

> In our institution, we take great care with the consent process. We approach each person slowly, carefully assessing ability to see, hear, and communicate, to understand, judge, and reason, and the level of comfort or discomfort. It is a slow process. We explain the consent, verbatim, if necessary. For one deaf, partially sighted man, we copied key parts of the consent onto poster board in large letters so he could read it for himself. We go back the next day or week if the [person] is unsure and wishes to talk with family or friends, or just wants to think it over. We also tell [people] how to reach us if they change their minds or have questions (P. Tabloski, Monroe Community Hospital, *personal communication*, 1984).

As to the important matter of contributing to a person's sense of control over her/his environment, this may come mainly through accretion of many small details—through consultation and agreement with each person on timing, on who the personnel will be, on whether one takes pains to leave things in the person's room as they were when found, whether one is careful to knock before entering, to ask permission to speak with the resident, or to return at a more convenient time; whether one remembers to sit down so that he/she is on the same eye level as the person being visited and to speak slowly, avoiding jargon and "medicalese."

A word about families, which I have so far neglected. All will agree that their understanding of the goals of the teaching and research are crucial, so time needs to be allowed for contacts with them. They will be needed as very important sources of backup, interpretation, and support to their institutionalized family members. There are varieties of families, carrying their own particular constellations of relationships to their sick older relatives living in the institution.

What of the person like Mrs. Eckland who, in effect, has no family? Again, on the basis of personal experience, any such person is so very vulnerable that it is essential that someone accept an advocacy role with and for him/ her. Mrs. Eckland, for example, needed frequent interpretation about what happened to her in the nursing home. She needed to be able to turn to someone outside the home for help and reassurance. My suggestion is that everyone who is without close family and friends have an advocate, who could be a volunteer trained much as the ombudsman is and who could be recruited from the community through churches, temples, and service organizations.

This discussion with the questions it raises has been presented to sensitize us to the possible pitfalls of introducing teaching and research to the home of the older person with chronic illness. In some of the institutions where these functions already exist, there are encouraging reports of positive results for the residents. For example, participation in a research project often does result in a welcome increase in attention and enrichment in relationships. It adds interest and sense of purpose to the individual's life. Results of some studies can bring about certain immediate improvements in care. And there is a positive spin-off in the added interest teaching and research may bring to the work of the staff if they are properly prepared for it and are not too overworked. One physician, highly experienced in research in long-term care facilities, reports that he does not set foot on a floor to talk to any resident until extensive meetings have been held with all nursing staff in which a full understanding of goals and procedures has been reached lest rumors and apprehensions abound (D. Bentley, University of Rochester, *personal communication*, 1984). When staffing ratios are poor, as I have known them to be at times in all institutions, but particularly in the smaller proprietary facilities, it is recommended that the teaching and research projects bring in some additional personnel. The good reports of successful teaching and research are always accompanied by this proviso: time must be spent to prepare the people participating as subjects as well as their family members, advocates, and staff at all levels.

We need to learn so much more about the health and well-being of people who live in chronic-care institutions and the diseases and systems that affect them. What about the system that emerges from the maternalistic attitude that pervades most nursing homes—is it beneficial to the people living there? They are, after all, adults and not kindergartners. We need research to learn how to protect those for whom a fall is dangerous without the sense of imprisonment and punishment restraints produce. We urgently need to know more about how to teach personnel successfully at all levels about those things that make for personalization, dignity, and a sense of worth, so that a nurse does not address all she cares for as "honey" or "dear," so that the dining room assistant in front of a person newly admitted doesn't call over to her supervisor in a loud voice, "Does Smith feed herself?" which brings the immediate, indignant response from Mrs. Smith, "Of course I feed myself!" And we need to learn ways of expanding the institution-bound social worker's understanding and creativity, possibly by providing work partly outside the institution. The list of questions regarding all aspects of care—medical, nursing, social, administrative—is unending.

It is my hope that as one explores these questions, he/she will include sensitivity to the person being studied as an essential component of research, education, and clinical care. By procedures that personalize, by our findings and their application, we will help to remove some of the bitterness from the question with which we began: "And *this* is home?"

PART IV
Specific Strategies

The Teaching Nursing Home, edited by Edward
L. Schneider et al. © 1985 The Beverly
Foundation. Raven Press, New York.

Rehabilitation and Nursing Homes

Stanley J. Brody

*Rehabilitation Research and Training Center in Aging, Department of Physical Medicine
and Rehabilitation, Medical Center, University of Pennsylvania, Philadelphia,
Pennsylvania 19104*

The orientation of care in the skilled nursing facility (SNF) is responsive
to societal values. Similarly, the presence, or more likely the absence, of
rehabilitation services reflects these same values as they are expressed by
inadequate public reimbursement policies, limited professional education,
and sparse research findings (1–4).

"Rehabilitation," as Williams observes, "is an approach, a philosophy, and
a point of view as much as it is a set of techniques." Its goal is "to restore
an individual to his/her former functional and environmental status, or al-
ternatively, to maintain or maximize remaining function" (5).

Within this general goal, the objectives are to restore patients to their
highest possible levels of physical, psychological, and social functions; to
prevent disability; to retard the rate of deterioration in progressively degen-
erating conditions; and to enable patients to function effectively and independently within their limitations. Tangible services include tests, meas-
urements, and various therapeutic modalities; among the latter are exercises
and physical agents such as heat and massage to increase range of motion
and relieve pain.

Rehabilitation procedures are directed toward improving such functions
of mobility and activities of daily living (ADL) as eating, using the toilet,
dressing, sitting, turning, standing, walking, wheeling, transferring, and the
use of prosthetic devices. Included too are the teaching of verbal and nonverbal communication, the redirection of interests, and motivating, encouraging, and keeping patients physically, mentally, and socially active.
These services are usually medically prescribed, often under the direction
of a physiatrist who specializes in physical medicine and rehabilitation. For
the most part, the services are given by physical, occupational, and speech
therapists, although nurses, social workers, and psychologists may be active
members of the rehabilitation team.

Historically, rehabilitation of the aging has received a low priority among
physiatrists and other rehabilitation professionals (6) and, until recently, it
has virtually been ignored as a societal goal (7).

The roots of the medical specialty of physical medicine and rehabilitation are traceable to the American Congress of Physical Therapy, X-Ray and Radium, founded in the early 1920s. (Later, "X-Ray" and "Radium" were dropped, and "Physical Medicine" was substituted for "Physical Therapy" in the name of the organization.) In 1947, the American Board of Physical Medicine was established, with "and Rehabilitation" added two years later.

In the decade of the 1940s rehabilitation was very much concerned with childhood diseases, poliomyelitis in particular. During the same period, rehabilitation skills were applied to modifying the disabilities that arose from the casualties of World War II. A third major concern was for spinal injuries resulting from traumata.

That first early stage was followed in the 1950s and 1960s by a new and expanded emphasis on vocational outcomes as measured by reentry into the labor force. This goal, too, was a reflection of social concerns—those relating to industrial trauma and the social cost of dependency.

The 1960s and 1970s witnessed a third period of rehabilitation. The developmentally disabled—another discrete target group—were recognized as not inevitably handicapped. For them, the rehabilitation intervention was many faceted. Physical medicine and the rehabilitation therapies advanced the expectation of independent living for this group. In'addition, vocational training was made available for the most seriously disabled. Society began to acknowledge its responsibility to provide barrier-free environments, transportation, and (to some degree) housing.

Throughout this period of evolution, assessment methodology, which is rehabilitation's major diagnostic, treatment, and evaluation tool, responded to these target populations by focusing on maximizing the level of functioning. Rehabilitation objectives consider the basic levels of Maslow's hierarchy of human needs (8) as the basis of the fundamental aim for rehabilitation to help patients achieve skill in the essential bodily functions—mobility, eating, and toileting.

Rehabilitation, in a sense, has come of age. The language of the most recent rehabilitation legislation has dropped the word "vocational" from its title, and to the past concern for independent living has been added focus on the "geriatric" population (9).

Although public policy changes have slowly evolved in rehabilitation and aging legislation, professional attitudes have lagged. Many leaders in the medical specialties of geriatrics and physical medicine have been unclear as to their objectives as well as their mutual concerns. Thus, Fowler, in his 1982 presidential address to the Academy of Physical Medicine and Rehabilitation considering medical school curricula, speculated that "it might be necessary and even desirable to consider an entry through expanding high interest areas such as geriatrics" (10). Libow, in his 1982 Kent lecture on education for geriatric medicine, described rehabilitation activities in detail, but physical medicine was not mentioned specifically as a related medical specialty (11).

Rather than rapprochement and collaboration between the geriatric and physical medicine specialties, competition for economic turf seems to be accelerating rivalry between the two groups. The physiatrist is rarely used in the few inpatient geriatric services which have been instituted in general hospitals. Prospective payment systems, currently in the form of the diagnosis-related groups (DRGs), put a premium on rehabilitation inpatient units by excluding them from the reimbursement constraint (12). The internists who direct inpatient geriatric units already have unsuccessfully attempted to include those units under the rehabilitation exemption (13).

There are three subgroups of elderly disabled who are increasingly utilizing rehabilitation services. First, many developmentally disabled people are now surviving past middle age for the first time. The introduction of antibiotics and the control of respiratory infections have enabled a large cohort of mentally retarded people (and their families) to face the problems of aging. Second, because of improved medical care, adults who have suffered trauma at an earlier time are also aging in large numbers. The third and largest group are those aged who have become disabled because of traumata (such as falls and other accidents) or those diseases and conditions that become more prevalent or intense in the eighth stage of life (aging). For this group, medical/surgical intervention has been effective, but patients have been left with residual impairments (14). These three groups of elderly constitute the new population that challenges rehabilitation and tests the therapeutic optimism characteristic of the field.

Rehabilitation services are concerned with preventing disability and handicap as well as improving the level of functioning of the disabled and handicapped. The major target population is made up of those suffering the residual of the disease or trauma in the process represented in Table 1. The distinctions among the terms (impairment, disability, handicap) have been recently clarified by the World Health Organization:

Impairment: Any loss or abnormality of psychological, physiological, or anatomical structure or function. **Disability:** Any restriction or lack (resulting from an impairment) of ability to perform an activity in the manner or within the range considered normal for a human being. **Handicap:** A disadvantage for a given individual, resulting from an impairment or disability, that limits or prevents the fulfillment of a role that is normal, depending on age, sex, social and cultural factors, for that individual (15).

The disabled and handicapped population is well represented in SNFs. One of the most important predictors of institutionalization is dependency in ADL, particularly in the personal care functions of eating, toileting, bathing, and dressing (16). Lawton has summarized the physical and mental conditions and functional capacities of nursing home residents in Table 2 (17).

TABLE 1. *Decision tree*

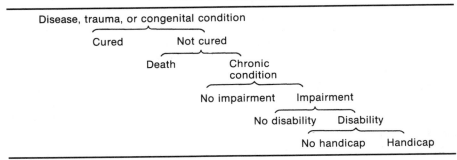

TABLE 2. *Selected physical and mental conditions and functional capacities of nursing home residents*

Condition	Percentage of residents
Arthritis	34
Heart trouble	34
Diabetes	13
Paralysis as result of stroke	11
Impaired vision	47
Impaired hearing	32
Impaired speech	26
Impaired ability to bathe	86[a]
Impaired ability to dress self	68[a]
Impaired mobility	65[a]
Impaired continence	45[a]
Impaired ability to eat	32[a]
Senility	58
Agitation or nervousness	42
Depression	39
Sleep disturbance	19
Abusiveness or aggressiveness	17
Other behavioral problem	5

[a] 1977 data; all other data from 1973 to 1974.
From Lawton (17), with permission.

Over the last 10 years, when limited to statutory language, Congressional perception of the need for rehabilitation services in SNFs has not changed. The category "skilled nursing facilities" was created for both the Medicare and Medicaid programs by the Social Security Amendments (SSA) of 1972 (18), which authorized "skilled care benefits for individuals in need of 'skilled nursing care and/or skilled rehabilitation services on a daily basis in a skilled nursing facility which it is practical to provide only on an inpatient basis'" (18, p.59). The specific language of the act defines the SNF in part with the following:

Sec. 1861 (h) The term "extended care services" means the following items and services furnished to an inpatient of a "skilled nursing facility". . . .

(3) physical, occupational or speech therapy furnished by the . . . "skilled nursing facility" or by others under arrangements with them made by the facility (18, p. 1025).

The rehabilitation role of the SNF was reinforced by the provision that requires transfer agreements between the hospital and the SNF, which

(1) is primarily engaged in providing to patients (A) skilled nursing care and related services for patients who require medical or nursing care, or (B) rehabilitation services for the rehabilitation of injured, disabled, or sick persons (18, p. 1026).

Prior to the passage of the 1972 SSA amendments, a 1968 survey reported that only 32% of nursing homes offered any rehabilitation services, including physical, occupational, speech, or any other therapies (19). A subsequent survey in 1975 found that:

many patients in skilled nursing facilities needed specialized rehabilitative services that they were not receiving, e.g., 47.9 percent needed physical therapy, 35 percent needed occupational therapy, and 13 percent needed speech therapy (20).

Two years later, the 1977 National Nursing Home Survey reported that among Medicare- or Medicaid-certified SNFs, 24.9%, 24.8%, and 27.1% routinely provided physical, occupational, or speech and hearing therapies, respectively (21). It further reported that 75% of the residents were dependent in one or more ADL activities; during the year prior to the survey, only 35% of the SNF population received any therapy service; of all the residents, 13.7% received physical therapy, 5.9% occupational therapy, and 0.9% speech or hearing therapy (21, p. 56).

The SNF population is not homogeneous. A significant number of residents are discharged within 90 days. According to the same 1977 report, 625,000 residents were discharged in less than 3 months. Of these, 127,000 died, 210,000 moved to another health facility, and 238,000 returned to a private or semiprivate residence (21, p. 63). A structural analysis of service intensity positively and significantly associates the frequency of admissions, a measure of turnover, with the offering of rehabilitation services (22). Moreover, 267,000 Medicare patients were reimbursed for a SNF stay (for stays of less than 100 days and for which charges were related to costs) (23). Rehabilitation services are positively related to costs (22). It is reasonable to assume, then, that most of the rehabilitation services in the SNF are received by the short-stay residents based on the factors of high turnover and high costs. Most of the long-term SNF residents are paid for by Medicaid, and their stays are associated with low reimbursement and low turnover (16, p. 4). (With the fiscal incentives provided by prospective payment systems, of which DRG is currently the most prevalent, the pressure on SNFs to accept short-term patients will increase.) The parallel conclusion is that the long-term resident in an SNF receives very few rehabilitation services.

Most long-term SNF residents suffer from senile dementia of the Alzheimer's type (SDAT). Since one-third of SNF residents are short term and half of residents have been identified as suffering from SDAT (20), at least two-thirds of those staying more than 90 days carry that diagnosis, among others. Thus, it would appear that a *de facto* policy exists that would exclude SDAT SNF residents from rehabilitation services.

One of the major responsibilities that rehabilitation has assumed is the restoration of the elderly to the roles they had prior to disease or trauma. For most, a vocational role is not appropriate. However, for the elderly widow living alone, the role of homemaker is appropriate, and for such women who spend a short term in the SNF, the rehabilitation intervention is significant. Even this objective may not be realistic, and independent living may not be a relevant or even desirable goal. For many elderly, some level of dependency must be accepted as a legitimate condition, and the goals of rehabilitation should be organized toward restoring the family's (or caregiving unit's) premorbid level of functioning. In many instances, the objective of treatment may be minimal but significant to the quality of life.

These goals anticipate a return to living in the community alone, with family, or with a substitute caregiver. Thus, for the older person who is admitted to the SNF for a short-term stay of less than 90 days, rehabilitation services are relevant, and there is some evidence that these modalities are available to them. Moreover, with the expansion of the prospective payment system to reimburse acute patient care, SNFs will be called on to increase their short-term, rehabilitation-oriented care (24).

The dilemma of setting rehabilitation goals for the disabled elderly, particularly for the long-term SNF resident, is value laden. Roles are determined by society and reflect the values of the community. The rehabilitation unit of a general hospital is evaluated by third-party payers on the basis of whether the elderly went to a SNF or returned to the community. Similarly, the entire debate and discussion of "alternatives" is couched in terms of success for community living and failure if referral is made to an SNF for permanent residence. Virtually all of the discussion is focused on cost: SNFs are expensive to the governmental body and therefore bad; community living is seen as less costly to the public and consequently good. Whether or not this is true, the value preference remains clear (25). The effect of values on rehabilitation services for the permanently disabled who live in SNFs is controlling (26). Values are expressed by three groups: the community, the caregivers, and the elderly themselves.

The Federal Survey of Long Term Care Facilities pointed out that since 1974, "Federal regulations for Medicare and Medicaid patients require that participating facilities not admit or retain patients in need of specialized rehabilitative services unless they are provided, either directly or under arrangements with outside resources" (20, p. 51). The survey concluded that this requirement was not being met and that the quality of the services was deficient. Safety rules were ignored, there was a lack of treatment objectives in the rehabilitation plan of care, there was no coordination of rehabilitation plans with the patient's total plan of care, and there was a lack of participation by nursing personnel in the patient's rehabilitative programs. The survey called for better-trained inspectors and for attention to be given to the financial reimbursement aspects of these services. It concluded that slow and inadequate reimbursement appears to affect the delivery of appropriate services, a conclusion that a Health Care Financing Administration review of long-term care confirms a decade later (22, pp. 665 ff.).

It would seem that Medicaid reimbursement rates, notwithstanding explicit rehabilitation regulatory and statutory requirements and the lack of appropriate supervision, have contributed to the virtual absence of rehabilitation services for needy long-term residents in SNFs. Since this state of affairs has been repeatedly reported in public documents, it must be assumed that the public value structure does not require other than custodial services for the SNF long-term resident. A specific confirmation of this conclusion may be found in those few states that restrict Medicaid coverage to skilled nursing care and specifically deny rehabilitation services (27).

In support of this conclusion, the 1983 GAO report on Medicaid and Nursing Home Care cites the HCFA Study of Skilled Nursing Facilities mandated by Congress in 1980 (28). It defines the SNF as "an institution (or distinct part of an institution) that provides skilled nursing care and related services to patients who require medical or nursing care. It *may* also provide rehabilitation services to injured, disabled, or sick persons" (25,29,30) (italics added). Thus, although the statutory language defining SNFs has not changed in over 10 years, the interpretation has, and rehabilitation services, insofar as the administering agency is concerned, are now optional.

The role of rehabilitation in the care of the aged has been largely overlooked by medicine (31). The two specialties specifically involved, geriatric medicine and physical medicine, each present educational curricula that appear to ignore the other despite the fact that both address the same elderly population (32). The literature of both gerontology and rehabilitation are oblivious to each other. Both fields espouse a multidisciplinary approach and, for more than two decades, both have used functional assessment as a key tool. However, reviews of assessment from the rehabilitation and gerontological literature concerned with similar measurement issues did not have a single common citation among their more than 150 references (33,34). The same observations may be made of the gerontological content in the educational programs of the overlapping professions that are key participants in the rehabilitation and geriatric teams. As Butler and Lewis observed 10 years ago, "medicine and the behavioral sciences have mirrored societal attitudes by presenting old age as a grim litany of physical and emotional ills. *Decline* of the individual has been the key concept, and *neglect* the major treatment technique" (35). There has been some positive change during the last 10 years in clinical practice, but with respect to those long-term residents in SNFs, the clinical practice remains therapeutically nihilistic. The societal and professional bias that Butler (36) described as "ageism" might well be revised to "age disabilityism."

The third group of value-setters are the aged themselves. As Butler has observed, "oppressed groups develop their own subculture in which values and behavior patterns are shared" (36, pp. 404–405). Provider and community attitudes that placement in an SNF represents failure are readily absorbed and shared by the elderly SNF resident group. The result is a sense of hopelessness and discouragement, which is adopted rather than countered by the health team (37).

The teaching nursing home (TNH) has a major responsibility to explore and define appropriate goals for the SNF. The maintenance of a positive therapeutic point of view should be a *sine qua non* to the training of all health workers. In-service training manuals and procedures must be developed so that:

> Each participant on the health care team must be able to see the connection between his and her own reaction and the patient's illness . . . a systematic management plan must be formulated through which the aged patient may recognize the way in which distress is dissipated in order to avoid the full impact of the disability. This recognition may help the patient focus on the pertinent issues, work toward adaptation, and allow the health care team to repair its lost therapeutic perspective (38).

The education of all health workers who are preparing to serve the elderly must integrate the knowledge of skills of the geriatric and rehabilitation professions. The TNH is an ideal setting for such a clinical educational process.

Formal research should be encouraged by the TNH to demonstrate the efficacy of rehabilitative interventions with the very old, disabled SNF long-term resident. Efficacy should be defined in terms of what "may seem to be small gains in function." As Williams points out, "such 'small gains' can make all the difference in the degree of independence that a person can achieve" (5). Specifically, the issue of rehabilitation services for SDAT residents in SNFs must begin to be addressed as a significant research question.

Although data and findings do not necessarily control or affect the values of a society, we have the responsibility as professionals and researchers to contribute to the knowledge and experimental base required for rational policy and program decisions. It would be dangerous and, at the least, inaccurate to assert that any one program can change the value structure of a society; it remains for the electorate and its representatives to affirm the role of rehabilitation for the long-term resident in SNFs.

REFERENCES

1. Kane RL, Kane RA (eds): *Values and Long Term Care.* Lexington, MA, DC Heath & Co, 1982, pp 3–25.
2. Vladeck BC: *Unloving Care: The Nursing Home Tragedy.* New York, Basic Books, 1980.
3. Brody SJ: Comprehensive health care for the elderly: An analysis. *Gerontologist* 1973;13:412–418.
4. Palmer HC, Vogel RJ: Models of the nursing home, in Vogel RJ, Palmer HC (eds): *Long-Term Care, Perspectives from Research and Demonstrations.* Washington, DC. HCFA, USDHHS, US Government Printing Office, 1983, pp 537–578.
5. Williams TF: *Rehabilitation in the Aging.* New York, Raven Press, 1984, p xiii.
6. Steinberg FU: Education in geriatrics and physical medicine residency programs. *Arch Phy Med Rehab* 1984;65(1):8–10.
7. Rusk HA: *Rehabilitation Medicine, ed 4.* St Louis, CV Mosby, 1977, p v.
8. Huizinga G: *Maslow's Need Hierarchy in the Work Situation.* Groninger, Wolters-Noordhuff, 1970.
9. Public Law 95-602, Rehabilitation Act of 1978.
10. Fowler WM: Viability of physical medicine and rehabilitation in the 1980s. *Arch Phys Med Rehab* 1982;63:4.
11. Libow LS: Geriatric medicine and the nursing home: A mechanism for mutual excellence. *Gerontologist* 1982;22:134–141.
12. *Federal Register:* Vol 48, No 171, September 1, 1983, p 39755.
13. *Federal Register:* Vol 49, No 1, January 3, 1984, p 240.
14. Greunberg EM: The failures of success. *Milbank Mem Fund Q* 1977 (Winter), pp 3–24.
15. World Health Organization: *World Programme of Action Concerning Disabled Persons.* Geneva, WHO, 1982.
16. General Accounting Office: *Medicaid and Nursing Home Care: Cost Increases and the Need for Services Are Creating Problems for the States and the Elderly.* Washington, DC GAO/IPE-84-1, US Government Printing Office, 1983, p 20.
17. Lawton MP: *Environment and Aging.* Monterey, CA, Brooks/Cole, 1980, p 110.
18. Social Security Amendments of 1972: Report of Committee on Finance, US Senate, to Accompany HR 1. Senate Report No 92-1930, 92nd Congress, 2nd Session, September 26, 1972.
19. *Services and Activities Offered to Nursing Home Residents, United States, 1968.* Rockville, MD, US DHEW, 1972.
20. Office of Nursing Home Affairs, PHS, DHEW: *Long Term Care Facility Improvement Study. Introductory Report.* Washington, DC, US Government Printing Office, pub. #0S-7650021, 1975.
21. National Nursing Home Survey: 1977 Summary for the United States, *Vital and Health Statistics,* Ser 13, No. 43. Washington, DC, National Center for Health Statistics, PHS, DHEW, DHEW Pub No (PHS) 79-2794, p 16.
22. Vogel RJ, Palmer HC (eds): *Long-Term Care, Perspectives from Research and Demonstrations.* Washington DC, HCFA, USDHHS, US Government Printing Office, 1983, p 690.
23. Muse DN, Sayer F: *The Medicare and Medicaid Data Book, 1982, Health Care Financing Program Statistics.* Baltimore, Maryland, DHHS, HCFA, 1982, p. 51.
24. Brody SJ, Persily NA: *Hospitals and the Aged: The New Old Market.* Rockville, MD, Aspen Press, 1984.
25. General Accounting Office: *The Elderly Should Benefit from Expanded Home Health Care But Increasing These Services Will Not Insure Cost Reductions.* Washington, DC, US Government Printing Office, 1982.
26. Kane RA, Kane RL: *Assessing the Elderly.* Lexington, MA, Lexington Books, 1981, p 267.
27. Study of Skilled Nursing Facilities Mandated by Section 919 of PL 96-499., Office of Research, Demonstrations and Statistics, HCFA, DHHS, July 9, 1982 [mimeographed].

28. Public Law 96-499, Omnibus Reconciliation Act of 1980, Sec 919, Study of Need for Dual Participation of Skilled Nursing Facilities, December 5, 1980.
29. Department of Health and Human Services, Health Care Financing Administration, Office of Research, Demonstrations and Statistics: Study of Skilled Nursing Facilities Mandated by Section 919 of Public Law 96-499. Washington, DC, US Government Printing Office, 1982.
30. Feder J, Scanlon W: *Medicare and Medicaid Patient's Access to Skilled Nursing Facilities* (*Working Paper 1438-02*). Cleveland, The Urban Institute, 1981.
31. Institute of Medicine: *Aging and Medical Education*. Washington, National Academy of Sciences, 1978.
32. Rickels B: Geriatric care in the future. *Phys Occup Ther Geriatr* 1983;2(4):1.
33. Brown M, Gordon WA, Diller L: Functional assessment and outcome measurement. In Pan EL, Backer T, Vesh CK (eds): *Annual Review of Rehabilitation, vol 3*. New York, Springer, 1983, pp 93–121.
34. Shaie KW, Stone V: Psychological assessment, in Eisdorfer C (ed): *Annual Review of Gerontology and Geriatrics*, vol 3. New York, Springer, 1983, pp 329–361.
35. Butler RN, Lewis MI: *Aging and Mental Health*. St Louis, CV Mosby, 1973, p 17.
36. Butler RN: *Why Survive? Being Old in America*. New York, Harper & Row, 1975.
37. Brody E: Tomorrow and tomorrow and tomorrow: Towards squaring the suffering curve, in Gaitz C (ed): *Aging 2000: Our Health Care Destiny Vol. 2*. New York, Springer (in press).
38. Breslau L: Problems of maintaining a therapeutic viewpoint. In Haug MR (ed): *Elderly Patients and Their Doctors*. New York, Springer, 1981, p 127.

The Teaching Nursing Home, edited by Edward
L. Schneider et al. © 1985 The Beverly
Foundation. Raven Press, New York.

Mental Health Aspects of Nursing Home Care

Gene D. Cohen

*Program on Aging, National Institute of Mental Health, National Institutes of Health,
Rockville, Maryland 20852*

That a problem of enormous proportions can be largely overlooked is not a new phenomenon. The confusing of diseases in later life with normal concomitants of the aging process has been the paradigm of this phenomenon for the field of geriatrics. Inattention to the mental health problems that affect 70% to 80% of nursing home residents represents a lingering variation of the same theme (1,2). Moreover, although the role of social factors in influencing nursing home placement is being recognized, less appreciation of psychiatric influences occurs. For example, the social factors of not having a spouse and living alone have been identified as contributing variables in nursing-home placement for those with serious physical illness; if these patients had someone at home to help, institutionalization might have been prevented or postponed. Psychiatric factors can assume a related role. A person with a debilitating cardiac condition who also has psychotic episodes may be too disorganized to manage his or her own illness through proper digitalis and diuretic regimens, thereby increasing the likelihood of needing placement in a more protective setting such as a nursing home. Mental problems, therefore, can be a primary or secondary factor in nursing home placement; they can also be a later development in those who initially entered the nursing home without such disturbance.

MENTAL HEALTH CONSIDERATIONS

Individuals enter nursing homes because of diminished capacities to function independently along with reduced reserves. Accordingly, they need to be assessed in terms of the portfolio of problems with which they present as well the portfolio of their strengths. A risk in a setting where one receives help is that the focus will be too much on what one cannot do and not enough on what one can do. This is an illness-versus-health dichotomy that requires consideration along mental- as well as physical-health parameters. From another perspective, a tension between dependency needs and the need for independence is at work. In emotional terms the proper balance of these psychodynamic variables speaks to better mental health, especially in an institutional environment. Unfortunately, there is no clear dependence/independence ratio to draw on, since the proportion of one to the other varies considerably with individuals. Thus, we are dealing here as much with the art as with the science of health care delivery.

Dependency matters are invariably complicated. First, external dependency needs must be separated from internal, intrapsychic ones. The dependency of a hard-of-hearing person on a hearing aid reflects, of course, an appropriate external dependency need; meeting this need can typically be better for the individual. If this person, however, feels that having to have a hearing aid means losing control of his or her own destiny and rebels against it, then we are witnessing an internal dependency conflict. The individual can be emotionally assisted by being helped to realize that by using a hearing aid one is actually *taking* control—an action that will enhance his or her ability to function more independently. To the extent that this individual does not feel that he or she is taking control of the situation, the likelihood increases that maladaptive efforts of control will begin to appear. At this point, a number of disturbing behaviors often enter the nursing home scene. Such behaviors, whether in the form of incessant demands or disruptive acts, may be the unconscious acting out of a desperate need to feel in control. Put differently, these behaviors may represent a desperate defense against feeling increasingly less in control.

The challenge for the nursing home staff in this area is multifold. Whenever any intervention is required for a nursing home resident, the resident's involvement in the planning and implementation for the intervention should be considered so as to enhance that individual's sense of influencing his or her own course. If a resident continues to lose capacity in one area, staff should explore with that person alternative avenues for exercising capacity in line with an existential need to exert one's being. Disturbing behaviors should be examined as symptoms or misrouted energy, with the aim of helping the resident to rechannel this energy in a more constructive direction that effects control. Nursing home staff are often required to deal with the consequences of deficit alone—to assist one resident to the bathroom, to help straighten up another in a chair, to assist someone else in walking, and so forth. But to overlook the emotional and psychodynamic consequences of the deficit in this setting is to overlook areas that potentially generate a myriad of even more taxing behavioral events. It would, in short, be overlooking the impact of overall functioning on mental health and the impact of mental health on overall functioning in the nursing home environment. This is ripe terrain for the researcher who endeavors to better delineate mental health considerations and consequences of deficit and decline in the nursing home environment (3,4).

DEPRESSION IN THE NURSING HOME RESIDENT

One aspect of illness in the elderly that commonly distinguishes it from a disease in earlier adulthood is its variability or atypical presentation. For example, infection in later life may present without fever or an elevated white blood cell count on laboratory study; hyperthyroidism can appear in a paradoxical form known as apathetic hyperthyroidism; depression can resemble dementia. Indeed, depression in the elderly, particularly in frail older persons in a nursing home, can present in a variety of masked or atypical forms. Whereas classical depression is characterized by a mood of serious and prolonged sadness, thoughts about hopelessness, and social withdrawal along with sleep and appetite disturbances, many of these typical symptoms may be masked by other symptoms in the depressed aged (5).

Multiple somatic complaints can represent a common illustration of a masked depression in the elderly. The nursing home resident who suffers serious loss of a sense of autonomy may experience consequent damage to his or her self-esteem. Instead of developing classical depressive symptomatology, this older individual may express the inner pain somatically. These somatic symptoms may not only signal an underlying depression but may reflect a maladaptive maneuver of attempting to compensate for feelings of lost autonomy by the control of others through complaints. This pattern relates to the earlier discussion on mental health considerations. Evaluating the complaints of such older patients can be difficult, since frail older persons by definition have physical problems. But it is important to question whether physical problems alone can explain the entire clinical picture. If some of the somatic concerns do not appear to have a physical basis, the solution is not in challenging their "legitimacy" but rather in acknowledging the person's discomfort and tactfully exploring emotional sources of trauma (6).

Whereas on the one hand the presence of depression in the older patient may be missed, on the other, the source of the disorder may be overlooked. Drug side effects are a case in point. Sometimes an elderly individual can have taken a drug over a considerable period of time without appearing to have developed any adverse effects, only to experience insidious difficulties later. The antihypertensive drug reserpine illustrates this phenomenon. It is estimated that 10% to 15% of older persons treated with reserpine develop depression (7). With some, the onset of depression occurs within a week; in others, more than a year goes by before the symptom manifests itself. In the latter group, it would be easy to dismiss the drug as the source of the problem by assuming that such symptoms would have become evident earlier. Hence, with those individuals the source of the depression would have been misdiagnosed.

PSYCHOSIS IN THE NURSING HOME RESIDENT

Certainly one of the most dramatic pictures of altered functioning in an individual is that which accompanies psychosis—the changes in a person's thought, affect, and behavior. The impact of psychosis on the nursing home resident and consequently on the nursing home staff is no exception. In psychosis the perception of reality is distorted; delusions and/or hallucinations alter the way the individual interacts with his or her environment. Reality for the nursing home resident is already difficult enough. Psychosis compounds the situation by making it more difficult for the resident to negotiate the environment and to seek or receive help.

Sometimes the problem is worse when the symptoms are more subtle. A borderline paranoid state, for example, may be marked by suspiciousness, negativism, uncooperativeness, anger, hostility, or nastiness on the part of the individual. Too often, nursing aides as well as family members interpret these displays personally or else see them as reflecting the real personality. In such cases, the service providers need to be educated or reminded that one sees not the real person but rather disturbing symptoms signaling great distress within. If displays of inner distress are not so recognized, they will result in conflict between the giver and receiver of care. Moreover, neglecting to counsel family members about the phenomenology of psychosis can leave them with a lingering unsettled feeling about their loved one should their relative die before the problem is understood or alleviated. Meanwhile, a number of psychotherapeutic, behavioral, and psychopharmacologic aproaches are available for treating psychosis in the elderly (8).

PSYCHIATRIC ASPECTS OF ALZHEIMER'S DISEASE

The clinical management of Alzheimer's disease is replete with opportunities for psychiatric expertise (9,10). This is because Alzheimer's disease is a brain disorder in which the major symptom clusters along its clinical course are mental, behavioral, and psychological—the terrain of the mental health professional. The mental symptoms are those of memory and intellectual dysfunction; the behavioral can include problems of agitation, wandering, and angry outbursts; the psychological can include depression and delusions. The latter clinical states reflect two of the ways Alzheimer's disease is classified in *ICD-9* (*International Classification of Diseases*, Ninth Edition) and *DSM-III* (*Diagnostic and Statistical Manual of the American Psychiatric Association*, Third Edition). Hence, Alzheimer's disease with depression and Alzheimer's disease with delusions are diagnostic entities in *ICD-9* and *DSM-III* (*ICD-9* refers to Alzeimer's disease as senile dementia, whereas *DSM-III* refers to it as primary degenerative dementia). Listing Alzheimer's disease in these two ways also identifies treatment opportunities. This is especially important in the nursing home setting, where so many residents have Alzheimer's disease.

Too often one hears the comment that Alzheimer's disease is untreatable. The statement would be accurate only if it said that one cannot cure, reverse, or stop the progression of the disorder. There is a state of the art, however, in treating the disorder in which interventions for many individuals with Alzheimer's disease can bring about an actual improvement in clinical status and overall functioning at a given time along the progression of the disease.

Consider the patient who has Alzheimer's disease with depression. Too often one asks "Is the problem Alzheimer's disease or depression?" instead of asking "Is it Alzheimer's disease *with* depression?" We know that depression by itself can interfere with concentration and memory. Thus, depression coupled with dementia is a double detriment to sound intellectual functioning. It is postulated that depression is a part of the clinical picture of those with Alzheimer's disease for two reasons—one psychodynamic, the other biologic. Psychodynamically, individuals in the early and middle stages of Alzheimer's disease observe the decline in their own intellectual functioning. Some come to terms with it, others grieve, and many are emotionally devastated or suffer serious depression. Biologically, it appears that the subcortical brain changes in Alzheimer's disease not only interfere with the cholinergic system that is claimed to influence memory but with the biogenic amines that affect mood as well. The resulting depression leads to what has been called "excess disability" in the Alzheimer patient. However, this excess disability can respond to treatment. Supportive psychotherapy alone or in combination with the judicious use of antidepressant medication can often lift the compounding depression, thereby improving the quality of life for the patient and the level of interaction between patient and staff. A similar scenario applies to Alzheimer patients whose excess disability is in the form of delusions that add to the intellectual disorganization caused by the dementia. Again, behavioral interventions, supportive psychotherapy, and the use of antipsychotic medication can make a therapeutic difference for the patient at that stage of the illness.

Mental health considerations apply even at an advanced stage of dementia. The double tragedy surrounding the personal history suffered by the institutionalized Alzheimer patient illustrates this point. Severely demented individuals have not only lost touch with their personal history but have lost the ability to convey their own history to others. In this sense we all have a compound history or two-faceted history—a history of ourselves as we know it and a history of ourselves as others perceive us. Not to be known by others, to be in effect without a history as a consequence of being unable to convey one's past, puts a person at a severe disadvantage in eliciting the understanding and empathy of others. The clinician can be enormously helpful here in conveying the individual's personal and dynamic history— the patient's clinical biography so to speak—to the various staff who will be working with the patient. With such an improved frame of reference for staff, the outcome is likely to be better interpersonal exchange despite the patient's marked cognitive impairment. It might be said in this regard that how the Alzheimer patient is viewed in late-stage dementia is as much a factor of biography as biology.

A problem that remains is how to effectively transmit this clinical biography. It is clearly difficult to do so dynamically by relying on the traditional chart history, since the necessary length would discourage many from reading it. An oral history is often more engaging and effective. But practical issues such as multiple shifts and substantial staff turnover can limit the life of or the audience for the oral history. A possible alternative is using audio or video cassettes to record the biography and clinical notes, told by a clinician who has followed the patient in the past, perhaps with participation by a family member who can recount the history well. Staff on all shifts might be more likely to review these histories because it is easier to listen to or watch a cassette presentation than to ponder a chart. Family members, especially if they have good information or stories about the patient's history, could assume an important role here and probably would derive much satisfaction from contributing to the presentation of the history. The experience could be rewarding for patient, family, and staff alike. Quality of life for the patient, family involvement, and staff morale might all be positively affected (11).

THE INTERFACE OF MENTAL AND PHYSICAL DISORDERS

As suggested earlier, it is risky with the older patient in general, and certainly with the nursing home resident in particular, to look only for a single cause for clinical symptoms. Quite often concurrent problems are interacting, and this interaction is frequently between concurrent mental and physical disorders. The resident who has a respiratory tract infection and fever while being depressed may, because of the depression, neglect proper fluid intake and become dehydrated as well, thereby aggravating the overall condition. Thus, the infection and the depression must be treated.

As another example, older patients with hearing problems are at increased risk of developing delusions, which then compound their already compromised ability to communicate. Similarly, older patients with impaired vision may be at greater risk of developing schizophreniform symptoms. There are a number of research questions surrounding the frequency of psychosis in these patients, the nature of the genesis of such symptoms, and optimal interventions. Auditory and visual problems affect a large number of older people as a whole—29% have trouble hearing, and 22% have difficulty seeing (12). Meanwhile, it is felt that the sensory deprivation with such disorders puts these individuals at greater risk for trouble. However, the question remains, why are some affected and not others?

MEDICATION ISSUES

Mental health considerations with respect to drug use in the elderly come from two directions (13). One needs to be aware of psychiatric side effects that can accompany the use of drugs for the treatment of physical disorders. Various antihypertensive and other cardiac medications, for example, can have depression as a side effect. One needs also to be aware of somatic side effects that can accompany the use of psychotropic drugs; for example, the tricyclic antidepressants can aggravate glaucoma or urologic functioning. Of course, it is important to keep in mind that most side effects are possibilities, not probabilities. Otherwise, the drug would generally not be used. As long as certain side effects are possible, however, their nature, frequency, and source should be under study.

SPECIAL CONSIDERATIONS: SUNDOWNER'S SYNDROME AND INDIRECT SUICIDAL BEHAVIOR

Any number of special mental-health-related conditions could be elaborated. Only two are presented here as examples of the myriad areas needing further research in the nursing home setting: sundowner's syndrome and indirect suicidal behavior.

Sundowner's syndrome is characterized by agitation and/or confusion that typically becomes more apparent or marked after the sun goes down. Not adequately understood, "sundowning" appears to reflect symptomatic expression in the face of lower central nervous system arousal and decreased sensory stimulation, as would accompany the reduction in light and sound in the evening after the sun goes down. If sedating medications are used to "treat" the agitation, the lowered CNS arousal can be further reduced, thereby resulting in a paradoxical worsening of the agitation. Interventions involve the search for medications the patient is already receiving that are too sedating and, if possible, cessation of the drug, reduction in its dosage, or substitution of another medication. Interventions also involve increasing the amount of sensory stimulus around the patient—providing more light, music, etc. Nonetheless, sundowner's syndrome remains a clinical problem in need of more research to help us to understand its frequency, genesis, manifestations, and management.

Indirect suicidal behaviors can assume a diversity of forms. The earlier example of the depressed nursing home resident with a respiratory tract infection could have been such an example; the failure to take adequate fluids might have represented a feeling of giving-up, a form of passive suicide response. Thus, any difficult-to-explain change in the patient should be examined not in terms of the natural course of the physical disorder alone but in terms of compounding psychiatric if not indirect suicidal influences as well.

CONCLUSION

Although we are witnessing advances in the diagnosis and treatment of mental disorders in general, this progress has been inadequately applied in the nursing home. The problem is multifold: too little research has been conducted specifically focused on mental health and mental illness in the nursing home setting; training of nursing home staff in this area is largely absent; there are currently no mental health standards for nursing homes; and limitations in the reimbursement of mental health services for the elderly as a whole have added to service delivery obstacles. But to the extent that the magnitude of mental health problems in the nursing home is recognized and the responsiveness of these problems to mental health interventions is acknowledged, then the likelihood for change should increase. The analogous understanding that many of the health problems in later life are not normal aging changes and can be alleviated by appropriate clinical interventions has led to the burgeoning of the field of geriatrics. These insights would do especially well if focused on mental health issues in the nursing home.

REFERENCES

1. Teeter RB, Garetz FK, Miller WB, et al: Psychiatric disturbances of aged in skilled nursing homes. *Am J Psychiatry* 1976;133:1430–1434.
2. Cohen GD: Prospects for mental health and aging, in Birren JE, Sloane RB (eds): *Handbook of Mental Health and Aging*. Englewood Cliffs, NJ, Prentice-Hall, 1980, pp 971–993.
3. Sherwood S, Mor V: Mental health institutions and the elderly, in Birren JE, Sloane RB (eds): *Handbook of Mental Health and Aging*. Englewood Cliffs, NJ, Prentice-Hall, 1980, pp 854–884.
4. Whanger AD: Treatment within the institution, in Busse EW, Blazer DG (eds): *Handbook of Geriatric Psychiatry*. New York, Van Nostrand Rheinhold, 1980, pp 453–472.
5. Roth M: The psychiatric disorders of later life. *Psychiatr Ann* 1976;6:57–101.
6. Pfeiffer E, Busse EW: Mental disorders in later life—affective disorders; paranoid, neurotic, and situational reactions, in Busse EW, Pfeiffer E (eds): *Mental Illness in Later Life*. Baltimore, Garamond/Pridemark Press, 1973, pp 107–144.
7. Cole JO, Davis JM: Reserpine-induced depression, in Freedman AM, Kaplan HI, Sadock BJ (eds): *Comprehensive Textbook of Psychiatry-II*, vol 2. Baltimore, Williams & Wilkins, 1975, p 1952.
8. Gaitz CM, Varner RV: Principles of mental health care for elderly inpatients. *Hosp Commun Psychiatry* 1982; 33:127–133.
9. Verwoerdt A: *Clinical Geropsychiatry*. Baltimore, Williams & Wilkins, 1976.
10. Miller NE, Cohen GD (eds): *Clinical Aspects of Alzheimer's Disease and Senile Dementia*. New York, Raven Press, 1981.
11. Cohen GD: The mental health professional and the Alzheimer patient. *Hosp Commun Psychiatry* 1984; 35:115–116.
12. Butler RN, Lewis MI: *Aging and Mental Health*. St Louis, CV Mosby, 1973.
13. Levinson AJ (ed): *Aging*, vol 9: *Neuropsychiatric Side Effects of Drugs in the Elderly*, New York, Raven Press, 1979.

The Teaching Nursing Home, edited by Edward
L. Schneider et al. © 1985 The Beverly
Foundation. Raven Press, New York.

Dementia in the Context of the Teaching Nursing Home

Robert Katzman

Department of Neurology, Albert Einstein College of Medicine, Yeshiva University, Bronx, New York 10461

Dementia is one of the most important contributors to the admission of the "frail elderly" to the skilled nursing facility, and, therefore, we must consider dementia a priority in regard to teaching, research, and medical care in a teaching nursing home.[1]

The term dementia is a technical one describing the syndrome characterized by deterioration of intellectual function of sufficient severity to interfere with occupational and/or social performance. The field was somewhat obscured for a number of years because psychiatrists referred to this syndrome as "chronic organic brain syndrome," whereas neurologists used the term dementia. In 1980, the American Psychiatric Association, in the third edition of the *Diagnostic and Statistical Manual* (1), abandoned "chronic organic brain syndrome" and adopted the term dementia. The description of dementia above is, in part, a paraphrase of this definition. Dementia involves loss of memory and other cognitive functions such as abstraction, learning, reasoning, and visuospatial ability.

Over the past 25 years, there have been a number of studies of the prevalence of dementia in persons over the age of 65. In most of these studies it was found that severe dementia, leading to impairment of independent functioning such that the individual must be cared for either in an institution or essentially full-time at home, occurs in about 5% of the elderly population (2). Mild to moderate dementia with the individual still semiindependent occurs in an additional 5% to 10% (2). In the United States, with over 26 million persons over the age of 65, about 1.3 million would be expected to have severe dementia. Moreover, within the group over the age of 65, the prevalence of dementia is age specific with a prevalence of less than 1% severe dementia at age 65, rising to a prevalence of 15% to 20% past age 80. Thus, one can extrapolate that many of the individuals with

---

[1]A useful series of review articles covering management of Alzheimer's disease both in the nursing home and in the community as well as clinical aspects may be found in the Fall 1982 *Generation*, Vol. 7, #1.

severe dementia, individuals in their 80s, will eventually be in a nursing home.

In our own experience in a skilled nursing facility in New York, a facility with over 500 residents, approximately 75% have dementia as measured on formal examination. In this nursing home, the average age is just over 85 years. Moreover, the dementias in the residents in this home did not first appear during institutionalization but were demonstrated at the time of admission. Similar results were found, although never reported, in two other New York City skilled nursing facilities (2).

Patients admitted to nursing homes most often have more than one disorder, and many of those admitted with dementia also have heart disease or other conditions common in the elderly. Nevertheless, the "straw" that finally necessitates admission is the cognitive impairment that prevents the individual from participating actively in his or her own care.

The concept of dementia has changed radically during the past 20 years as it has become recognized that dementia is a syndrome complex that can be produced by a number of diseases and disorders. Over 50 diseases that produce dementia have beem listed, and that number is certainly incomplete (3). However, there have been a number of clinical pathological reports in which autopsy findings in the brain and the premortem clinical status of patients with dementia have been analyzed. In each of these series, approximately 50% of individuals with dementia (in one series rising to 65%) were found to have the disorder known as Alzheimer's disease (4–6). Another 10% to 20% have a dementia of vascular origin, usually the result of multiple strokes. A variety of other disorders ranging from thyroid disease to B_{12} deficiency to head trauma, brain tumor, neurosyphilis, and hydrocephalus are also important causes of dementia, although the numbers of these patients are small. Thus, in Jellinger's series (4), undiagnosed brain tumors accounted for about 4% of patients with dementia; today, with the CT scan, such patients would be readily identified. In addition, a very important subset of patients with clinical dementia are found not to have obvious pathology at the time of postmortem examination. An important question is whether these patients have as yet undefined disorders with brain changes not evident by current histopathological techniques or whether such patients in face had metabolic disorders during life that were not diagnosed.

During the past several years, a consensus has developed as to the best obtainable workup or assessment for the differential diagnosis of dementia. This assessment includes a careful history, mental status examination, physical and neurological examination, and neuropsychological tests. An important constituent of the workup is the CT scan to rule out mass lesions and hydrocephalus as well as to help identify some cases of multiinfarct dementia. A comprehensive biochemical screen is required to rule out such disorders as thyroid dysfunction, B_{12} deficiency, and a variety of other metabolic diseases that may present with cognitive impairment. Tests for neurosyphilis and other evidence of infection should be done. This type of workup is very useful but at present still incomplete, since differential diagnosis during life is not yet optimum. With the expected addition of nuclear magnetic resonance (NMR), additional improvement in diagnostic techniques may become possible. However, an important area of research is identification of simpler methods of diagnosing dementia, particularly development of a test specific for Alzheimer's disease.

Since Alzheimer's disease (originally described in 1907) is the most important cause of dementia, it has attracted the interest of a number of investigators (7–9). Alzheimer first discovered the presence of specific changes on microscopic examination of sections of the brain of a relatively young patient (in her 50s) with a progressive dementia. Applying newly discovered silver stains, he discovered the presence of groups of abnormally staining silver spots forming a rough circle, a phenonemon that he described as the neuritic plaque, and abnormal nerve cells that appeared to have tangles of fibers within them, the so-called neurofibrillary tangles.

In 1964, electron microscopy revealed that the neuritic plaque consists of degenerative nerve endings surrounding a core of an abnormal fibrillar protein called amyloid (10,11). The neurofibrillary tangle was found to consist of a large array of abnormal very fine filaments, approximately 100 Å in diameter, present in pairs wound around each other and termed a paired helical filament.

In 1968, Blessed et al. reported on the results of a prospective study in which they demonstrated a significant correlation between the degree of dementia during life and the number of plaques and tangles in the cerebral cortex at autopsy in a population that included elderly (12).

In 1976, three groups in Great Britain independently described the marked loss of choline acetyltransferase, an enzyme required for the synthesis of acetylcholine, one of the important neurotransmitters within the brain (8,13). Strikingly, the plaques, tangles, and cholinergic abnormality occur in the outer mantle of the brain, that is, the cerebral cortex and in a deeper structure in the temporal lobe, the hippocampus, which is known to be an important site of memory. Quite recently it has been found that the cholinergic deficit results from the loss of cells deep in the forebrain, in the basal nucleus of Meynert (14). These cholinergic cells project diffusely throughout the cerebral cortex, and an adjacent set of cells in the diagonal band of Broca and the septal regions of the brain project to the hippocampus. The loss of these cells appears to be an important factor in Alzheimer's disease. There is evidence that some of the nerve endings in the neuritic plaque are the endings arising from this cholinergic projection system.

There has also been important research on the nature of the protein forming the paired helical filament. Selkoe (15) has shown that these filaments are very tightly bound, that is, covalently bonded, and are resistent to a large number of solvents that dissolve most proteins (15). Because of this stability, it has been possible to dissolve away most other brain structures and to obtain very pure preparations of paired helical filaments. Antibodies raised to these paired helical filaments do not interact with normal nerve filaments present in nerve cells (15). This is a very exciting finding, for it raises the possibility that the paired helical filament may contain a protein not normally present in nerve cells. This protein may be the result of altered gene expression or perhaps the incorporation of a slow virus within the nerve cell. These areas of research are moving forward at a rapid rate, and more specific data should replace speculation within the next 2 years. Such on-going research is part of a major effort to identify the pathogenetic mechanisms in Alzheimer's disease in the hope of finding a clue to its etiology.

There have also been studies trying to identify risk factors in this disorder. As previously indicated, Alzheimer's disease is strongly age related. There is some question as to whether women may be more susceptible to Alzheimer's disease than men. The apparent greater number of women than men could merely reflect the increased ratio of women to men in older population groups, or women could be intrinsically at greater risk. In one study of 400 80-year-olds, the incidence per 100 person-years appears to be increased in females in the population as compared to males, but this disparity may represent a selection bias, since the men in the sample appeared to be cognitively more intact than the women when initially enrolled (R. Katzman, *unpublished data*, 1984).

An interesting new discovery is the occurrence of head injury as a risk factor. In two studies, it has been found that a history of head injuries was reported in 15% to 25% of patients with Alzheimer's as compared to 5% in age-matched controls. This unexpected finding brings to mind the reports from England that "punch-drunk" fighters with so-called "dementia pugilistica" are found to have numerous neurofibrillary tangles at postmortem examination. Although at present there has been no evidence that stress per se is a precipitating factor for Alzheimer's disease, it appears that perhaps the true "knocks" that one receives during life may be important.

There is an intriguing relationship of Alzheimer's disease to inheritance. Approximately 10% of Alzheimer patients have clear-cut family histories of dementia in prior generations, suggesting a simple autosomal dominant defect. However, there are also many Alzheimer patients in whom there is no apparent family history. Even more common are patients with a single relative with reported Alzheimer's disease. A problem inherent in such studies is the fact that Alzheimer's is a disease of late life, and until recently, few persons lived to advanced age. Thus, family histories are often incomplete. Nevertheless, it is unlikely that the majority of patients with Alzheimer's develop this disease on the basis of a simple gene inheritance.

An exciting discovery is that all individuals with Down's syndrome develop Alzheimer changes both pathologically and biochemically if they live past the age of 40. This becomes important since it demonstrates that a genetic change may be a sufficient although not a necessary cause of the development of Alzheimer's late in life. With the marked improvement in technology in molecular biology and genetics, it may become possible within the next decade to identify the specific gene that predisposes to Alzheimer's disease in some families and in Down's syndrome patients.

The teaching nursing home can play a very important role in Alzheimer research. Most of the important research that relates to the biology of Alzheimer's has depended on clinical pathological correlation and on the microscopic or biochemical examination of pathology samples of affected brains obtained at autopsy. Many of the most important studies, including those carried out in Newcastle in the late 1960s (12) and the more recent studies of Davies, Terry and others (9,10,13), have utilized autopsies obtained from nursing home patients (12,13,16). This should be expected, since so many patients with Alzheimer's disease are admitted to and die in nursing homes.

In our own work, we have had the opportunity of studying the residents in a large skilled nursing facility on a yearly basis to provide a clinical counterpart to correlate with findings at autopsy. However, in the Newcastle study and our own studies, clinical evaluation was limited to an appraisal of mental status and function using relatively simple scales. With the advent of the teaching nursing home, it now becomes possible to carry out a much more detailed assessment of a subset of the patients, including a relatively complete workup for dementia and serial neurological examinations as well as serial neuropsychological tests in individuals involved in these studies.

A very important limitation of studies of patients in the nursing home is the problem of informed consent. This problem has already been dealt with by a special task force of the National Institute on Aging (17). Individuals early in the course of an Alzheimer process can give informed consent, and there is no problem in clinical investigation. Frequently clinical investigation is simple and does not involve invasive procedures, for example, clinical examination, mental status test, or when it can be performed without additional hardship as with the drawing of an additional ounce of blood at a time when routine blood chemistries are done by the doctors at the nursing home. In a meeting hosted by NIA,[2] the consensus of research scientists, clinicians, ethicists, lawyers, family members, and others was that it is appropriate in these situations for permission to be obtained from the next of kin. Such procedures must be stopped if the patient shows by word or deed that he or she objects. Further along the scheme are procedures that might have therapeutic value. For example, because of the existence of the cholinergic deficit, there are now important studies being carried out trying to

---

[2] Conference on Senile Dementia of the Alzheimer's Type and Related Diseases: Ethical and Legal Issues Related to Informed Consent.

identify drugs that may overcome this deficit. Among such drugs, for example, is physostigmine, a compound that does enhance memory in some Alzheimer patients early in the course of the disease (18). Physostigmine is a drug that has been in intermittent clinical use since 1840; its disadvantage is that it has significant side effects in doses only slightly higher than that used in current clinical studies.

Under what conditions can such drugs be used in patients who are unable because of their own condition to give informed consent? Obviously, with informed consent of next of kin, one must proceed very cautiously using small doses of such medicines to make sure that side effects of a serious nature do not occur. There is an inherent dilemma if one is unable to carry out any research on patients with Alzheimer's, a disease for which there is no adequate model in animals. Finally, there might indeed be a need for an invasive procedure that would provide some answers that could lead to an effective treatment of Alzheimer's. Is some mechanism needed for determining which research project can be attempted? One mechanism is a decision by a patient early in the course of Alzheimer's to volunteer for such procedures, perhaps through delegation of power of attorney to a person whom the individual trusts. Nevertheless, this approach may be so difficult as to produce a chilling effect on vital research. How can society preserve the integrity and autonomy of Alzheimer patients and yet achieve the goal of treating and preventing this disorder?

The same ethical issues can also be raised in regard to the everyday management of Alzheimer patients. Many patients with Alzheimer's disease go through a stage in which they become very agitated, restless, pace incessantly, have sleep disrupted, and, at times, scream and yell. It is precisely such agitation that often leads to institutionalization. The agitated, ambulatory Alzheimer patient can be very disruptive on the floor of a nursing home, and even if not ambulatory, the cries and screams may be disruptive to other patients. Agitation can be easily overcome if one were willing to use neuroleptic medications such as haloperidol. Haloperidol, however, has many side effects, particularly in the very old, and may produce not only parkinsonian changes that interfere with mobility of patients but may also produce a severe bradykinesia such that the patient is much less responsive and in fact appears more confused than when not on haloperidol.

There is now universal acceptance in such cases of the need for drug therapy, yet such therapy is almost invariably rendered not only with the absence of informed consent by the patients but sometimes against the patient's instinctive reaction to refuse any kind of medication. So one is forced to seek management techniques that do not require such medications. One important approach developed quite independently in many nursing homes is that of an environment that minimizes the effects of agitation such that these disturbing behaviors can be ignored by staff. In essence, this requires establishing an environment similar to that of a "childproof" situation so that the Alzheimer patients cannot hurt themselves: an environment in which patients could wander freely but would have difficulty in leaving the premises. At the same time, it is imperative to provide a high staff-to-patient ratio in order to maximize social interaction. The patients who are actively engaged in the Einstein Alzheimer's group and other socialization activities are less prone to develop episodes of agitation.

It is important to establish a diagnosis of the patient with dementia. That subset of demented patients without pathology at postmortem represents an important challenge, since they potentially could have been rehabilitated in life if the etiology of their disease had been discovered. In a series of autopsies from a nursing home, there was found among the patients with dementia one patient with treatable hydrocephalus, undiagnosed during life, as well as a patient with a brain tumor (*unpublished data*). Neither patient had received a CT scan during life. Thus, although the yield may be only 2% to 6% of truly treatable conditions in patients in their 80s, a full evaluation for the differential diagnosis of dementia must be conducted on every patient entering a nursing home.

What is the relationship of dementia to teaching in a nursing home setting? Is the nursing home an adequate place to teach medical students and junior house officers who perhaps learn best when dealing with a patient early in the course of a disease, a patient more likely to be seen in an office or clinic setting than in a nursing home? It is evident that the patient with dementia must be well understood by the staff of nursing homes, by geriatricians who deal with these patients, and by social workers and others who counsel the family. The objective of every physician–specialist, certainly of every research physician, is to eliminate the disease that interests the investigator. Those involved in nursing homes should also have as a goal the elimination of the most important disorder that causes the elderly to seek institutionalization, dementia.

REFERENCES

1. American Psychiatric Association: *Diagnostic and Statistical Manual-III*. Washington, DC, American Psychiatric Association, 1980, p 494.
2. Katzman R: The prevalence and malignancy of Alzheimer disease. A major killer. *Arch Neurol* 1976;33:217–218.
3. Haase GR: Diseases presenting as dementia, in Wells CE (ed): *Dementia*, ed 2. Philadelphia, FA Davis, 1977, pp 27–67.
4. Jellinger K: Neuropathological aspects of dementias resulting from abnormal blood and cerebrospinal fluid dynamics. *Acta Neurol (Belg)* 1976;76:83–102.
5. Sjorgren T, Sjogren H, Lindgren AGH: Morbus Alzheimer and morbus Pick: A genetic, clinical, and pathoanatomical study. *Acta Psychiatr Scand [Suppl]* 1952;82:1–152.
6. Tomlinson BE, Blessed G, Roth G: Observations on the brains of demented old people. *J Neurol Sci* 1970;11:205–242.
7. Katzman R: *Biological Aspects of Alzheimer's Disease*. Banbury Report # 15. New York, Cold Spring Harbor Laboratory, 1983, p 495.
8. Katzman R, Terry RD, Bick KL (eds): *Aging*, vol 7: *Alzheimer's Disease: Senile Dementia and Related Disorders*. New York, Raven Press, 1978, p 595.

9.   Terry RD, Katzman R: Senile dementia of the Alzheimer type. *Ann Neurol* 1983;14:497–506.

10. Terry RD, Gonatas NK, Weiss M: Ultrastructural studies in Alzheimer's presenile dementia. *Am J Pathol* 1964;44:269–297.

11. Kidd M: Paired helical filaments in electron microscopy in Alzheimer's disease. *Nature* 1963;197:192–193.

12. Blessed G, Tomlinson BE, Roth M: The association between quantitative measures of dementia and of senile change in the cerebral grey matter of elderly subjects. *Br J Psychiatry* 1968;114:797–811.

13. Davies P, Maloney AJF: Selective loss of central cholinergic neurons in Alzheimer's disease. *Lancet* 1976;2:1403.

14. Whitehouse PJ, Price DL, Clark AW, et al: Alzheimer disease: Evidence for selective loss of cholinergic neurons in the nucleus basalis. *Ann Neurol* 1981;10:122–126.

15. Selkoe DJ, Ihara Y, Salazar FJ: Alzheimer's disease; Insolubility of partially purified paired helical filaments in sodium dodecyl sulfate and urea. *Science* 1982;215:1243–1245.

16. Davies P, Katzman R, Terry RD: Reduced somatostatin-like immunoreactivity in cerebral cortex from cases of Alzheimer disease and Alzheimer senile dementia. *Nature* 1980;288:279–280.

17. Senile Dementia of the Alzheimer's Type and Related Diseases: Ethical and Legal Issues Related to Informed Consent, Conference at the National Institute on Aging, Bethesda, MD, November, 1981.

18. Thal LJ, Fuld PA, Masur DM, et al: Oral physostigmine and lecithin improve memory in Alzheimer disease. *Ann Neurol* 1983;13:491–496.

The Teaching Nursing Home, edited by Edward
L. Schneider et al. © 1985 The Beverly
Foundation. Raven Press, New York.

Urinary Incontinence: Opportunities for Research, Education, and Improvements in Medical Care in the Nursing Home Setting

Joseph G. Ouslander* and Gwen C. Uman†

*Multicampus Division of Geriatric Medicine, UCLA School of Medicine and †University
of Southern California School of Education, Los Angeles, California

Urinary incontinence (UI) is a common, disruptive, potentially disabling, and costly health problem. Defined as the involuntary loss of urine sufficient in amount or frequency to be a social and/or health problem, UI affects between 5 and 10 million Americans and millions of others throughout the world. Several different treatment modalities can be used to manage UI, but affected individuals and health professionals often ignore or deny the problem and underevaluate it or manage it suboptimally. Despite its prevalence and impact, very little systematic research has addressed the causes and most efficacious management strategies for UI, especially in the nursing home setting. This chapter reviews what is known about UI in nursing homes and explores opportunities for research, education and improvements in the care of incontinent patients in a teaching nursing home (TNH) program.

TYPES AND CAUSES OF INCONTINENCE

British geriatricians, who have been investigating UI for several decades, distinguish between "transient" and "established" forms of UI [1,2]. Urinary incontinence has been shown to be a transient phenomenon in up to one-third of affected persons [3,4]. Although differentiating UI on the basis of easily reversible versus more fixed causes has some merit, distinguishing between "acute" and "persistent" forms of UI may be more clinically useful [5,6].

Acute UI refers to incontinence that is sudden in onset and resolves with appropriate management of an acute medical condition, drug side effect, or other reversible factor. Common causes for acute UI include: acute urinary tract infection with bladder inflammation, urinary frequency, urgency,

173

TABLE 1.　*Types and causes of persistent urinary incontinence*

Type	Definition	Common causes
Stress	Involuntary loss of urine (usually small amounts) with increases in intraabdominal pressure (e.g., cough, laugh, exercise)	Weakness and laxity of pelvic floor musculature Bladder outlet or urethral sphincter weakness
Urge	Leakage of urine (usually larger volumes) because of inability to delay voiding after sensation of bladder fullness is perceived	Unstable bladder,[a] isolated or associated with the following: Local genitourinary condition such as cystitis, urethritis, tumors, stones, diverticuli, and mild outflow obstruction Central nervous system disorders such as stroke, dementia, parkinsonism, spinal cord injury
Overflow	Leakage of urine (usually small amounts) resulting from mechanical forces on an overdistended bladder	Anatomic obstruction by prostate stricture, cystocele Acontractile bladder Diabetes Spinal cord injury
Functional	Urinary leakage associated with inability (because of impairment of cognitive or physical functioning), psychological unwillingness, or environmental barriers to toilet	Severe dementia and other neurological disorders Psychological conditions such as depression, regression, anger, hostility Inaccessible toilets (or toilet substitutes) Unavailable caregivers

[a] See text for definition.

and dysuria; acute medical illnesses, especially when associated with delirium, immobility, and environmental barriers, fecal impaction; drug side effects, such as urinary frequency and urgency caused by diuretics, and sedation and immobility caused by sedative and hypnotic agents; urinary retention, precipitated by an anticholinergic drug or acute spinal cord injury; and polyuria caused by a metabolic condition, such as the osmotic diuresis associated with hyperglycemia when diabetes is poorly controlled.

Persistent UI implies incontinence that continues after an acute problem has resolved or UI that is unassociated with an acute medical condition and gradually worsens over time. Individuals with persistent forms of UI should have a thorough diagnostic evaluation in order to determine the most appropriate treatment(s).

Persistent UI can be subdivided into four broad categories: stress, urge, overflow, and functional (Table 1). Stress UI almost always occurs in women and is generally related to previous childbirth, pelvic surgery, and postmenopausal estrogen deficiency. Occasionally elderly men experience stress UI after transurethral resection of the prostate (TURP).

Urge UI, either alone or in combination with symptoms of stress UI, is probably the most common type of UI in the elderly population (2,7–12). Usually associated with a urodynamically unstable bladder (see *Diagnostic Evaluation*), urge UI can be caused by local inflammatory or irritant conditions in the lower genitourinary tract such as chronic cystitis, atrophic urethritis, mild outflow obstruction, bladder diverticuli, stones, or tumors or by neurologic disorders that impair central nervous system control over voiding (stroke, dementia, and parkinsonism).

Overflow UI occurs when the bladder cannot empty completely. In elderly persons, this is usually caused by anatomic obstruction (most commonly by the prostrate or urethral stricture in men; occasionally by a large prolapsed cystocele in women) or to inadequate bladder contraction (as can occur with a diabetic neuropathic bladder). Drugs with anticholinergic activity, which are used frequently in the elderly population, can contribute to urinary retention and overflow UI.

Functional UI refers to incontinence that is related primarily to the physical or mental inability to reach a toilet or to psychological conditions associated with unwillingness to use a toilet appropriately (such as depression and hostility). Environmental factors (such as physical barriers and unavailable caregivers) can also contribute to this type of UI. Several studies have indicated that UI in nursing home patients is commonly associated with impairment of cognitive function and mobility (2,3,13,14). Thus, functional type UI, which requires very different approaches to management than other forms of persistent UI, may be a major cause of UI in the nursing home setting.

PREVALENCE

Several studies have examined the prevalance of UI in various settings (Table 2) (3,4,13–20). Although the population samples differ, and the definitions of UI and methods of data collection are not consistent among these studies, several findings are worth noting. Studies done in mainly noninstitutionalized populations indicate that between 6% and 15% of elderly men (aged 65 and over) and 11% to 50% of elderly women have some problem with UI. Most of these incontinent persons have occasional episodes of UI (at least twice per month), whereas 5% to 10% have more severe UI with at least daily episodes of UI and require frequent clothing changes.

Urinary incontinence is extremely common in nursing homes, where 40% to 60% of patients are reported to have some degree of incontinence (Table 2). In contrast to community-dwelling incontinent persons, most incontinent nursing home patients have several episodes per day of UI, and 50% to 64% also have episodes of fecal incontinence (13,20,21). The high prevalence of fecal incontinence in patients with UI probably relates to common pathophysiologic mechanisms (especially severe neurological disorders such as stroke and end-stage dementia) and to functional causes such as fecal

TABLE 2. *Prevalence of incontinence*

Study[a]	Population sample	Definition of incontinence	Method of data collection	Prevalence (%)			Comments
				Female	Male	Overall	
Studies done in mainly noninstitutionalized populations							
Yarnell and St. Leger (4)	Random sample of elderly (over 65), practices in Wales (N = 388)	Any leakage of urine in the previous 12 months	Personal interview and question- naire given at home to subject, next of kin, or personal attendant	17	11	14	One-third had become continent 6 months after original interview; close to half of severely incontinent expressed reluctance to approach their physician with the problem
Feneley et al. (15)	Persons aged 5 and older from one group practice in Britain (N = 7,000)	Involuntary excretion or leakage of urine in inappropriate places or times at least twice a month, regardless of quantity	Postal questionnaire	All subjects 8 ... Those over age 65 14	3 ... 6	5 ... —	20% of those with urinary incontinence also had fecal incontinence

Study	Population	Definition/Question	Method	Results	Findings
Thomas et al. (17)	Persons aged 5 and older from 12 general practices in Britain (N = 18,084)	Leakage of urine in inappropriate places, at inappropriate times, regardless of quantity	Postal questionnaire; personal interviews conducted with 237 subjects	% with 2 or more episodes per month: All subjects 8 3 6 Those over age 65 11 7 10 % with fewer than 2 episodes per month All subjects 25 9 17 Those over age 65 25 15 21	Fewer than one-third were getting health or social services for the incontinence
Vetter et al. (18)	Elderly (aged 70 and older) from two general practices in Wales (N = 1,280)	"Do you ever wet yourself if you are unable to get to the lavatory as soon as you need to, or when you are asleep at night, or if you cough or sneeze?"	Structured interview	18 7 14	Five percent of the incontinent persons reported episodes daily or more frequently One-third of the incontinent persons used no aids or treatment
Yarnell et al. (19)	Random sample of women aged 18 or older from Wales (N = 1,060)	Loss of urine on the way to the toilet or with cough, laugh, sneeze, etc.	Personal interview by a nurse using a standard questionnaire	Age 18–64 42 65–74 43 75 + 59 All ages 45	Most had infrequent loss of small amounts of urine. Only 3% had to change clothes daily, and 3% felt the incontinence interfered with social or domestic life. Of the latter, only one-half sought medical advice

TABLE 2. (continued)

Study[a]	Population sample	Definition of incontinence	Method of data collection	Prevalence (%)			Comments
				Female	Male	Overall	
Studies done in nursing homes							
US DHEW (14)	15 randomly selected patients in each of 288 nursing homes in Medicare/ Medicaid program (N = 4,320) (total nursing home population, 283,914)	Involuntary loss of urine or feces at least occasionally	Assessment form completed by nursing home staff	—	—	56	6% had an indwelling or external device
Jewett et al. (16)	New geriatric (65 and older) admissions to a long-term care facility in Canada (N = 277)	Involuntary loss of urine that was a social or hygenic problem and that could be objectively demonstrated	Research nurse completed a questionnaire	36	40	38	Another 20% of the 277 admissions had a urinary diversion device. Thirty percent of the subjects could not give an adequate health history
Ouslander et al. (13)	Patients aged 65 and older in 7 U.S. nursing homes (4 proprietary, 3 nonprofit) (N = 842)	Any uncontrolled leakage of urine regardless of amount or frequency	Incontinent patients identified by nurses and verified by interviews with patients and nurses	50	48	50	Of the incontinent patients: 34% had more than one episode per day 28% had an indwelling catheter 10% wore an external catheter continuously

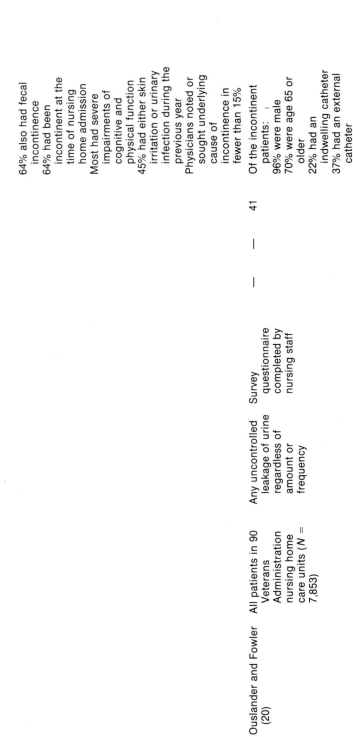

| Ouslander and Fowler (20) | All patients in 90 Veterans Administration nursing home care units (N = 7,853) | Any uncontrolled leakage of urine regardless of amount or frequency | Survey questionnaire completed by nursing staff | — | — | 41 | 64% also had fecal incontinence
64% had been incontinent at the time of nursing home admission
Most had severe impairments of cognitive and physical function
45% had either skin irritation or urinary infection during the previous year
Physicians noted or sought underlying cause of incontinence in fewer than 15%
Of the incontinent patients:
96% were male
70% were age 65 or older
22% had an indwelling catheter
37% had an external catheter (continuous)
only 10% had fewer than one episode per day
55% also had episodes of fecal incontinence |

---

a This table does not include all published reports of the prevalence of incontinence. More recent studies and those that had substantial elderly populations were included.

impaction and the overuse of laxatives. The causes and management of fecal incontinence are beyond the scope of this chapter and are reviewed elsewhere (2,5).

COSTS

Incontinence is a costly condition, in terms of both dollars and adverse effects on patients, families, and caregivers. Skin irritation or breakdown and urinary tract infection, most commonly secondary to the inappropriate use of catheters to manage incontinence, are common medical complications of incontinence.

There are many potential adverse psychosocial effects of UI. Embarrassment because of odor, wetness, and the need for frequent visits to the bathroom can lead to social isolation and predispose to depression. The physical, emotional, and economic burden of caring for incontinent relatives or friends is among the most frequently cited reasons for nursing home admission (1,2,22). Although no studies have carefully documented its precise contribution to the need for nursing home care, UI clearly plays a pivotal role in many decisions to enter the nursing home. One study has documented that most incontinent nursing home patients were incontinent at the time they were admitted (13). In an analysis of stress on caregivers of frail community-dwelling elderly, problems with toilet activities were found to be among the most stressful (23). Thus, research designed to improve the management of UI must include developing strategies to appropriately evaluate and treat the condition before admission in addition to exploring the most cost-effective approaches in the nursing home setting.

Very little research has addressed the economic impact of UI. The entry of several large companies into the incontinence care product line indicates that the potential market in this area is considerable (6). The Surgeon General of the United States estimates that $8 billion per year is spent in this country on the management of UI (24). A few studies have considered the costs of various components of incontinence care in nursing homes such as nursing time, laundry, and supplies (6,25–29). One recent analysis examined the overall costs of incontinence in the nursing home setting (6). With simple formulas to calculate the cost of daily care (first-order costs) and the cost of complications (second-order costs) of managing UI (see Fig. 1), incontinence was calculated to add $3 to $11 to the daily cost of caring for an incontinent nursing home patient depending on the method of management (6). In some states this may represent as much as one-quarter to one-third of the daily reimbursement rate. Interestingly, the daily costs that administrators are concerned with appear lowest when incontinence is managed by indwelling catheterization. When the costs of complications (those costs that are generally borne by third-party payers) are considered, savings in daily costs are greatly reduced. In addition, the cost calculations do not

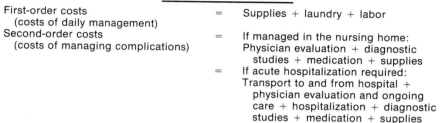

FIG. 1. Calculating the economic impacts of incontinence in the nursing home setting. (From ref. 25, with permission.)

take into account the potential morbidity and mortality associated with indwelling catheterization (30–32).

The potential savings in cost that could result from optimal diagnostic evaluation and treatment of incontinent nursing home patients are unknown. The net economic impact would depend on several factors, including the extent and cost of the diagnostic evaluation and the type and effectiveness of the treatment prescribed (Fig. 1). Although complete cure of UI in a majority of incontinent nursing home patients is probably unlikely even after intensive evaluation and treatment, substantial amelioration of the UI is possible for many (1,2,5,10,22).

Analyses of the cost effectiveness of diagnostic evaluation and treatment of UI in nursing home patients should go beyond monetary considerations. The potential impacts of ameliorating or curing UI on the ability of these patients to interact socially, the emotional status of the patients and their families, and the job satisfaction of nursing home staff should be considered.

DIAGNOSTIC EVALUATION

Despite the potential adverse effects of UI on physical and psychological health, patients and health professionals do not appear to evaluate the condition thoroughly. Studies in Great Britain, where incontinence clinics and incontinence nurses are available, indicate that one-third to one-half of incontinent persons, even those with severe UI, do not seek the help of health professionals (4,17–19). In this country, one study of UI in nursing homes revealed that the condition was infrequently mentioned in physicians' notes and that fewer than 5% of incontinent nursing home patients have any type of diagnostic evaluation (13).

TABLE 3.   *Components of the diagnostic evaluation of urinary incontinence*

All patients
History
Physical examination
Postvoid residual determination
Urinalysis
Urine culture
Selected patients[a]
Urological evaluation
Cystoscopy
Voiding cystourethrography (VCUG)
Urodynamic tests[b]
Cystometrogram (CMG)
Urine flowmetry
Urethral pressure profilometry (UPP)
Sphincter electromyography (EMG)

[a] Patients in whom, after the initial diagnostic evaluation, (a) a treatable condition has not been identified, (b) a condition has been treated, but the incontinence persists, (c) findings indicate the need for urologic evaluation (e.g., urinary retention, hematuria).
[b] The appropriate use of these tests in elderly incontinent patients is controversial (see text).

All patients with incontinence that persists after an acute illness or that is unrelated to an acute condition, a drug effect, or environmental factors should have a thorough diagnostic evaluation. The components of the evaluation of incontinent patients are shown in Table 3. There is considerable controversy over the optimal extent of the diagnostic evaluation for UI, especially with regard to urodynamic tests. Urodynamic testing requires expensive equipment and personnel experienced in the performance and interpretation of the tests (12,33,34). These tests can clearly help to define precisely the underlying pathophysiology of UI and lead to specific treatment recommendations (10,33,34). However, they are expensive, relatively uncomfortable, and invasive (requiring repeated catheterizations), time-consuming, and inconvenient for many elderly persons (often requiring a trip to a hospital and 2 to 3 hr to perform). Lack of data on urodynamic abnormalities and their significance in elderly patients and age-related changes in lower genitourinary function can complicate the interpretation of these tests (35).

Some experts state that most incontinent elderly patients can be diagnosed and treated without urodynamic tests (9). Others indicate that treating UI without urodynamics is like "treating an arrhythmia without an electrocardiogram" (8). Diagnostic algorithms for UI have been described (5,9,10); they have been designed mainly for women and have not been tested prospectively. One was tested retrospectively in 100 elderly women, and the investigators claim that 60% of invasive urodynamic studies could have been avoided if the alogrithm had been used (9).

Although several investigators have begun to address questions about the optimal diagnostic evaluation of UI in the elderly, and some experience with urodynamics and incontinence clinics has been reported (8,9,11,12), insufficient data are available to allow us to draw any conclusions. Virtually no data relevant to these questions in elderly incontinent nursing home patients are available.

TREATMENT

Figure 2 depicts the various treatment options available to manage UI. In general, optimal treatment depends on the identification of the specific causes(s) of the UI. Nonspecific supportive measures are often helpful, especially in the nursing home setting. Table 4 lists the primary and secondary treatment options for the different types of UI. The treatments and evidence for their efficacy are reviewed extensively elsewhere (1,2,5,6,10,22,35–39). The major types of treatment relevant to the elderly incontinent population are briefly discussed below.

Surgery

Surgery is probably the treatment of choice for women with stress UI (39). Newer techniques of bladder neck suspension can be done under spinal anesthesia in less than an hour and require only 2 to 4 days of hospitalization (40). Cure rates of over 90%, even in elderly patients, have been reported in several series (39,41–43).

Surgery is essential in the management of overflow incontinence caused by anatomic obstruction such as prostatic hyperplasia or carcinoma and urethral strictures in men and the relatively unusual occurrence of obstruction in women associated with a large prolapsed cystocele (5,10,39). In addition to persistent UI, patients with overflow UI can develop recurrent urinary tract infections and chronic renal failure unless the obstruction is relieved.

Surgery is also essential for those patients whose incontinence is related to specific pathologic conditions in the lower genitourinary tract such as bladder tumors, stones, and diverticuli. Other surgical procedures for UI, such as bladder denervation, bladder distention under anesthesia, bladder neck transection, and total urinary diversion (ureteroileostomy), are less commonly performed (39,44,45).

Drugs

Several types of drugs can be used to manage incontinence (Table 5). Although a great deal is known about the neuropharmacology of the lower urinary tract (37,38), few carefully designed drug trials for UI have been

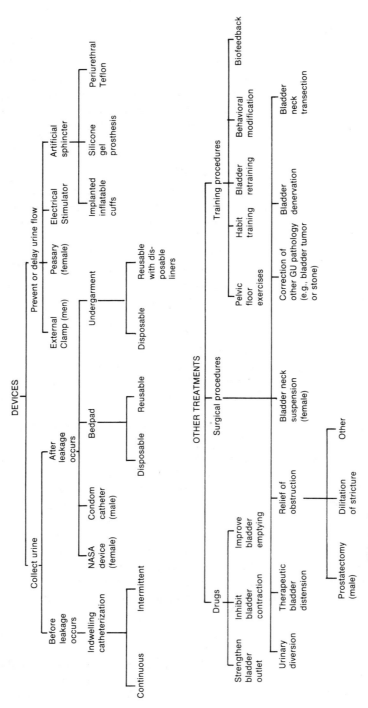

FIG. 2. Treatment options for urinary incontinence. (From ref. 6, with permission.)

TABLE 4. *Treatment options for different types of urinary incontinence*

Type of incontinence	Primary treatment	Other treatments
Acute	Manage acute illness, modify drug regimen, or alter the environment	Bladder retraining Habit training Incontinence undergarments or bedpads
Persistent		
Stress	Surgery	Drugs (α-adrenergic agents) Pelvic (Kegel) exercises Artificial sphincter Electrical stimulation
Urge[a]	Drugs (anticholinergics, bladder relaxants) Training procedures	Bladder deneivation Bladder distention Electrical stimulation
Overflow[b]	Surgery Intermittent catheterization	Continuous catheterization
Functional	Habit training Incontinence undergarments or bedpads	Environmental alterations

[a] Certain types of urge incontinence require other treatments such as surgical removal of a tumor or stone or estrogen treatment for atrophic urethritis.
[b] Cholinergic agents (e.g., bethanechol) are sometimes used but have limited effectiveness and bothersome side effects.

done in the elderly (10,35,46,47). Most studies have involved only small numbers of elderly subjects, have been poorly controlled, and have imprecisely defined the subjects in terms of clinical characteristics, lower genitourinary pathology, and outcome measures (35). In addition to the lack of data on efficacy, drugs used to treat UI in the elderly can have bothersome or potentially dangerous side effects (Table 5) (10,35,48). Thus, despite their effectiveness in properly selected patients, drugs currently available to manage UI must be used carefully in the elderly.

Training Procedures

A wide variety of techniques, often lumped under the term "bladder training," are used to manage UI (Fig. 2). The nosology and effectiveness of these techniques were recently reviewed at a workshop sponsored by the National Institute on Aging (36).

Pelvic floor (or "Kegel") exercises, which involve repetitive contraction of muscles around the vagina and urethra, can be helpful in women with stress UI who are able and willing to perform on an ongoing basis (22,49).

"Bladder retraining" is a term often used by nurses in acute hospitals and nursing homes to describe a heterogeneous group of techniques to manage UI (20,22,36,50–60). In many instances they are not retraining the bladder but training the staff to manage the incontinence. The latter techniques

TABLE 5. *Examples of drugs used to treat incontinence*

Drugs	Type of incontinence	Mechanism of action	Potential adverse reactions
Anticholinergic bladder relaxants Propantheline (Probanthine®) Imipramine (Tofranil®) Flavoxate (Urispas®) Oxybutinin (Ditropan®)	Urge	Inhibit bladder contraction	Dry mouth Constipation Blurry vision Exacerbation of glaucoma Tachycardia Urinary retention
α-Adrenergic agonists Pseudoephedrine (Sudafed®) Phenylpropanolamine (in Ornade®)	Stress	Increase tone in bladder outlet and urethra	Headache Palpitations Hypertension Tachycardia
Cholinergic Bethanechol (Urecholine®)	Overflow	Promotes bladder contraction	Gastrointestinal cramping Diarrhea Bronchoconstriction Bradycardia
Estrogens[a] (intravaginal or oral)	Urge or stress	Diminish inflammation Strengthen periurethral tissues	Uterine cancer Hypertension Cardiovascular complications[a]

[a] See Judd et al. (48) for a detailed discussion of the risks and benefits of estrogen therapy.

are better labeled "scheduled voiding" or "habit training." True bladder retraining is most applicable in patients who have had an acute or subacute insult to bladder function such as overdistention caused by urinary retention, inflammation resulting from the temporary placement of an indwelling catheter, or a stroke, which has disrupted central nervous system control of urination. The procedure involves careful timing of fluids intake, medication, and voiding, complete bladder emptying, techniques designed to inhibit or stimulate voiding, and gradual lengthening (or in some cases of overdistention injury, shortening) of the interval between voidings. The ultimate objective of bladder retraining is to restore a normal pattern of voiding. In order for bladder retraining to succeed, patients must have adequate mental and physical functioning.

Two major features distinguish scheduled voiding and habit-training procedures from bladder retraining. The objective of scheduled voiding and habit-training procedures is to keep the patient dry rather than to restore a completely normal pattern of voiding, and these procedures can be successful even in patients with substantial impairment of cognitive and physical functioning. Similar to bladder retraining, habit training involves the timing of voiding, fluids, and medications. Many nursing homes use a fixed interval (usually every 2 hr during the day), whereas others modify the voiding interval based on the patient's response (20).

Behavior modification and biofeedback have been used infrequently in the management of UI. The latter technique requires specialized equipment and trained personnel. It has been reported to be effective for both stress and urge UI as well as fecal incontinence in small numbers of elderly patients (57,59).

Although several training procedures have been reported to be effective, none has been rigorously tested in elderly incontinent nursing home patients (20,22,36).

Mechanical Devices

Several devices have been developed to manage UI, ranging from the relatively unsophisticated pessary and external penile clamp to highly technologic devices such as the artificial sphincter and the intravaginal electric stimulator (61–64).

Artificial sphincters consist of a soft cuff, which is surgically implanted to surround the bladder neck in women or the urethra in men. A balloon reservoir regulates the pressure in the cuff, and the patient or a caregiver can deflate the cuff by pressing a bulb implanted under the skin in order to allow urine to pass. These devices are generally implanted in women whose stress incontinence persists despite previous surgical and drug treatment, in men with surgical or traumatic damage to the urethral sphincter mechanism, and in persons with severe neurological disorders (e.g., myelomeningocele). Several series have shown these devices to be successful in 60% to 90% of cases (6).

Intravaginal electrical stimulation (IVS) is a newer technique employing pessary-like devices with electrodes, which are inserted into the vagina. Battery packs are worn around the waist or in the bra, and electrical impulses are discharged in a regular intermittent pattern (64). Extensive studies in animals have shown that these devices work by stimulating nerve endings rather than by directly causing muscle contraction (65). Higher-frequency impulses (e.g., 40 Hz) cause contraction of muscles around the bladder outlet and urethra and can be used for stress UI. Lower frequency (e.g., 10 Hz) stimulation causes reflex bladder relaxation and can be used for urge UI (66). Very few studies of the use of these devices in humans have been reported, and none has been adequately controlled (6).

Catheters

Catheters are probably overused in the management of UI (67,68). Between 10% and 30% of incontinent elderly patients in nursing homes are managed by continuous indwelling catheterization (13,20). Given the substantial risks and costs associated with the use of indwelling catheters (21,25,30,31,32,69), they should be used only when absolutely necessary. Indwelling catheters can be justified for a brief period during an acute illness when accurate measurement of urine output is critical to overall management, when skin breakdown or surgical wounds are not healing because of frequent contamination with urine, and when urinary retention severe enough to cause recurrent infections and/or impairment of renal function cannot be corrected surgically or by other means.

Intermittent catheterization has been shown to be safer than continuous catheterization in young patients with urinary retention resulting from neurological disorders (such as paraplegia) (70). It requires the patient and/or caregiver to be able to perform the technique regularly. In addition, no studies have documented its efficacy in elderly patients—either community-dwelling ones or those in nursing homes.

External catheters (condom catheters) are commonly used to manage UI in elderly males. Thirty-seven percent (37%) of incontinent males in Veterans Administration nursing homes wear external catheters continuously (20). Although they may be safer than indwelling catheters, these devices commonly require frequent changing, can cause severe skin irritation, may be associated with an increased risk of UTI, and may promote dependency.

Proper techniques can reduce the risk resulting from the use of catheters (31,32,71). Several studies have shown that overly intensive perineal care, bladder irrigations, and prophylactic antimicrobials are ineffective in preventing catheter-related UTIs and may in fact increase the risk or predispose to infection with resistant organisms (72,73). Recent studies involving the installation of small amounts of antiseptic solutions into catheter drainage bags have shown promise in preventing infections but have not been carried out in incontinent nursing home patients with long-term indwelling catheters (74,75).

Nonspecific, Supportive Treatments

A wide variety of supportive measures can be useful as adjuncts to other more specific forms of treatment; they are especially relevant for the management of UI in the nursing home setting. These measures include appropriate attitude and response toward the incontinent patient, the timely use of toilet substitutes such as urinals, bedpans, and portable commodes, environmental alterations such as making bathrooms accessible and safe with carefully placed railing, good skin care, and specially designed incontinence undergarments and bed pads.

Several types of incontinence undergarments have been developed and are becoming increasingly available in the United States (1,6,22,76,77). Some are completely disposable, some are completely launderable, and others are launderable briefs into which a highly absorbent disposable pad is

TABLE 6. *Examples of important research directions in the nursing home setting*

Precise definition of the causes of incontinence
Development of cost-effective diagnostic strategies
Design and testing of outcome measures for treatment trials
Treatment studies
   Effectiveness: Surgery, drugs, training procedures
   Relative efficacy
      Surgical vs. drug treatment of stress UI
      Drug treatment vs. habit training for urge UI
   Improved treatment techniques
      Prevention of catheter-induced infections
      Testing of intravaginal electrical stimulators
   Cost effectiveness
      Incontinence undergarments vs. habit training
Techniques to improve nursing home staff knowledge and attitudes on incontinence

inserted. Many supervisory nurses in nursing homes are reluctant to use these products because their high absorbency makes the patients appear dry, and nurses' aides then do not change the patients' garments frequently enough. In addition, the undergarments may foster dependency by allowing patients to wet themselves rather than attempt to succeed at a habit-training regimen. The undergarments should not be considered a "simple solution" to UI. Patients should be evaluated and specific treatment prescribed whenever possible. Although the manufacturers claim that these products are cost effective in the nursing home setting by diminishing labor and laundry costs, few carefully designed studies have been published that support this assertion (26–28,78,79).

PROMISING DIRECTIONS FOR RESEARCH AND EDUCATION

There is clearly a need for innovative research and educational efforts designed to improve the management of incontinence. Most health professionals have little understanding of the pathophysiology, diagnostic evaluation, and treatment of incontinence. This may explain in part the infrequent mention of incontinence or any specific diagnostic evaluation for the condition in physicians' notes in nursing home records (13). More than 90% of nursing supervisors in 90 Veterans Administration nursing homes have indicated that in-service educational programs and written or audiovisual educational materials would be helpful (20).

Despite the vast literature on incontinence reviewed above, there is a dearth of well-designed research on this condition in the nursing home setting. Table 6 lists several examples of important areas for research. Studies that carefully characterize the incontinent nursing home population are critical for developing further research questions and improved care. Most incontinent nursing home patients have severe impairments in other functional abilities such as mobility or cognitive function (2,3,13). Since UI associated with these impairments requires quite different therapeutic approaches than does UI primarily related to lower genitourinary disorders, studies designed to determine the role of functional disability versus lower genitourinary dysfunction in the pathogenesis of UI would be of value.

Studies designed to determine the most practical and cost-effective diagnostic evaluation strategies are critical to the improvement in care of UI in the nursing home setting. Because urodynamic testing is relatively expensive and invasive and requires special equipment and trained personnel, determining the most efficient use of these procedures in the nursing home setting would be especially valuable.

Well-designed, properly controlled treatment trials are probably the most important directions for research. Subject populations must be carefully defined and treatment groups stratified along characteristics that are relevant to incontinence and its management such as specific lower genitourinary pathologies, mental and functional status, severity of UI, and concomitant medical conditions and medications. Treatment studies should address not only effectiveness but the relative efficacy of different treatments for the same type of UI, the improvement of existing treatments and testing of new ones, and the relative cost effectiveness of various treatment options (Table 6). Severity of the UI, its complications and therapy, changes in cognitive, functional, and psychosocial status of patients, stress of nursing home personnel, and economic costs are all important outcomes to consider in these treatment trials.

A special consideration in research on UI in the nursing home setting is the measurement of changes in severity of UI. As in any other clinical research, reliable and valid measurement tools must be developed. Many "incontinence charts" and "bladder records" have been described (1,2,5,22,50), but none has been tested for practicality and reliability for research in a nursing home setting. The low educational level, non-English-speaking status, and high turnover rate of a substantial proportion of the nurses' aides who would be completing the records makes the design and testing of these tools critical. Pilot studies being carried out at UCLA in conjunction with Beverly Enterprises are addressing this issue by testing an "incontinence monitoring record." The testing of this type of tool will not only be of value for research but will enable licensed nurses and nurses' aides to become more involved and knowledgeable in the management of UI, which, in turn, may lead to substantial improvements in care.

Finally, research on effective strategies to improve knowledge about and attitudes toward UI and its management are needed. These research and educational efforts should not be directed only at licensed nurses, administrators, and physicians who work in nursing homes; they must also be directed at improving the knowledge and attitudes of nurses' aides who are

TABLE 7. *Advantages and limitations of the nursing home setting for studies on UI*

Advantages	Limitations
Most nursing home staff indicate interest in learning more about incontinence and techniques to improve its management	Most nursing homes have not had experience with teaching and research programs
Large and "captured" pool of incontinent patients	Nursing home administrators may view education and research as add-on costs to already constrained budgets
Opportunity to institute uniform: environmental manipulations timing of administration of fluids and medications toileting schedules	Logistical considerations in evaluating incontinent patients, e.g. Do expensive equipment and trained personnel come to the nursing home, or are frail incontinent patients transported to the medical center?
Availability of nursing personnel to monitor treatments	Many patients may not be competent to sign informed consent or refuse to participate, thus limiting sample size
Nursing home can facilitate the logistics of: assessment of outcomes data collection	Nursing home staff may view research on improved incontinence management as added work with few tangible benefits
	Carryover ("Hawthorne") effects may bias results in controlled trials, especially those involving training procedures
	Pressure from companies marketing incontinence care products may interfere with the design and implementation of controlled studies

responsible for changing clothes and beds, caring for patients, and emptying urinals, bedpans, and catheter bags.

ADVANTAGES AND LIMITATIONS OF THE NURSING HOME SETTING

The nursing home is in many ways a hybrid setting. Some nursing homes are like small hospitals, some resemble large convalescent homes, and many are somewhere in between (80). Most are run for profit, although most nursing home care is financed by state welfare programs. They offer several unique advantages and limitations for the design and implementation of research and teaching programs. Table 7 lists some of the key advantages and limitations for research on UI in a nursing home setting.

Although few nursing homes have had active research and education programs, many are interested in both. Most nursing home personnel express an interest in educational and research efforts designed to improve the management of UI (20). Despite the interest, however, economic, logistical, cognitive, and attitudinal considerations may limit these efforts.

Nursing staff may have a difficult time perceiving the potential impact of research on UI and may consider these efforts added work with little tangible benefit. Administrators may perceive research and teaching as potential add-on costs to already constrained budgets.

Researchers should be sensitive to the costs of staff involvement in scheduling and preparing patients for research appointments as well as to the costs of minor supplies that may be used during the study. The numerous companies now marketing incontinence care products may also influence the NH administrator's assessment of the potential costs and benefits of research. Logistical considerations may pose difficult problems, especially when urodynamic testing is involved. Unless equipment is purchased for the nursing home, patients must be transported to a medical center. This could involve considerable effort on the part of nursing home staff and raises questions about who should be responsible for arranging and paying for such transportation. Because of impairments of cognitive function, multiple medical problems and medications, depression, and cultural beliefs and attitudes, many patients may be unable or unwilling to sign informed consent and/or to participate in the study. This may create difficulties in obtaining adequate sample sizes and thereby bias study results.

Despite these limitations, nursing homes provide several potential advantages for the implementation of research and teaching programs. They provide a large conveniently gathered pool of subjects for incontinence research. Additionally, they could institute standard protocols relevant to incontinence research such as appropriate timing of medications, fluids, and toilet habits, and innovative environmental alterations. The constant availability of nursing personnel provides an opportunity to insure compliance with assessment and treatment protocols and monitor outcomes of treatment, especially when compared with a protocol carried out in ambulatory clinic setting with community-dwelling elderly. The relatively small size of the nursing home compared to an acute-care hospital may provide substantial advantages for data collection. Advances in computer technology might make it possible to install "user-friendly" terminals in nursing homes into which all levels of personnel could input research data for storage and analysis.

In addition to these potential limitations and advantages, several critical questions arise regarding the transfer of research findings on incontinence and its management carried out in a TNH setting into the over 18,000 nonteaching facilities in this country. Will strategies of diagnostic evaluation and management shown to be effective in a TNH be effective in the standard nursing home setting? Will staff in the nonteaching nursing home be willing and able to implement these strategies? Will owners of proprietary nursing homes consider these strategies cost effective? Consideration of these types of questions is essential in order to conduct teaching and research programs that will ultimately improve the health and well-being of the increasing numbers of elderly persons in our nation's nursing homes.

CONCLUSIONS

Incontinence is one of the most prevalent, disruptive, and costly conditions that affects nursing home patients and the staff that care for them. Very few well-designed research and teaching efforts have been carried out on this condition in the nursing home setting. Thus, incontinence offers a good model for the development of research and teaching activities designed to improve nursing home care. Although the nursing home setting has several potential limitations that could affect such efforts, it offers several advantages that could greatly facilitate research and teaching. The impact of research and teaching carried out in TNHs on the health and well-being of the resident population in general will depend on our ability to effectively transfer research findings and successful educational programs into the over 18,000 nonteaching nursing homes in this country.

ACKNOWLEDGMENT

This work was supported by an Academic Award from the National Institute on Aging, Beverly Enterprises, the Geriatric Research Education and Clinical Center at the VA Medical Center, Sepulveda, CA, and the VA Office of Academic Affairs.

REFERENCES

1. Willington FL (ed): *Incontinence in the Elderly*. San Francisco, Academic Press, 1976.
2. Brocklehurst JC: The genitourinary system, in Brocklehurst JC (ed): *Textbook of Geriatric Medicine and Gerontology*. New York, Churchill Livingstone, 1978, pp 291–337.
3. Isaacs B, Walkey FA: A survey of incontinence in the elderly. *Gerontol Clin* 1964;6:367.
4. Yarnell JWG, Stilegar A: The prevalence, severity and factors associated with urinary incontinence in a random sample of the elderly. *Age Ageing* 1979;8:81.
5. Kane RL, Ouslander JG, Abrass IB: *Essentials of Clinical Geriatrics*. New York, McGraw-Hill, 1984, pp 107–135.
6. Ouslander JG, Kane RL, Vollmer S, et al: *Medical Devices for Urinary Incontinence: A Case Study*. Prepared for the Office of Technology Assessment, Washington, 1983.
7. Brocklehurst JC, Dillane JB: Studies of the female bladder in old age II. Cystometrograms in 100 incontinent women. *Gerontol Clin* 1966;8:306–319.
8. Castleden CM, Duffin HM, Aswer MJ: Clinical and urodynamic studies in 100 elderly incontinent patients. *Br Med J* 1981;282:1103–1105.
9. Hilton P, Stanton SL: Algorithmic method for assessing urinary incontinence in elderly women. *Br Med J* 1981;282:940–942.
10. Williams ME, Panill FC: Urinary incontinence in the elderly. *Ann Intern Med* 1982;97:895–907.
11. Overstall PW, Rounce K, Palmer JH: Experience with an incontinence clinic. *J Am Geriatr Soc* 1980;28:535.
12. Eastwood HDH: Urodynamic studies in the management of urinary incontinence in the elderly. *Age Ageing* 1979;8:41.
13. Ouslander JG, Kane RL, Abrass IB: Urinary incontinence in elderly nursing home patients. *JAMA* 1982;248:1194–1198.
14. US DHEW, PHS, Office of Nursing Home Affairs: *Long-Term Care Facility Improvement Study* (Publ # PHS 588–459). Washington, Government Printing Office, 1975.

15. Feneley RCL, Shepherd AM, Powell PH, et al: Urinary incontinence: Prevalence and needs. *Br J Urol* 1974;51:493–496.
16. Jewett MAS, Fernie GR, Holliday PJ, et al: Urinary dysfunction in a geriatric long-term care population: Prevalence and patterns. *J Am Geriatr Soc* 1981;29:211–214.
17. Thomas TM, Plymat FR, Blannin J, et al: Prevalence of urinary incontinence. *Br Med J* 1980;281:1243–1245.
18. Vetter NJ, Jones DA, Victor CR: Urinary incontinence in the elderly at home. *Lancet* 1981;2:1275–1277.
19. Yarnell JWG, Voyle GJ, Richards CJ, et al: The prevalence and severity of urinary incontinence in women. *J Epidemiol Commun Health* 1981;35:71–74.
20. Ouslander JG, Fowler E: Incontinence in VA nursing home care units: Epidemiology and management. *Gerontologist* 1983;23(Special Issue):257.
21. Garibaldi RA, Brodine S, Matsumiya S: Infections among patients in nursing homes—policies, prevalence, and problems. *N Engl J Med* 1981;305:731–735.
22. Wells TJ, Brink CA: Urinary incontinence: Assessment and management, in Burnside IM (ed): *Nursing and the Aged*. New York, McGraw-Hill, 1981, pp 519–548.
23. Noelker LS. Incontinence in aged cared for by family [Abstract]. *Gerontologist* 1983;23:258.
24. Brazda JF: Washington report. *The Nation's Health* March, 1983. p 3.
25. Ouslander JG, Kane RL. The costs of urinary incontinence in nursing homes. *Med Care* 1984;22:69–79.
26. Smith B: A dry bed—and save on costs. *Nurs Mirror* 1979;149:26–29.
27. Williams TF, Foerster JE, Proctor JK, et al: A new double-layered launderable bed sheet for patients with urinary incontinence. *J Am Gerontol Soc* 1981;29:520–524.
28. Grant R: Washable pads or disposable diapers? *J Geriatr Nurs* July–August, 1982, p 248.
29. Weissert WG: Long-term care: Current policy and directions for the 80s. Presented at the 1981 White House Conference on Aging, Long-Term Care Session, Washington, DC, 1981.
30. Garibaldi RA, Burke JP, Dickman ML, et al: Factors predisposing to bacteriuria during indwelling urethral catheterization. *N. Engl J Med* 1974;291:215–219.
31. Stamm WE: Guidelines for prevention of catheter associated urinary tract infections. *Ann Intern Med* 1975;82:386–390.
32. Warren JW. Muncie HL, Berquist EJ, et al: Sequelae and management of urinary infection in the patient requiring chronic catheterization. *J Urol* 1981;125:1–7.
33. Abrams P, Fenely R, Torrens M: *Urodynamics*. New York, Springer-Verlag, 1983.
34. Blaivas JG: Urodynamic testing, in Raz S (ed): *Female Urology*. Philadelphia, WB Saunders, 1983, pp 79–103.
35. Ouslander JG: Lower urinary tract disorders in the elderly female, in Raz S (ed): *Female Urology*. Philadelphia, WB Saunders, 1983, pp 308–325.
36. Hadley E: Bladder training and related therapies. Prepared for the National Institute on Aging's Workshop on Bladder Training, Washington, DC, April, 1983.
37. Williams ME: A critical evaluation of the assessment technology for urinary continence in older persons. *J Am Geriatr Soc* 1983;31:657–664.
38. Raz S: Pharmacologic treatment of lower urinary tract dysfunction. *Urol Clin North Am* 1978;5:323–334.
39. Raz S: *Female Urology*. Philadelphia, WB Saunders, 1983.
40. Raz S: Modified bladder neck suspension for female stress incontinence. *Urology* 1981;17:82–85.
41. McDuffie RW, Litin RB, Blundon KE: Urethrovesical suspension (Marshall–Marchetti–Krantz)—experience with 204 cases. *Am J Surg* 1981;141:297–298.
42. Stanton SL, Cardozo LD: Results of the colosuspension operation for incontinence and prolapse. *Br J Obstet Gynaecol* 1979;86:693–697.
43. Stanton SL, Cardozo LD: Surgical treatment of incontinence in elderly women. *Surg Gynecol Obstet* 1980;150:555–557.
44. Dunn M, Smith JC, Ardan GM: Prolonged bladder distention as treatment of urge incontinence of urine. *Br J Urol* 1974;46:645–652.
45. Pengelly AW: Effect of prolonged bladder distention on detrusor function. *Urol Clin North Am* 1979;6:279–281.

46. Castleden CM, George CF, Renwick AG, et al: Imipramine—a possible alternative to current therapy for urinary incontinence in the elderly. *J Urol* 1981;125:318–320.

47. Castleden CM, Duffin M, Briggs RS, et al: Clinical and urodynamic effects of ephedrine in elderly incontinent patients. *J Urol* 1982;128:1250–1252.

48. Judd HL, Clearly RE, Creasman WI, et al: Estrogen replacement therapy. *Obstet Gynecol* 1981;58:267–275.

49. Kegel AH: Progressive resistence exercise in the functional restoration of the perineal muscles. Am J Obstet Gynecol 1948;56:238–248.

50. Clay EC: Incontinence of urine: A regime for retaining. *Nurs Mirror* 1978;146:23–24.

51. Fantl JA, Hunt WG, Dunn LJ: Detrusor instability syndrome: The use of bladder retraining drills with and without anticholinergics. *Am J Obstet Gynecol* 1981;140:885–890.

52. Frewen WA: A reassessment of bladder training in detrusor dysfunction in the female. *Br J Urol* 1982;54:372–373.

53. Jarvis GJ: A controlled trial of bladder drill and drug therapy in the management of detrusor instability. *Br J Urol* 1981;53:565–566.

54. Jarvis GJ, Millar DR: Controlled trial of bladder drill for detrusor instability. *Br Med J* 1980;281:1322–1323.

55. Mahady IW, Begg BM: Long-term symptomatic and cystometric cure of the urge incontinence symdrome using a technique of bladder reeducation. *Br J Obstet Gynecol* 1981;88:1038–1043.

56. Pengelly AW, Booth CM: A prospective trial of bladder training as treatment for detrusor instability. *Br J Urol* 1980;52:463–466.

57. Pollock DD, Liberman RP: Behavior therapy of incontinence in demented patients. *Gerontology* 1974;14:488–491.

58. Svigas JM, Mathews DC: Assessment and treatment of female urinary incontinence by cystometrogram and bladder retraining programs. *Obstet Gynecol* 1971;50:9–12.

59. Engle BT: *Using Biofeedback with the Elderly* (National Institute on Aging Science Writer's Seminar Series NIH # 79-1404). Washington, DC, National Institute on Aging, 1979.

60. Sogbein SK, Awad SA: Behavioral treatment of incontinence in geriatric patients. *Can Med Assoc J* 1982;127:638.

61. Furlow WL: Artificial sphincter, in Stanton SL, Tanagho EA (eds): *Surgery of the Female Incontinent.* New York, Springer-Verlag, 1980, 119–134.

62. Hager T: New surgical techniques ease incontinence. *JAMA* 1983;249:3284–3287.

63. Kaufman JJ: The silicone-gel prosthesis for treatment of male urinary incontinence. *Urol Clin North Am* 1978;5:393–404.

64. Suhel P, Kralj B: Treatment of urinary incontinence using functional electrical stimulation, in Raz S (ed): *Female Urology.* Philadelphia, WB Saunders, 1983, pp 189–228.

65. Fall M, Erlandson BE, Carlsson CA, et al: The effect of intravaginal electrical stimulation on the feline urethra and urinary bladder: Neuronal mechanisms. *Scand J Urol Nephrol* 1977;44(Suppl):19–30.

66. Erlandson BE, Fall M, Carlsson CA: The effect of intravaginal electrical stimulation on the feline urethral and urinary bladder electrical parameters. *Scand J Urol Nephrol* 1977;44(Suppl):5–18.

67. Kunin CM: The incontinent patient and the catheter. *J Am Geriatr Soc* 1983;31:259–260.

68. Maron KR, Fillit H, Peskowitz M, et al: The nonuse of urethral catheterization in the management of urinary incontinence in the teaching nursing home. *J Am Geriatr Soc* 1983;31:278–281.

69. Priefer BA, Duthie EH, Gambert SR: Frequency of urinary tract infection: Study in hospital based, skilled nursing home. *Urology* 1982;20:141–142.

70. Lapides J, Diokno AC: Clean, intermittent self-catheterization, in Raz S (ed): *Female Urology.* Philadelphia, WB Saunders, 1983. pp 344–348.

71. Wong ES: *Guidelines for Prevention of Catheter-Associated Urinary Tract Infections.* Philadelphia, WB Saunders, 1974.

72. Burke JP, Garibaldi RA, Britt MR, et al: Prevention of catheter associated urinary tract infections: Efficacy of daily meatal care regimens. *Am J Med* 1981;70:655–658.

73. Warren JW, Platt R, Thomas RJ, et al: Antibiotic irrigation and catheter-associated urinary tract infections. *N Engl J Med* 1978;299:570–573.

74. Maizels M, Schaeffer AJ: Decreased incidence of bacteriuria associated with periodic installations of hydrogen peroxide into the urethral catheter drainage bag. *J Urol* 1980;123:841–845.

75. Southhampton Infection Control Team: Evaluation of aseptic techniques and chlorhexidine on the rate of catheter-associated urinary tract infection. *Lancet* 1982;2:89–91.
76. Beber C: Freedom for the incontinent. *Am J Nurs* 1980;80:483–484.
77. Broughten N: The Kylie. *Nurs Times* 1979;75:1140–1141.
78. Thomas S. Hubbard JU: A lab evaluation of incontinence underpads. *Nurs Times* 1979;75:1136–1139.
79. Mendelson HS, Ouslander JG: Effectiveness of a specially designed undergarment for urinary incontinence [Abstract]. *Gerontologist* 1983;23(Special Issue):257.
80. Kane RL, Kane RA: Care of the aged: Old problems in need of new solutions. *Science* 1978;200:913.

The Teaching Nursing Home, edited by Edward
L. Schneider et al. © 1985 The Beverly
Foundation. Raven Press, New York.

Drug Therapy in the Teaching Nursing Home

Marcus M. Reidenberg, Rosanne M. Leipzig, Harriet
Goodman, Geri Gray, and Henry Erle

*Departments of Pharmacology and Medicine, Cornell University Medical College and The
Supportive Care Service of The New York Hospital, New York, New York 10021*

Patients in a nursing home tend to be elderly and to receive multiple drugs for multiple conditions. The results of the National Nursing Home Survey emphasize the aging of the nursing home population and the increasing burden of multiple medical diseases in this group (1). Eighty-eight percent of patients in nursing homes in the New Haven, Connecticut area in 1966 were receiving regularly scheduled medications in addition to those prescribed to be taken as needed (2). Eighteen percent were receiving five or more different medications regularly (2). Fifty-eight percent of patients in skilled nursing homes were reported by Lamy to be taking three to seven different prescribed medications regularly, and 57% were taking five or more different drugs (3). These surveys indicate that the therapeutic situation for many patients in nursing homes is very complex and can lead to inappropriate responses to drugs.

Examples of some of these drug effects illustrate the complexity of the therapeutic situation. The research used to define the therapeutic and toxic concentrations of digoxin in serum focused on cardiac toxicity. The adverse drug effects on the central nervous system (anorexia, nausea, vomiting, headache, fatigue, malaise, disorientation, confusion, and even delirium) were not really considered in much of this research. There is some clinical experience that the elderly are sensitive to the central nervous system (CNS) effects of digitalis and that these effects can occur with digoxin levels within the "therapeutic" range. It can be difficult to tell the extent to which digitalis effects on the CNS contribute to the confusion, malaise, or disorientation of an elderly person, and one can be misled by the measurement of a glycoside level that is below the "toxic" range.

There is now good evidence that very large doses of scopolamine can impair recent memory in healthy young subjects because of the drug's central anticholinergic action. The elderly may be more sensitive to the recent memory impairment effects of centrally acting anticholinergic drugs. Patients with Alzheimer's disease may be particularly sensitive to the impairment of what little cognitive performance capacity they have left. Yet many of the drugs we give the elderly have central anticholinergic activity. These include the antidepressants and the antihistamines (even when used as bedtime hypnotics and not for their antihistaminic effects) as well as drugs given for their anticholinergic effect. One wonders if drugs with central anticholinergic activity contribute to the impairment of cognitive performance in some of the elderly who are receiving them.

Hearing can be impaired by many drugs including aspirin, the nonsteroidal antiinflammatory drugs, the potent loop diuretics, aminoglycoside antibiotics, and cisplatin. These pharmacologic effects on hearing may interact with the presbycusis of the elderly to further impair their perception of speech. This is another problem for study and another example of the complexity of the medical situation in the elderly.

In addition to the complexity of the medical situation, much of the information about the actions of drugs, and particularly the dose–response relationships, may not be applicable to the majority of patients in nursing homes. Most of the information about the actions of drugs is obtained in clinical research and clinical trials in patients who are much younger than those in nursing homes. Yet aging is an important biological variable influencing dose–response relationships. Aging can change aspects of drug absorption, distribution, metabolism, and excretion and in this way modify the amount of drug that reaches its site of action for any given dose. Aging can also alter the sensitivity of the cells of the body so that the intensity of effect produced is changed for any given amount of drug that reaches its site of action. Clearly, the effects of aging on dose response must be known if information obtained in young and middle-aged people is to be utilized to treat the elderly.

Much has been learned about how aging affects drug absorption, distribution, metabolism, and excretion (4–7). Absorption of most drugs is not affected by aging, since they are absorbed by passive diffusion. Drugs absorbed actively, such as iron or calcium, have their absorption slowed in the elderly. Drug distribution is also not affected, in general, if allowance is made for the smaller body size of the elderly compared to the young. Drug metabolism is slowed in the elderly, with the average older person metabolizing drugs at one-half to two-thirds the rate of the average young and middle-aged adult. Some drugs, including the barbiturates, can cause an increase in the amount of drug-metabolizing enzymes in the liver and thereby increase the rate of metabolism of drugs. This effect is named "enzyme induction." The elderly seem to have less induction of drug-metabolizing enzymes when given inducing drugs than do younger people (8,9).

Overall kidney function declines with aging (10,11). This leads to a marked decline in the excretion of drugs as people age. An example of this is the decline in the renal clearance of cimetidine as a function of age (Fig. 1)

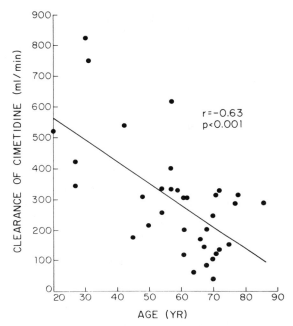

FIG. 1. Effect of age on renal clearance of cimetidine. Clearance of cimetidine (ml/min) = 709 − 7.09 age in years. *r* = −0.63; *p* < 0.001. (From ref. 12, with permission.)

(12). This decline in cimetidine excretion rate leads to accumulation of this drug in the elderly and is one of the reasons why the elderly are predisposed to the development of delirium from this drug. Appropriate dosage reduction of excreted drugs is necessary to compensate for this decline in renal function with aging. Renal function in the elderly can best be estimated by the method of Cockcroft and Gault (11). For men:

$$\text{Creatinine clearance (ml/min)} = \frac{(140 - \text{age in years}) \times \text{weight in kg}}{72 \times \text{serum creatinine in mg/dl}}$$

For women, this result is to be multiplied by 0.85.

Some drugs excreted by the kidney that require individualization of dosage based on glomerular filtration rate are acyclovir, amikacin, cimetidine, clycloserine, digoxin, ethambutol, 5-fluorocytosine, gentamicin, lithium, methotrexate, procainamide, radiographic contrast media, streptomycin, sulfonamides, tobramycin, trimethoprim–sulfamethoxazole, and vancomycin.

Although enough is known to make these generalizations about drug disposition in the elderly, many important details are missing. A major omission is data on a large enough sample of people over the age of 81 to be able to permit generalizable conclusions to be drawn. Most drug disposition studies appear to use age 65 as the beginning of "the elderly" and include few if any patients over 81 years of age. Yet half the people in nursing homes in the United States in 1977 were over 81 (1). Whether the changes in drug disposition observed as people age from their 30s into their 70s can be simply extrapolated into the 80s and 90s is not known and must be learned for rational drug dosage decisions to be made for the nursing home population.

Studies of drug disposition are easier to do than studies of drug sensitivity. Drug disposition can be studied by measuring drug concentrations in plasma and urine at various times after a dose of the drug. Studies of drug sensitivity require a measure of intensity of drug effect as well. This can be difficult to do in a clinically useful way. Studies have found that the elderly are sensitive to benzodiazepines and that this sensitivity results from a more sensitive central nervous system and not from slowed metabolism of the drug (13,14). Kaiko has observed that elderly people have a longer duration of pain relief than younger people after an injection of morphine for post-operative pain. He also observed a marked difference in effect of 8-mg doses compared to 16-mg doses in 40- to 60-year-olds and no difference in effect (pain relief) between these two doses in 70- to 89-year-olds (15). This difference in dose–response relationships must be the result of more than an age-related change in drug disposition, since what was observed was a change in the relationship between two different doses rather than simply a parallel change in intensity of effect of both doses as a function of age. Meyer et al. (16) observed a greater intensity of antiemetic effect of metoclopramide given to block cisplatin-induced emesis in people over 65 than that observed in younger patients at doses that produced identical drug levels in serum of both groups of patients.

Drug research relevant to patients in nursing homes will have to be done on patients in nursing homes. This cannot be accomplished in hospitalized patients, since many of the problems in need of study require repeated observations over a period of time when most aspects of a patient's condition and care are stable. This period of general stability is missing during acute-care hospitalizations. Thus, only limited types of research relevant to the problems of patients in nursing homes can be carried on outside of nursing homes.

One of the major issues to be faced in doing relevant research in this patient population is to identify, in operationally meaningful terms, the drug effects that are really desired and those that are undesired. Then one must develop acceptable ways to measure the intensity of these effects. Symptom control for patients with advanced cancer on the Supportive Care Service at The New York Hospital is presented as an example of how to develop practical ways to measure the intensity of important drug effects. The focus of this research has been on the problems related to drug therapy for the control of pain and, particularly, to the adverse effects of the drugs used.

Emphasis was placed on assessing the patient's intensity of pain, cognitive performance, psychomotor function, and mood to see how these functions are altered by treatment.

In a modification of the method of Kremer, Atkinson, and Ignelzi (17), the patient is asked to describe the intensity of pain at the primary pain site as being none, mild, moderate, severe, or the worst possible. Because cancer pain intensity varies with activity, this description of pain intensity is done for the patient lying still in bed, moving in bed, and, when relevant, when weight bearing and when walking. This five-point intensity scale at four levels of physical activity is a successful approach to measure pain intensity in these patients at a particular time. Treating cancer pain with narcotic drugs reduces the level of pain intensity on this scale.

Three different tests of cognitive performance were used to evaluate mental status (18–20). These were found to be either too long or too simple for our clinical needs. For these reasons, the individual questions were analyzed and three selected that seemed to have discriminatory power in our patient population. The first is registration, the ability to name three objects such as a pen or a watch displayed by the interviewer. Most patients could name these correctly, but an occasional patient could not. The second is attention, the ability to spell a five-letter word such as "world" backwards. Twenty-one of the initial patients could do this; nine could not. The third is recall, for which the patient repeated the names of the three objects named earlier. For the first object, 24 named it correctly, and seven did not. For the second object, 20 named it correctly, and 11 did not. For the third object, 17 named it correctly, and 14 did not in preliminary testing. Since there are three objects to name, five letters in the word spelled backward, and three objects to recall, one can achieve a maximum of 11 points on this test. The distribution of scores for the 10 patients assessed most recently was:

Test scores:	11	10	9	5
No. of patients:	4	2	3	1

Thus, this test appears to readily discriminate among degrees of cognitive performance impairment in these patients. The test cannot discriminate between impaired mental status and depression as the cause of the impaired cognitive performance.

Three out of 39 patients treated during the past 8 months had marked cognitive performance impairment detected by this assessment method but not recognized clinically prior to formal assessment. Two of these patients subsequently had brain metastases detected, and the third had lung cancer but no physical signs of brain metastases prior to death. In these cases, the narcotic analgesics were initially blamed for the impaired mental state even though the doses were not excessive. The brain metastases were likely to be either the primary cause of the delirium or a factor that increased the brain sensitivity to delirium induction by the narcotic for two of the patients,

TABLE 1. *Mood assessment scale for interview*

Engagement (distinguishes how socially engaging/cheerful vs aloof, down, or withdrawn one finds the patient)
   1 = Very withdrawn, little or no eye contact, dwelling on death and/or suffering, frequent crying
   2 = Little social engagement, does not initiate conversation but responds to interview; (non)verbally sad or depressed
   3 = Moderate social engagement but some sad or depressive statements; may occasionally withdraw
   4 = Appears spontaneous; initiates interactions during interview; may inject humorous comments

Irritability (prevalence and severity of sarcasm, irritability, or anger)
   1 = All or most verbal or nonverbal communication hostile or bitter; object of anger diffuse
   2 = Directed annoyance most of the time, most (non)verbal communication hostile or sarcastic
   3 = Some irritability or curtness expressed but willing to reconcile
   4 = No evidence of anger or irritability

Calmness (emphasizes indications of tension, anxiety, or restlessness)
   1 = Panicky, agitated, tearful
   2 = Apprehensive, restless, preoccupied with worries or fears
   3 = Some verbal or nonverbal expression of tension; can be diverted from worries or fears
   4 = Calm, peaceful; may not be cheerful but without evidence of worries or fears

and perhaps the patient with advanced lung cancer had brain metastases as well. Another patient with prostatic cancer taking narcotics developed delirium whenever he developed fever. The fever did not increase the analgesic intensity of the narcotic. When the fever subsided, the delirium remitted. Thus, in this patient, fever caused a change in dose response for production of delirium but not of analgesia. These cases raise the question of whether there are different relative potencies for different responses to a single drug (desired compared to side effects, for example) in sick elderly compared to the relative potencies described in younger, medically less complicated patients.

Psychomotor function is assessed by the tapping test (21,22): how many times the patient can click a Clay-Adams laboratory counter in 10 sec. Normal healthy subjects can record 52 ± 5 (SD). Cancer patients in this study did 41 ± 8. Six tested within a month of death did 26 ± 11 (statistically significantly different from other patients). There was no detectable clinical clue at the time of testing that these six patients had a shorter life expectancy than the others.

Mood is assessed on the basis of rating the patient's behavior during the assessment interview on a four-point scale in each of three areas: engagement, irritability, and calmness [after Dush (23)]. These are described in Table 1.

There is a maximum of 12 points on this assessment, with the low values indicating disturbed mood. The 10 most recent patients had the following distribution of mood scores:

Mood scores:	12	11	10	9	8	7
No. of patients:	0	3	1	3	2	1

Thus, this test discriminates degrees of mood disturbance among patients with advanced cancer.

To determine interrater agreement of mood assessment, two people witnessed 10 interviews and independently rated the mood scales. Since each interview assessment included the three mood scales, a total of 30 pairs of observations were compared. The two raters scored 28 identically, and the remainder were one point apart.

This entire assessment for pain intensity, psychomotor performance, mental status, and mood is practical to do with these very sick and old patients. It can be repeated daily if desired to follow changes in the functions tested. Used properly, changes in these functions can be used to assess drug action on mood, cognitive performance, and psychomotor function in the very sick and very old as well as in less sick or less complicated patients. These assessment methods are a practical way to give a quantitative assessment of the patient. The methods may be useful to address a number of problems related to the effects of drug therapy in patients in nursing homes. It is an illustration of how one can develop methods to measure clinically relevant factors related to disease and drug action. Feinstein has written extensively about this and named such methodology "clinimetrics" (24–26).

The nursing home is a unique site to enlarge our knowledge base about drug action in the sick elderly population, since the nursing home is where many of these patients are and where they reside for a long enough period of time to allow comparative studies. To do this sort of research in a nursing home requires developing an attitude of inquiry in the staff, gaining acceptance of the idea that the patients are proper subjects for ethical research, developing methodology for obtaining voluntary and informed consent, and obtaining the resources needed to conduct the research.

Drugs are being used extensively in the nursing home population. Usually, data on dose–response and time–action relationships and therapeutic efficacy obtained in younger patients with less complex illnesses are generalized to the nursing home population because of ignorance about drug effects in the elderly. For the nursing home population, there is little specific or quantitative information about risks or benefits, and there is no reason to assume that these are the same as they are in younger, healthier people. If the best care possible based on present standards is practiced with a spirit of inquiry in a teaching nursing home, and proper and meaningful research is done, useful knowledge about drug action can be obtained. With more knowledge about drug action, patients' responses will be more predictable, and in that way, therapeutics for patients will be safer and more effective.

ACKNOWLEDGMENTS

We thank Mary Grossi and Elyse Seidner for their assistance in some of the methodology development. This work was supported in part by N.I.H. Grant AG 03280, The Newtown Fund, The James Picker Foundation Program in the Human Qualities of Medicine, the Murray M. Rosenberg Trust Fund, The Melville Corporation, and other friends of The Supportive Care Service.

REFERENCES

1. The National Nursing Home Survey: 1977 *Summary for the United States*. DHEW Publication No. (PH5)79-1794. Washington, DC, Government Printing Office, 1979.
2. Pastore JO, Winston FB, Barrett HS, et al: Characteristics of patients and medical care in New Haven area nursing homes. *New Engl J Med* 1968;279:130–136.
3. Lamy PP: *Prescribing for the Elderly*. Littleton, MA, PSG Publishing, 1981, p 102.
4. Ouslander JG: Drug therapy in the elderly. *Ann Intern Med* 1981;95:711–722.
5. Greenblatt DJ, Sellers EM, Shader RI: Drug disposition in old age. *N Engl J Med* 1982;306:1081–1088.
6. Vestal RE, Dawson GW: Pharmacology and aging, in Finch CE, Schneider EL (eds): *Handbook of the Biology of Aging*, 2nd ed. (in press).
7. Reidenberg MM: Drugs in the elderly. *Bull NY Acad Med* 1980;56:703–714.
8. Salem SAM, Rajjayabun P, Shepherd AMM, et al: Reduced induction of drug metabolism in the elderly. *Age Aging* 1978;7:68–73.
9. Cusack B, Kelly JG, Lavan J, et al: Theophylline kinetics in relation to age: The importance of smoking. *Br J Clin Pharmacol* 1980;10:109–114.
10. Davies DF, Shock NW: Age changes in glomerular filtration rate, effective renal plasma flow, and tubular excretory capacity in adult males. *J Clin Invest* 1950;29:496–507.
11. Cockcroft DW, Gault HM: Prediction of creatinine clearance from serum creatinine. *Nephron* 1976;16:31–41.
12. Drayer DE, Romankiewicz J. Lorenzo B, et al: Aging and the renal clearance of cimetidine. *Clin Pharmacol Ther* 1982;31:45–50.
13. Reidenberg MM, Levy M, Warner H, et al: Relationship between diazepam dose, plasma level, age, and central nervous system depression. *Clin Pharmacol Ther* 1978;23:371–374.
14. Casteden CM, George CF, Marcer D, et al: Increased sensitivity to nitrazepam in old age. *Br Med J* 1977;1:10–12.
15. Kaiko RF: Age and morphine analgesia in cancer patients with postoperative pain. *Clin Pharmacol Ther* 1980;28:823–826.
16. Meyer BR, Lewin M, Drayer DE, et al: Optimizing metoclopramide control of cisplatin induced emesis. *Ann Intern Med* 1984;100:393–395.
17. Kremer E, Atkinson JH, Ignelzi RJ: Measurement of pain; Patient preference does not confound pain measurement. *Pain* 1981;10:241–248.
18. Folstein MF, Folstein SE, McHugh PR: Mini-mental state. *J Psychiatr Res* 1975;12:189–198.
19. Jacobs JW, Bernhard MR, Delgado A, et al: Screening for organic mental syndromes in the medically ill. *Ann Intern Med* 1977;86:40–46.
20. Pfeiffer E: A short portable mental status questionnaire for the assessment of organic brain deficit in elderly patients. *J Am Geriatr Soc* 1975;23:433–441.
21. Epstein CL, Lasagna L: A comparison of the effects of orally administered barbiturate salts and barbituric acid on human psychomotor performance. *J Pharmacol Exp Ther* 1968;164:433–441.
22. Salzman C, Shader RI, Harmatz J, et al: Psychopharmacologic investigation in elderly volunteers: Effect of diazepam in males. *J Am Geriatr Soc* 1975;23:451–457.

23. Dush DM, Ozga D, Ford D, et al: Psychosocial needs of the hospice patient: A health adjustment scale. Presented at the National Hospice Organization 1983 Annual Meeting.
24. Feinstein AR: Clinical biostatistics. XLV. The purposes and functions of criteria. *Clin Pharmacol Ther* 1978;24:479–492.
25. Feinstein AR: Clinical biostatistics. XLVI. What are the criteria for criteria. *Clin Pharmacol Ther* 1979;25:108–116.
26. Feinstein AR: An additional basic science for clinical medicine IV. The development of clinimetrics. *Ann Intern Med* 1983;99:843–848.

The Teaching Nursing Home, edited by Edward
L. Schneider et al. © 1985 The Beverly
Foundation. Raven Press, New York.

Nutrition

Robert B. McGandy

*Tufts University, Schools of Medicine and Nutrition, USDA Human Nutrition Research
Center on Aging, Boston, Massachusetts 02111*

Age-related nutritional problems have come to current attention for three reasons. First, nutritional status surveys directed at elderly populations— both institutionalized and noninstitutionalized—have shown a low-to-moderate risk of either overt or potential nutrient deficiencies (1). Secondly, nutritional status is a regulatory factor in the rate of functional decline in a number of body organ systems, decrements that are markers of the aging process (2). Nutrient status and energy balance may also modify the progressive losses of both lean body and bone mass and the increase in adipose tissue that occur throughout adult life (2). Third, many of the chronic diseases that are major forces of morbidity and mortality in older adults and elderly persons have substantial dietary components in their pathogenesis. Atherosclerotic and hypertensive vascular disease, several major sites of neoplasia, diabetes, mellitus, osteoporosis, and dental diseases are important examples.

CLINICAL STATE OF THE ART

Current recommended dietary allowances (RDA) for the elderly are categorized in a group "50 years and above" (3). These caloric and nutrient RDAs are based on research and survey findings in young adult populations—they are extrapolations. To date, there have been few thorough nutrition studies of elderly groups which include clinical and biochemical components as well as measurement of food intake. Data are particularly limited among populations over age 75 or 80.

There are three components to the assessment of nutritional status: evaluation of energy and nutrient intake; measurement of biochemical indices; and a clinical examination including both a search for the presence of signs of nutrient deficiencies and the measurement of height, weight, and other parameters of adipose and muscle mass.

There still remain problems in quantifying the "usual" or "typical" daily intake of energy and nutrients. Day-to-day variability in intake may be considerable. There are clearly errors in reporting and in quantitating consumption of individual foods as well as limitations in food-table analytical values and errors in our assumptions about the bioavailability and absorption of nutrients. Thus, in surveys of elderly populations based on short observation periods (1 to 3 days), the proportion of individuals at the low end of the distribution of intakes is invariably exaggerated. In any event, a low intake of one or another nutrient (low in comparison to some arbitrary proportion of the RDAs) does not "prove" deficiency. More accurately, these may be characterized as intakes increasing the risk of deficiency.

Biochemical evaluation also presents problems of interpretation. For unless a level is zero, there is a question of the functional utility of the standards of comparison. Levels labeled "borderline or low" or "suboptimal" have been reported in surveys of elderly persons (1), but without clinical evidence of a frank deficiency or some other quantifiable, functional impairment, it is difficult to interpret a measurement in terms of health or well-being.

Although measurement of height and weight are simple enough, estimation of adipose and lean body mass is less certain. Ideal weights for height specifically applicable to elderly populations have not been developed (4).

The techniques of nutritional assessment and the criteria by which they are evaluated will need substantial honing before the nutritional status of elderly individuals can be related to function, health, and well-being. At present, these kinds of health linkages have been much better established in earlier phases of the life cycle: growth and development; pregnancy; lactation; and energy and nutrient deficiencies in developing countries of the world.

These limitations are the basis for the central mandate of the USDA Human Nutrition Research Center on Aging: "to determine optimal nutrient requirements for adults and elderly."

The RDAs for energy and many nutrients (protein, some vitamins, and minerals) are developed for "healthy" individuals and apply to presumably homogeneous population groups. Allowances are set high enough to meet the requirements of 95% of individuals. For energy, the allowances proposed are average needs, adequate to maintain a desirable weight and to provide enough total intake to assure sufficiency of both protein and micronutrient consumption.

The heterogeneity of the group "50 and above" is becoming well documented. There are many sources of variability that can affect the requirements of older individuals—effects on digestion, absorption, and metabolism. Among these are age-related changes in digestive tract and organ functions, presence of concomitant chronic diseases, drug–nutrient interactions including the effects of alcohol and level of physical activity. Additionally, an overall nutritional evaluation of the elderly should examine social circumstances, isolation, apathy, physical and mental disabilities, and factors affecting food choices (taste, smell, and dentition, for example).

Consistently reported in surveys of elderly populations are low levels of total energy intake—averages and ranges well below the current RDAs (5).

The deficits are particularly marked among elderly noninstitutionalized females and among institutionalized populations of both sexes. It is well known that the decrement in energy needs with aging is based both on the decline in lean body mass (and therefore of basal metabolic rate) and on the diminished level of discretionary energy expenditure. But the extremely sedentary life style of so many free-living older persons and the disability-imposed inactivity of many institutionalized patients reduce energy needs into an area in which it becomes very difficult to insure protein and micronutrient adequacy. Food choices must be carefully made. Further restrictions related to special therapeutic dietary constraints often impose considerable problems in insuring acceptable and adequate diets.

PROMISING RESEARCH DIRECTIONS
Nutrition and Age-Associated Diseases
Atherosclerotic Vascular Disease

Although there has been a 25% to 30% decline in mortality from this form of cardiovascular disease over the past 15 years (6), a decline reported even among the elderly, atherosclerotic vascular disease remains the leading cause of death. Relationships among dietary fats, circulating lipoproteins, and the clinical complications of atherosclerosis are best understood in middle-aged populations. The relative predictive importance of the risk factors operative in younger adults (blood lipoprotein levels, blood pressure, smoking, physical activity, obesity, and so forth) is not known in older individuals. The preventive potential of dietary and life-style changes in elderly groups will require further study. On the other hand, since the disease progresses over the entire adult lifespan, it seems reasonable that acquisition of good dietary and personal health practices should commence in early life and continue into the elderly years.

Hypertensive Vascular Disease

Although the determinants of essential hypertension remain unknown, many dietary factors may play important roles in blood pressure regulation. Among these are obesity, the minerals sodium, potassium, and calcium, and dietary fatty acids. The potential of diet in the prevention or non-pharmacological management of hypertension requires further study.

Neoplasia

The relationships between nutrition and cancer of several important sites have been intensively studied over the past decade. There are two aspects to this field. First, the nutritional support and management of patients with advanced cancer or with cancer of sites interfering with food intake or digestion is now recognized as extremely important to their response to surgery and radio- or chemotherapy. Second, there is developing interest in the role of diet in the pathogenesis of cancer and, therefore, in the development of dietary guidelines that might actually reduce the incidence of this disease (7).

Among the dietary–nutritional factors are obesity, the proportions of total calories from fats and carbohydrates, fiber, vitamins A, C, and E, and minerals—particularly selenium and zinc. In addition, the roles of various food additives as well as several naturally occurring food chemicals remain to be clarified by experimental and epidemiological studies. Since the induction time ("incubation period") of human cancers is a matter of decades, the potential for prevention in elderly populations would reflect dietary changes made much earlier in life.

Diabetes Mellitus

The importance of obesity in the disturbance of glucose homeostasis and in the incidence of diabetes that occurs with advancing age is well known. Attention to energy balance—caloric restriction and increased energy expenditure—can often help control this disease and may even eliminate the need for pharmacologic management. Since diabetics have a much increased risk of atherosclerotic cardiovascular disease, fat-modified diets may also be prudently recommended.

Osteoporosis

Fractures of the hip and forearm and compression lesions of the vertebral skeleton are an enormous cause of disability among the elderly, particularly women. The importance of nutritional factors, particularly of dietary calcium, of hormonal factors, and of the role of physical activity, have been areas of intense recent research (8). The observation that increased calcium intake (a nutrient already consumed well below the RDA by most Americans of middle and older ages) can prevent osteoporosis needs further confirmation. The loss of skeletal bone salts occurs over adult life; thus, the potential for intervention by diet or by increasing physical activity in older individuals represents a very important research opportunity.

Dental Disease

The roles of diet (particularly of carbohydrates), oral bacterial flora, oral hygiene, and age changes in salivary flow are being examined in relation to the type of dental caries and periodontal disease that afflict the elderly. Since the state of oral health is assumed to be an important determinant of nutritional status of many older individuals, this too is an area of substantial research opportunity.

Nutrition and Age-Related Changes in Organ or System Functions

The rate of loss of bone mass with age is known to be regulated by diet and by physical activity. Whether these same factors can significantly modulate loss of lean body mass, particularly of muscle, is unknown. Not only does adipose tissue increase as muscle mass is lost, but the relentless net positive energy balance that characterizes many American adults of middle age leads to rather marked increases of total body fat stores and to a high prevalence of obesity.

Whereas excess body fat is well known to increase the morbidity and mortality rates of a variety of chronic and degenerative diseases in middle-aged adults, there is little data on older age groups.

Perhaps even modest increases in physical activity would allow for diets providing more calories and micronutrients without concomitant weight gain. The improvements from greater activity and better diets may significantly benefit health and well being.

Many of the age-related changes in the gastrointestinal tract, particularly in the stomach and small bowel, may well influence nutrient absorption and thus become factors to consider in setting RDAs for elderly populations (2). A particularly important research area is the problem of maintaining adequate calcium intake. Many elderly have decreased milk consumption because of abdominal discomfort, bloating, or even diarrhea following ingestion of milk. The basis for this is the age-related decrease in the activity of the enzyme which leads to the milk sugar (lactose) not being completely digested. The extent of this problem and the possible benefits of newer milk products need investigation. Another substantial area for research concerns the possible role of dietary fiber in constipation, diverticulosis, hiatus hernia, and hemorrhoidal disease.

Dietary factors have also been suggested as playing a role in the loss of cognitive function and in some behavioral changes noted in the elderly (9). This too presents many significant opportunities for clinical investigations.

The recognition that many of the diseases of the elderly are determined in part by a decline in immune function (2) and the knowledge that nutrients may regulate some important facets of this system offer many research possibilities in studying nutritional interventions in optimizing the competency of the immune system.

NUTRITION IN TEACHING AND MEDICAL CARE: SOME CAUTIONS REGARDING THERAPEUTIC DIETS

Greater awareness of the importance of adequate nutrition will depend in part on greater expertise in nutritional science among physicians, nurses, and attendant staffs. Familiarity with dietary assessment techniques (not merely the measurement of body weight), recognition of specific deficiencies, the use of appropriate diagnostic laboratory tests, and close cooperation among physicians, nurses, and dietitians must all be improved.

Along with the complex decision factors in setting treatment priorities for individuals with a variety of coexistent medical problems, the implications of dietary modifications must be taken into account. Food choices are a reflection of the cultural and socioeconomic backgrounds and of a lifetime of acquired individual preferences. They are a part of a patient's heritage that must often be left behind when she/he enters a nursing home.

The costs and logistics of delivering attractive, palatable, and nutritionally balanced diets create a difficult task. The low energy requirements of relatively sedentary elderly have already been mentioned. Levels of energy intake of 1,200 to 1,600 kcal per day are observed among institutionalized elderly (1). It becomes extremely difficult to meet recommended nutrient allowances in this range; food choices must be very carefully made, and actual consumption of meals must be assured. Further constraints imposed by therapeutic dietary modifications, alterations that usually translate into "taking away" rather than adding foods or seasonings, may well put the patient at nutritional risk: appetite and intake may decrease; nutrient adequacy may be more difficult to assure; and reactive, noncompliant food habits may result.

In order to keep a patient's mealtime as positive an experience as possible, therapeutic dietary modifications should be imposed only when indicated by periodic medical reviews. Particularly for diabetic and sodium-restricted diets, the regimens should be as liberal as possible consistent with realistic medical goals. Allowance should be made for occasional foods from family or friends, and, whenever possible, the patient must be involved in decisions regarding food choices.

REFERENCES

1. Young EA: Evidence relating selected vitamins and minerals to health and disease in the elderly population in the United States: Introduction. *Am J Clin Nutr* 1982;36:979–985.
2. Munro HN: Nutrition and Ageing. *Br Med J* 1981;37:83–88.
3. Food and Nutrition Board: *Recommended Dietary Allowances*, ed. 9. Washington, DC, National Academy of Sciences, 1980, pp 8–9.
4. Russell RM, McGandy RB, Jelliffe D: Reference weights: Practical considerations. *Am J Med* 1984;76:767–769.
5. Munro HN: Nutritional requirements in the elderly. *Hosp Pract* 1982 August;143–154.
6. Levy RI: The decline in cardiovascular disease mortality. *Annu Rev Publ Health* 1981;2:49–70.
7. Pariza MW: A perspective on diet, nutrition, and cancer. *JAMA* 1984;251:1455–1458.
8. Heaney RP, Gallagher JC, Johnston CC, et al: Calcium nutrition and bone health in the elderly. *Am. J Clin Nutr* 1982;36:986–1013.
9. Goodwin JS, Goodwin JM, Garry PJ: Association between nutritional status and cognitive functioning in a healthy elderly population. *JAMA* 1983;249:2917–2921.

The Teaching Nursing Home, edited by Edward L. Schneider et al. © 1985 The Beverly Foundation. Raven Press, New York.

Communication Disorders with Age

George Moushegian and Anna Morgan-Fisher

School of Human Development and Callier Center for Communication Disorders, University of Texas at Dallas, Dallas, Texas 75235

The primary mode of human communication occurs through spoken languages, which are centered on the sense of hearing. The smoothness and facility of language and speech belie the enormous complexity of the brain and the receptors that mediate the communicative processes. Psychological, physiological, and anatomical changes accompany aging but do not follow the same time course in every person. A major consequence of the inexorabilities of aging is that the complex systems of the brain become less able to handle normal communication effectively.

The purpose of this chapter is to describe communication disorders that are most common in the elderly population and to generate and establish guidelines for research, education, and clinical care for residents with these disorders in teaching nursing homes (TNHs). An overview of certain central and peripheral aging processes is provided, and some of the more common disorders of speech and hearing that accompany these changes are discussed. This is followed with a summary of recent advances in research that may bear directly on communication disorders in the elderly and suggestions for creating an environment that fosters effective and satisfying communication.

Communicative handicaps often provoke psychological or interpersonal problems or, conversely, may be the result of these impairments. A progressive decrement in hearing acuity or effective speech production, for example, may cause fear and embarrassment and precipitate a withdrawl from social situations. Although communication disorders of aging have captured the attention of only a few investigators in the past, there has been an increasing interest in recent years in the aging process and its impact on communication. This is timely and welcomed, since 54% of the 24 million people with communication disorders are 65 years or older [1].

Speech, language, and hearing impairments to which older adults are highly susceptible may appear primarily in the following dysfunctions: neurological disorders that affect vocal mechanisms, aphasia, Parkinson's disease, dysarthria, confusion–disorientation, and hearing loss [1]. All of these produce communication deficiencies that are etiologically and prognostically multidimensional. Since appropriate care, habilitation, and remediation are critically dependent on correct diagnoses, nursing home staff must be knowledgeable about the anatomy, physiology, and psychology of communication disorders prevalent in elderly adults.

AGING PROCESSES OF THE AUDITORY NEURAXIS

The biological aging of auditory function is termed presbycusis. The four types of peripheral pathology associated with presbycusis are:

(a) *sensory presbycusis*, which is characterized by atrophy and degeneration of hair cells in the basal coil of the organ of Corti in the cochlea and results in high-frequency loss with negligible effects on speech-range frequencies; (b) *mechanical presbycusis*, which is distinguishable by atrophic changes in the basilar membrane and results in hearing loss for all frequencies, some improvement being possible with proper sound amplification; (c) *strial presbycusis*, which is marked by atrophy of the stria vascularis, results in a uniform hearing loss across all frequencies, and is indicated by a flat audiogram; and (d) *neural presbycusis*, which is attributable to atrophy of cochlear nerve fibers and possibly to degeneration in the auditory pathway and results in impaired speech comprehension without apparent parallel impairment of pure-tone discrimination (2).

These age-related degenerative phenomena within the cochlea produce unquestionable diminutions of hearing acuity and speech understanding. Concomitant structural and functional alterations also occur within the central auditory pathways and nuclei. The changes take the form of cell loss and degeneration along with accumulation of the age pigment, lipofuscin. The combined effects of the various peripheral and central pathophysiologies introduce considerable variability in the resulting communication disorder. For this reason, evaluation of hearing loss and communication skills in the aged must be performed with extreme care, particularly in those circumstances in which heterogeneous factors contribute to diverse central and peripheral degenerative processes.

An example of peripheral presbycusis is shown in Fig. 1. The audiometric pattern of loss is profound at high frequencies (3 kHz and above) and moderate at lower frequencies. Histologic analysis of the patient's temporal bone revealed extensive atrophy of the hair cells and supporting cells in the basal end of the cochlea and a parallel loss of cochlear (VIII nerve) neurons from the same area. The patient had a discrimination score of 64% and functioned well with amplification. Neither this example, however, nor any other is typical, since the audiometric deficiencies with age are as varied as the physiological and structural ones that cause them. For these reasons, it is impossible to describe a classic presbycustic configuration because there may be a plethora of other etiologies along with it.

Certain drug therapies, physical trauma, noise exposure, fever, and familial history of hearing loss are among a host of other circumstances that can contribute to communication disorders. Despite such difficulties, a few studies have attempted to control for these effects in order to ferret out the

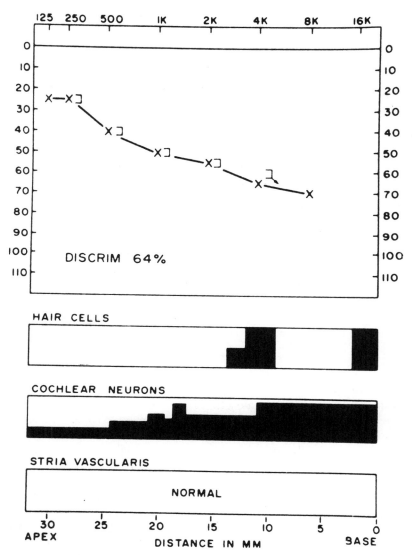

FIG. 1. Presbycusis of 81-year-old male. Histograms reveal normal stria vascularis with hair cell and extensive cochlear nerve loss from basal end of cochlea. (From ref. 3, with permission.)

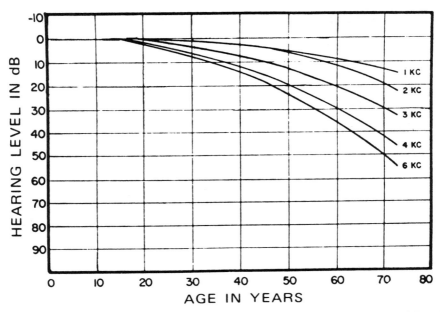

FIG. 2. Hearing levels as a function of age for 328 men with no history of high noise exposure or otologic disease. (From ref. 4, with permission.)

extent to which hearing deteriorates with age. In one study, 328 men with no history of otological disease, trauma, or exposure to gunfire or high noise levels were screened and tested (4). The results are displayed in Fig. 2 for hearing levels as a function of age for five frequencies. The data show that loss of sensitivity begins at age 30 for all frequencies and continues throughout the life span. The decrease is greater for higher than for lower frequencies. At 1.0 kHz, for instance, the loss is 3 dB for every 10 years of age through 70 years, and at 6.0 kHz, it is 10 dB for every 10 years. The pure-tone sensitivities of women reveal a similar but less severe pattern of loss.

When a patient, particularly an elderly one, presents with a mixed etiology, the audiometric consequences are often much more severe and the communication problems more resistive to remediation and treatment because of central nervous system pathology along with receptor and nerve dysfunction. Figure 3 illustrates results from an 82-year-old patient with a history of excessive noise exposure, vertigo, and recently diagnosed diabetes mellitus. The patient had a severe sensorineural hearing loss for high frequencies, extreme difficulty in phonemic discrimination, and poor speech-reading ability. Use of a hearing aid was not very successful. Such examples appear frequently in the elderly population, and extensive studies of them have demonstrated that: there is no classic presbycusic pattern; usable residual hearing varies considerably among the elderly; the effectiveness of

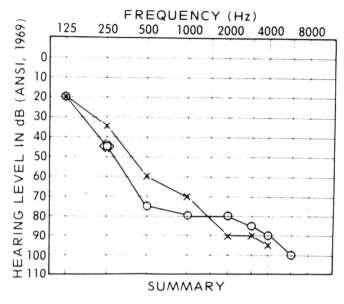

FIG. 3. Audiometric findings from 82-year-old patient with mixed etiologies. (From ref. 5, with permission.)

oral habilitation depends on multiple factors; and pure-tone thresholds alone are not predictive of suprathreshold performance with or without a hearing aid (5).

A number of testing materials are available for assessing the suprathreshold speech perception of the elderly. These may be syllables, words, and sentences, which are presented to the person in a variety of ways, e.g., written, oral, with headphones, or speakers (6). When most variables are held constant, it is generally acknowledged that "syllables are less intelligible than words, which in turn are less intelligible than sentences. As a general rule, the greater the linguistic and contextual information available to the listener, the greater the intelligibility" (7). Furthermore, in evaluating an elderly person's hearing, it is of considerable importance to bear in mind that speech reception is greatly affected by talker and listener variability (6).

A significant number of elderly adults can have deficits in communication that are severe enough to cause them problems in daily living. Any physiological time degradation, interruption, or alteration in speech generation greatly affects its understanding because hearing is a temporal sense. Along with memory loss and diminution of contextual redundancy, these probably are the major factors leading to poor speech reception with age. Imagine the difficulty an elderly person would have in comprehending the following sentence rapidly spoken: "The mill-*wright* on my *right* thinks it *right* that some conventional *rite* should symbolize the *right* of every man to *write* as he pleases" (8).

AGING PROCESSES OF THE SPEECH MECHANISM

Sensory modalities and nervous tissue are characterized as having organizational complexity, interdependence, redundancy, and environmental modifiability. For these reasons, it is suspected that increasing isolation or disengagement by the elderly can result in functional and structural alterations in the sensory links that initiate, maintain, and guide adaptation and behavior (9).

Speech is the audible expression of language and involves the generation of sound through the interactive participation of respiratory, phonatory, and articulatory physiological systems (10). Its execution is mediated by segmental, suprasegmental, and the neocortical portions of the nervous system. Collectively, these structures provide the anatomical and physiological bases for language, a system of symbols for communicating thoughts, desires, ideas, and emotions among persons for whom the symbols have meaning (10). The division of language and auditory comprehension into receptive and expressive communication provides a means for revealing its complexities. The diversity and multiplicity of these higher functions require that all speech-generating mechanisms, peripheral and central, perform smoothly, as faulty timing and integration can produce receptive, expressive, or both types of communication problems.

Noll's four-level hierarchical model of human communication clearly exhibits the multimodality of language. The levels are: language ideation, a generalized cortical function; symbolization, a process that is mediated at fronto–parietal–temporal and parieto–temporal–occipital areas of the dominant hemisphere (usually left); translation, an operation in Broca's area (Noll does not include Wernicke's area but should have); and execution, an interaction of upper- and lower-motor-neuron systems, cerebellum, and peripheral speech system with feedback (10).

Viewed physiologically or psychologically, the speech mechanism is obviously multidimensional by nature and for appropriate expression requires integration of its respiratory–phonatory, supralaryngeal, neuromuscular, and psychomotor components. The aging process affects each of these differently.

The aging person exhibits differences in oral communication as a result of the normal aging process, neurological disease, or both (10). Characteristic changes in manner and style of speaking, as well as physiological alterations, produce predictable variations in the acoustic parameters of speech, perhaps a result of susceptibility to neurological degeneration and disease that interrupt normal language processing and execution of speech (11).

The driving force for speech production is initiated by the respiratory system. It provides air flow through the human vocal tract, which results in vibration of the vocal folds in the larynx or turbulence at some point in the vocal tract and serves as a sound source for speech (12). With age, increased rigidity of collagenous tissue in the lungs and rib cage with simultaneous atrophy of muscles, glands, and soft tissue leads to progressive declines in ventilatory function. There is not only a reduction in vital capacity and vascular supply but a weakening and stretching of alveolar septal membranes and endocrine-induced disturbances of mucus secretion (11,13,14). The aging laryngeal cartilages become rigid and lead to changes in phonation because of increased ossification and calcification. These processes collectively alter the speech performance of the aging adult by affecting maximum vowel phonation, vocal fundamental frequency, vocal intensity, and vocal fold vibrations (10,11).

The supralaryngeal component of the speech mechanism consists of the vocal tract and articulators lying above the larynx. Complex vocal tract alterations induce distinct resonant changes in the acoustic signals (10). A host of insults and conditions often associated with age can disrupt the efficiency of many speech components. A few of the more common are: loss of teeth, malocclusion, and consequent resorption of alveolar bone which alters the structural integrity of the temporomandibular joint and the shape of the oral cavity involved in the articulatory and coarticulatory aspects of speech production (14); morphologic changes in facial bones (which shift the points of attachment of the facial muscles) that disrupt the oral resonatory characteristics and mandibular movements of speech; deterioration in peripheral neuromuscular control and reduced sensory feedback and central processing that decrease the speed and accuracy of oral gesturing; and mild loss of velar control and reduced rates of lip and tongue movements that result in hesitant and unclear speech (13,15).

Sensory, motor, and central factors collectively influence the processing time for expression of the neuromuscular component of speech. Integrity of the muscular and nervous systems is a *sine qua non* for meaningful and effective expression (12). Aging can affect the functional and structural ingredients of the nervous system as well as the integrity of muscles and glands (16). Subtle changes therefore may occur simultaneously in sensorimotor, vascular, and cognitive components of speech before any change in speech performance is noticed. It was once thought that speech production was minimally affected by aging because it is a well-rehearsed and automated function. Evaluations of speech reveal, however, that with age situational demands requiring speed and accuracy provoke decrements in performance and automaticity (16).

Cognition and psychomotor responses refer to the information-processing system of sensory coding, learning, and memory. They include modality-specific sensory memories and the important converging polysensory integrative processes that are distributed throughout the cortex. Of all the brain functions susceptible to decline, short-term memory, which crosses all sensory modalities, is most prey to the inevitable manifestations of aging (16). Age of onset and rate of deprivation differ sharply within and among sensory modalities and individuals. It is characterized more by the slowing of decision-making processes than the execution of movements (13,16,17). Other confounding factors include: increase in random neural (brain) activity, which blurs sensory perception and decision making; after-images, which contribute to interference; diminished signal strength and functional capacity, which lead to difficulties in manipulating mental data, particularly multiple-step processing and multimodal integration; excessive caution and emphasis on accuracy without commensurate concern for speed; rigidity in responding with an unwillingness to alter original percepts; and elevated thresholds for many sensory stimuli (13,16,17). An accelerated reduction in one or an increase in the number of other components will substantially alter communication processing. For all of these reasons, accurate predictions of cognitive and motor variations in senescence cannot be made.

COMMUNICATION DISORDERS AS SEQUELAE OF NEUROLOGICAL DISEASE

The natural aging process with its highly individualized variations of lifestyles and types of stress alters vocal acoustics. These changes may not appear to deter an elderly person's communication, but there often are accompanying psychological, social, and emotional influences that accentuate sensory and motor slowdown. Although mild alterations in sensory perceptions do not produce pathology or interfere severely with information acquisition, the disruption in balance of perceptual input can lead to diminution of integrative capabilities. Environmental demands, vocal abuse, stress, and fatigue also adversely affect the integrity of centrally and peripherally mediated performances. When complexity of processing increases, the accumulation of small changes begins to have a synergistic effect and produces a noticeable decline in proficiency, especially for the speech mechanism. This type of alteration in performance is the reason it is difficult to differentiate pathology from natural aging (12).

Although there is an increased prevalence of neurological disorders in the elderly population, not all communication disorders are a result of age or age-related disorders. Some communication deficits are acquired at younger ages, whereas most adult communication problems probably result from disruptions in the integrity of the nervous system and the consequent influences on speech and hearing mechanisms.

The number of persons with hearing impairments increases tenfold during the fifth, sixth, seventh, and eighth decades (1). Over half of the individuals 65 years of age are hearing impaired to some degree, and 1.2 million of them wear hearing aids. The elderly present with a variety of symptoms, which include auditory discrimination difficulties and disorders of auditory processing and synthesis (1). Whether amplification will be helpful depends on the amount of reduction, if any, in the dynamic range and the etiology of the presbycusis.

A large number of neurological disorders in old age can be attributed directly to changes in the arterial blood supply to the brain (17). Susceptibility to a cardiovascular accident (CVA) or stroke increases with arteriosclerosis, decreased cerebral blood circulation, and increased blood pressure, which collectively weaken blood vessel walls. The peak age for incidence of stroke occurs between 40 and 70 years (75% over 65 years) (15,18). Or those who have a stroke, 50% survive, but many do not escape brain injury (15). Although stroke is only one of three etiologies of aphasia, it is responsible for 78% of aphasia cases that occur at 55 years. It is believed by some that the age-related increases in prevalence of stroke are probably a direct function of physiologic processes that occur throughout the life span (15). The slowed articulation rate with natural aging often precedes the neuropathology in speech disorders such as aphasia and dysarthria.

Aphasia is a language disorder resulting from damage to speech and language centers in the dominant cerebral hemisphere of the central nervous system. The disorder crosses all modalities to produce a deficit for processing symbolic materials in audition, speech, reading, writing, and especially within the grammer system and lexicon (13). The site of the lesion determines the type, extent, and prognosis of the aphasia. Severity of the disorder and probable effectiveness of therapy depend not only on the type of aphasia and age of the patient but on home and work environments. The variabilities in prognosis are influenced by the medical, social, educational, and psychological histories of the stroke victim.

The major language symptoms of aphasia are characterized as fluent, nonfluent, or global. The fluent type is distinguished by rapid, flowing speech with semantics and syntax disrupted; nonfluent aphasia includes those with impaired prosody and difficulty in producing connected utterances; the global-type patients have little if any language output and appear not to comprehend what is said.

Nonlanguage problems that frequently accompany aphasia are facial paresis or weakness, visual sensation deficit, loss of touch, right hemiplegia, loss of balance, inappropriate laughing or crying, lower defense thresholds, reduced attention span, impaired short-term memory, and loss of geographic orientation (13). Because of reduced abilities to carry out essential social roles, the patient needs family intervention, involvement, and an awareness of the dysfunctions associated with aphasia (15). The communication process involves all aspects of human existence, and therapy should be a means for teaching a patient how to function maximally.

Apraxia in speech is a disturbance in phonologic programming in the absence of aphasia and dysarthria. Some of the hesitancy behaviors, reduced speech rate, and dysfluency patterns of the elderly may reflect subtle apraxic disturbances. Typical symptoms include variable articulatory patterns, disturbed prosody, oral struggle behavior, and inappropriate phonemic sequencing (13). Unlike aphasia, apraxia is modality specific with a disruption of motor planning that is frequently associated with articulation inconsistency. Oral apraxia can also affect nonspeech functions such as whistling, protruding the tongue, and blowing. This latter disorder, although a disorder within itself, frequently accompanies Broca's aphasia.

As presented above, age-related changes in the supraphonatory component produce diminished efficiency, integrity, and shape of the oral cavity needed for free-running discourse. The hesitant and unclear speech sometimes associated with aging can become more difficult to understand with neurological insult, stroke, or disease.

Dysarthria is a neurogenic disorder that results in poor speech intelligibility caused by impaired innervation of speech musculature. This includes lack of control in production of speech sounds and improper breathing or control of the voice because of paresis, weakness, or incoordination. With the exception of cerebral palsy, multiple sclerosis, and congenital malformations, most motor speech disorders are associated with age-related neuropathologies (19). The disturbed muscular control may result from damage to the central or peripheral nervous system following multiple strokes, injury, or amyotrophic lateral sclerosis (ALS).

Parkinson's disease is representative of hypokinetic dysarthria with onset usually after 50 years of age. It is the result of pathology in the basal ganglia and etiologically is viral, drug-induced, or idiopathic. The idiopathic etiology may possibly result from the increasing ratio of serotonin to dopamine in the caudate nucleus that occurs with advancing age (20). The articulation and vocalization of speech sounds in this disease progress from slowed articulation to increased inaudibility. One in every 1,000 individuals over age 50 will be afflicted with parkinsonism, and the incidence increases fivefold after age 60 (13).

Reduction in memory and cognitive functions provokes withdrawal from social activities to reduce stimuli and stress. This is unfortunate because continued involvement, and not withdrawal, is needed. Environmental stimulation of sensory systems is essential for normal functional and structural organization of afferents, intercomponents, and efferents (16). It is well known that rehearsal or practice improves the reaction time of the elderly because continued exposure to stimuli helps develop compensatory strategies to the greatest degree possible.

Cerebral damage leads to reduction in intellectual capacity and impairment of memory. Benign memory impairment, or inability to recall certain relative aspects of an experience with information later recalled, is common as well as natural with age. Malignant memory dysfunction occurs when complete events of the recent and remote past are totally forgotten. This type of intellectual and memory deficit is characteristic of dementia, a group of diseases that are discussed in another chapter (see R. Katzman, Chapter 19, *this volume*). Because of impaired cognitive abilities, there is a poverty of speech resulting from inaccessibility of vocabularies ordinarily utilized (13). The word-finding problems and impaired recognition, especially for rarer words, are a result of central nervous system delays. The reduction in quantity of all mental, speech, and motor activity is usually characterized by brisk replies to simple questions (21). Prominent impairments in memory, particularly of recent events, impoverished concrete thinking, and emotional and personality alterations are well-known symptoms (13). Language skills may appear to be highly automatized, but in actuality they are complex operations that are usually affected first when the health status of an elderly person changes (18).

Confusion–disorientation (nonaphasic) is viewed as an acquired cognitive disorder with confusion and reduced ability to use language skills; it is not always associated with a specific lesion or disorder (1).

An elderly person is confronted with a critical organic voice problem if removal of a malignant larynx, *laryngectomy*, is required. The ensuing difficulties are immense but the ability to learn esophageal speech is less disrupting for personalities who are aggressive, alert, and mechanically inclined (19). Each laryngectomized patient should have postsurgical counseling and speech therapy for reorientation into meaningful communication (12).

Each component of the speech mechanism has certain pathologies that can affect the elderly person. When more than one disease or affliction is present, effective communication is placed in jeopardy. It does not matter whether the onset is swift or insidious, communication disorder is inevitable and harsh to that population for whom any change is uncomfortable and difficult.

SOME RESEARCH DIRECTIONS IN COMMUNICATION SCIENCES

Research advances related to hearing aids, speech synthesis, and electrical measures (EEG) would provide better knowledge than presently exists for effective intervention and remediation in communicative illnesses associated with the elderly. These three research areas certainly are not the only ones in the communication and neurological sciences that can be pursued advantageously within nursing homes, but they are among those that collectively address many of the problems associated with age.

Hearing Aids

Hearing assessment and hearing aid fitting continue to improve because of increased knowledge of normal and pathological ears and improved characteristics of certain components in conventional aids, e.g., amplifiers, filters, and microphones. Significant advances can occur if modern technologies are brought to bear on hearing measurement (or hearing loss) and aid fitting of the patient. The key technological ingredients are a digital hearing aid and computer-based programs for assessment. The singular advantage of an adjustable digital hearing aid is that one and only one type of transducer will be available to all patients. The same instrument is employed during testing and, once fitted with adjustments and tests of parameters, may be immediately assigned to the patient. Subsequent parameter adjustments of the aid can be tested to optimize the acoustic input to the wearer when the environment is changed, e.g., from a quiet room to a noisy or reverberant one. Since the digital aid will contain a probe microphone, the acoustic sound pressure level at the eardrum can be constantly monitored and adjustments made in the output characteristics to conform closely to the wearer's residual hearing. The advantages of computer-assisted audiological assessment and service are that fewer visits will be necessary to fit the patient with the instrument and that essentially only one aid (a master aid) need be tailored to provide the most effective amplification for any kind of audiometric loss.

Speech Synthesis

Speech synthesis is beginning to provide understanding as well as practical applications concerning human speech perception. Speech synthesis and analysis should be central in the pursuit of understanding speech mechanisms and associated cognitive functions. Since one can now generate and selectively control the parameters of an acoustic stimulus, aspects of information that are most important in normal and aging language comprehension can be identified. For example, analysis of speech breathing could ascertain what adaptations an elderly person employs to accommodate for laryngeal and respiratory changes. The data could be related to histological studies of the larynx, tongue, pharynx, and velopharyngeal mechanisms.

Alterations in the characteristics of the vocal tract and larynx as a consequence of aging can also be related to speech generation and would provide a reliable prognosis for intervention and remediation strategies. There are few acoustic studies on aging speech, and most have utilized gross measures and have not provided any poignant insights. Although speech is a motor behavior that is continuously in use and presumably produces a redundant message, subtleties in speech generation occur because aging un-questionably affects all aspects of speech production to varying degrees. Therefore, the cognitive strategies that elderly adults adopt in certain tasks become difficult to evaluate. Presumed deficits in cognitive function may be no more than an adaptive way of maintaining communication under certain life situations. One wonders whether age per se is a ubiquitous or minor factor in the etiology of speech and language disorders. History of illness, severity, and the many indefinable psychological characteristics may be, separately or collectively, essential ingredients in the etiologies of hear-ing, speech, and language disorders.

Voice and language disorders, whether functional or organic, introduce considerable difficulties in communication. Voice disorders associated, for instance, with laryngectomies, dysarthrias, spastic dysphonia, and aphasia have high incidences of occurrence among older adults. In each of these, meaningful remediation requires an awareness and understanding of bio-logical, sociological, psychological, and environmental influences without which effective care would be impossible. A TNH would be an ideal setting to pursue this problem if trained professionals with knowledge of higher cortical function were available for collaboration.

Electrical Measures

The electroencephalographic (EEG) and event-related potentials (ERP) provide records of the electrical activities of the brain. The EEG is evaluated in terms of voltage oscillations converted to frequency. There are studies that suggest that some deviations of the EEG appear to be age related. Decreases in the α waves, increases in β waves, a diffuse slow activity in a few normals (about 20%) above the age of 75 years, and a high incidence of episodic high-voltage activity in the temporal region of the left hemisphere have been reported. These changes in the EEG in aging have poor prog-nostic value primarily because the physiological basis of electroencephal-ography, an utterly complex phenomenon, is poorly understood.

Event-related potentials, in contrast, are more amenable for correlation with sensory, behavioral, cognitive, and attentional processes. These po-tentials are a sequence of waveforms that are evolved by a click stimulus or tone bursts. There is probably no better noninvasive technique than the ERP to study the aging brain with its fairly high incidence of cognitive dysfunctions (22).

Consideration and thought should be given to the appropriateness and timeliness of research in a TNH on auditory implants, known also as coch-lear prostheses. Technological advances in microsurgical procedures have led to a relatively widespread application of such devices on profoundly deaf persons. The aim is to bypass the initial transducer (cochlea) and electrically stimulate the auditory nerve, or what remains of it. A number of implant programs exist throughout the country and world. Each utilizes different systems, approaches, and techniques of electrical stimulation, and the results vary accordingly. The reported results are that: patients receive comfort in having auditory contact of some sort with the environment; multichannel are better than single-channel implants; the best implant performance is not much better than performance by a well-practiced subject using a multichannel tactile speech receiver; and simple cochlear implant devices provide a select group of patients with the benefits of detecting some common environmental sounds and assistance in lip reading.

Auditory prosthesis research and application are presently very much in the experimental stage. None of the prostheses provide adequate speech discrimination; and those that are multichannel introduce the risk of producing neural and sensory damage to remaining tissue. Since speech cannot be transmitted with these devices, and the range of stimulus intensity, frequency, and tonal quality are limited, prosthesis research would be untimely and should not be conducted within a TNH.

SUMMARY AND RECOMMENDATIONS

Rapid structural changes within the nervous system can precipitate distortion in sensations and perceptions. Because the senses link man with his external and internal environments, nervous system malfunctions result in an increase of poor judgment. Along with becoming weaker, slower, and easily fatigued, an individual delays or hesitates and is unaware or denies his/her limitations.

Successful communication is very important throughout the life span and is most effective when both speaker and listener share information. Individual thoughts, beliefs, and actions provide impetus for the exchange. As age-related changes in the sensory system reduce stimulus strength and processing capacity, some elderly may disengage from society. Nursing homes should provide activities that promote social interaction to counteract social atrophy from lack of use. Resident education about sensory and memory changes that bring decline in acuity might provoke compensatory strategies toward use and improvement of existing sensory capabilities. Learning is facilitated through active subject choice, practice, and a self-paced schedule compensating for loss in speed and accuracy.

The activities of the TNH could also include instructions about use and care of hearing aids, speech discrimination, and speech gestures. Hearing aid amplification should be presented gradually with the limit determined by an individual's dynamic range. Regular inspection for impacted cerumen as well as periodic aid reevaluation is imperative for optimum care.

Those who work in a nursing home are urged always to talk to the hearing-imparied individual face to face at eye level and not shout but have voice raised slightly. Visual and gestural cues, slowed speech rate, and distinct articulation, without exaggeration, are needed in discourse with any communicatively impaired person. Also encouraged is the use of situational, visual, and tactual cues during conversation while avoiding abstract, emotional, and controversial subjects or a sudden shift in topics. Knowledge of the type of communication deficit, i.e., receptive, expressive, or confusion–disorientation, helps to compensate for deficiency and improve communication between staff personnel and nursing home resident. It offers the opportunity to learn effective and suitable coping strategies.

It is important to understand the patient's perception of his/her sensory impairment and communication difficulties, as this can affect the content of any messages. Sometimes it is necessary to ask questions or repeat a statement in order to determine whether the patient's intended communication is understood.

Short concise phrases high in visible terms to simplify and reduce complexity should be emphasized. Repetition of information may be necessary when organizational complexity requires stimulation and realistic message redundancy. Whenever understanding does not occur even after repeated tries, an alternate communication form should be chosen. Liberal use of verbal and visual demonstrations helps to clarify instructions or directions.

Speech therapy in conjunction with physical therapy to improve posture, strength, and muscle tone can increase intelligibility for the dysarthric patient. Some postural adjustments include turning the patient's head to one side or supporting the neck with a collar or the trunk with overhead slings (all adjustments should have physician approval) (23). Muscle tone improvement can be achieved through medication, i.e., L-DOPA for parkinsonian rigidity, and relaxation exercises can improve posture as well as control of articulators subject to spasms. Continual medical management should be employed in order to keep each patient's general health at its best possible level.

Alteration in personality and behavioral reactions are often manifestations of disease. Special attention, therefore, should be given in the nursing home to the following:

1. Frequent complaints, irritability, agitation, and possible volatile behavior are common with dementia.
2. Perseveration is frequent in aphasic and demented patients.
3. Parkinson's disease can produce immobility of facial muscles that leads to unimpressive facial expression so often misunderstood as aloofness or lack of interest in conversation.
4. Emotional lability may at times accompany the dysarthric or confusion–disoriented patients.
5. Those with loss in memory capacity suffer attention deficits and are particularly vulnerable to interference in noisy settings, e.g., ambient noise produced by a constantly playing radio or television.
6. Most older people prefer a routine schedule with control over a familiar environment, as adjustment to change is often difficult.

7. When patient "wanders," attention span and reality orientation can be fostered through touching.
8. Communication boards or some type of signing may be needed for severely dysarthric or glossectomized patients.
9. Although contexual redundancy is usually beneficial for successful message comprehension, caution is needed to prevent sensory overload during discourse with a generalized intellectually impaired person.
10. Staff and family of the demented resident should conduct discussions concerning the resident in privacy since the severely impaired have intermittent bursts of comprehension.

ACKNOWLEDGMENTS

We are grateful to Tami Shimatsu for her patient and constructive assistance and to M. A. Whitcomb for review of the manuscript.

REFERENCES

1. Hull RH: Demography and characteristics of the communicatively impaired elderly in the United States. *Semin Speech Lang Hear* 1981;2:137–148.
2. Ordy JM, Brizzee KR, Beavers T, et al: Age differences in the functional and structural organization of the auditory system in man, in Ordy JM, Brizzee KR (eds): *Sensory Systems and Communication in the Elderly*. New York, Raven Press, 1979, p. 161.
3. Nadol JB: The aging peripheral hearing mechanisms, in Beasley DS, Davis GA (eds): *Aging: Communication Processes and Disorders*. New York, Grune & Stratton, 1981, pp 63–86.
4. Glorig A, Nixon J: Distributions of hearing loss in various populations. *Ann Otol Rhinol Laryngol* 1960;69:502.
5. Kopra LL: The auditory–communicative manifestations of presbycusis, in Hull RH (ed): *Rehabilitative Audiology*. New York, Grune & Stratton, 1982, pp 243–270.
6. Pickett JM, Bergman M, Levitt H: Aging and speech understanding, in Ordy JM, Brizzee KR (eds): *Sensory Systems and Communication in the Elderly*. New York, Raven Press, 1979, pp 167–186.
7. Pickett JM, Bergman M, Levitt H: Aging and speech understanding, in Ordy JM, Brizzee KR (eds): *Sensory Systems and Communication in the Elderly*. New York, Raven Press, 1979, p 170.
8. Lashley KS: The problem of serial order in behavior, in Jeffress LA (ed): *Cerebral Mechanisms in Behavior*. New York, John Wiley, 1951, pp 112–146.
9. Ordy JM, Brizzee K: Sensory coding: Sensation, perception, information processing and sensory–motor integraton from maturity to old age, in Ordy JM, Brizzee KR (eds): *Sensory Systems and Communication in the Elderly*. New York, Raven Press, 1979, pp 1–11.
10. Hutchinson JM, Beasley DS: Speech and language functioning among the aging, in Oyer HJ, Oyer EJ (eds): *Aging and Communication*. Baltimore, University Park Press, 1976, pp 155–174.
11. Kent RD, Burkard R: Changes in the acoustic correlates of speech production, in Beasley DS, Davis GA (eds): *Aging: Communication Processes and Disorders*. New York, Grune & Stratton, 1981, pp 47–62.
12. Meyerson MD, Shanks SJ: Voice disorders in adulthood, in Beasley DS, Davis GA (eds): *Aging: Communication Processes and Disorders*. New York, Grune & Stratton, 1981, pp 191–206.
13. Schow RL, Christensen JM, Hutchinson JM, et al: *Communication Disorders of the Aged: A Guide for Health Professionals*. Baltimore, University Park Press, 1978.

14. Kahane JC: Anatomic and physiologic changes in the aging peripheral speech mechanism in Beasley DS, Davis GA (eds): *Aging: Communication Processes and Disorders*. New York, Grune & Stratton, 1981, pp 21–46.
15. Davis GA, Holland AL: Age in understanding and treating aphasia, in Beasley DS, Davis GA (eds): *Aging: Communication Processes and Disorders*. New York, Grune & Stratton, 1981, pp 207–228.
16. Ordy JM, Brizzee KR, Beavers T, et al: Age differences in the functional and structural organization of the auditory system in man, in Ordy JM, Brizzee KR (eds): *Sensory Systems and Communication in the Elderly*. New York, Raven Press, 1979, pp 153–165.
17. Exton-Smith AN, Overstall PW: *Geriatrics: Guidelines in Medicine*. Baltimore, University Park Press, 1979.
18. Groher ME: Neurologically based disorders of speech and language among the older adults. *Semin Speech Lang Hear* 1981;2:149–156.
19. Rosenbek JC, LaPointe LL: Motor speech disorders and the aging process, in Beasley DS, Davis GA (eds): *Aging: Communication Processes and Disorders*. New York, Grune & Stratton, 1981, pp 159–174.
20. Timiras PS, Segall PE, Walker RF: Physiological aging in the central nervous system: Perspectives on 'interventive' gerontology, in Dietz AA, Marcum VS (eds): *Aging—Its Chemistry: Proceedings of the Third Arnold O. Beckman Conference in Clinical Chemistry*. Washington, DC, The American Association for Clinical Chemistry, 1979, pp 46–61.
21. Adams RD: Altered cerebrospinal fluid dynamics in relationship to dementia and aging, in Amaducci L, Davison AN, Piero A, (eds): *Aging of the Brain and Dementia*. New York, Raven Press, 1980, pp 217–225.
22. Galambos R: Maturation of auditory evoked potentials, in Chiarenza GA, Papakosto-poulous D (eds): *Clinical Application of Cerebral Evoked Potentials in Pediatric Medicine*. Amsterdam, Excerpta Medica, 1982, pp 323–343.
23. Wertz RT: Neuropathologies of speech and language: An introduction to patient management, in Johns DF (ed): *Clinical Management of Neurogenic Communicative Disorders*. Boston, Little, Brown, 1978, pp 1–102.

The Teaching Nursing Home, edited by Edward
L. Schneider et al. © 1985 The Beverly
Foundation. Raven Press, New York.

Mobility

Carol C. Hogue

Center for the Study of Aging and Human Development, Duke University, Durham, North Carolina 27710

This chapter will discuss the meaning of the concept of mobility and its significance for the health of the elderly, describe approaches to the measurement of mobility, and indicate sources of relevant data. A conceptual model of mobility will be offered to help guide care, enrich teaching, and stimulate research in the teaching nursing home (TNH).

MEANING

The term mobility, which generally means ability to move, also has many specialized meanings. For example, at the cellular level, mobility refers to the movement of ions across cell membranes. At the level of body parts, one can speak of the mobility of a joint, and at the level of the whole person, one can consider the movement needed for performance of activities of daily living. Additionally, beyond a person's immediate environment, mobility may refer to transportation; and from a sociological perspective, it may be related to moving from one geographical area to another or from one social status to another.

This chapter focuses on the mobility of whole persons in their immediate environments. Immobility as well as mobility is considered for two reasons. First, just as information about disease has often been used to describe health, most of the data related to mobility are in fact data about limitations of mobility. Secondly, although there is an emphasis on maintaining and enhancing mobility, this discussion also has implications for care, teaching, and research about persons with considerable immobility.

Several questions will help clarify the meaning of mobility used in this chapter. Is walking synonymous with mobility? On the surface, the concrete term "walking" has much shared meaning with the more abstract concept "mobility," but the two are not the same. A person in a wheelchair who is unable to walk may be more mobile than someone who walks only with assistance. For that very reason Linn and Linn (1) include in their revised Rapid Disability Rating Scale, the RDRS-2, a separate category called mobility, in addition to the category walking.

Is mobility an aspect of physical health? Assessment of gait is part of the neurological examination performed in a comprehensive assessment of physical health, but evaluation of mobility is not usually included in such an examination. Although there are many ways to evaluate physical health, the traditional history and physical examination are based on body systems and the presence of signs and symptoms indicating disease. Therefore, although mobility depends, in part, on physical health, it is not usually considered an aspect of physical health.

Is mobility an activity of daily living? We currently think of activities of daily living as bathing, dressing, using the toilet, eating, and so on. Mobility does not easily fit that scheme conceptually despite the fact that the National Nursing Home Survey included it as an activity of daily living (2) and some ADL scales include it. Leering suggested that mobility includes "bed activities, rising and standing, walking, or wheelchair management" (3, p. 315). If the focus is broadened from activities of daily living to functional health or physical functioning, which includes some of the more complex behaviors considered instrumental activities of daily living, then mobility more easily fits into that category.

Thus, in this chapter mobility is viewed as a dimension of functional health. This provides an orientation, if not a conceptual definition, for examining mobility issues of relevance to older people in both institutional and community settings. This is especially important because nursing home residents come from the population at large, and because over half of those admitted to nursing homes are discharged in less than 3 months (4) with an estimated 41% of the short stayers discharged to private residences, 24% to hospitals, and 13% to other health facilities (4).

SIGNIFICANCE

Maintenance of mobility is crucial for the health and well-being of the elderly in any setting. It may be more important in institutional settings because of environmental constraints and because of interaction with the factors that led to the institutionalization in the first place. Kane and Kane (5) note that "the most common problems seen in long-term care are immobility and falls, incontinence, and mental confusion."

Several decades ago, Dietrick (6) studied the biochemical and physiologic effects of prolonged immobilization on healthy, young, male volunteers. Subjects were immobilized in casts in bed for 6 weeks. A control period of similar length preceded the experimental treatment, and a recovery period of 4 to 6 weeks followed. A dramatic hypercalciuria and nitrogen loss were among the important findings of that study. At about the same time, Powers (7) surprised the medical community with his reports of clear benefits of early ambulation in a controlled study of 200 patients recovering from common abdominal or gynecological surgical procedures. Not only was the length of hospital stay and at-home recovery time less in experimental sub-

TABLE 1. *Consequences of limitations of mobility in the elderly*

Falls/fracture
Disuse osteoporosis/hypercalcemia
  Anorexia, malaise, nausea, vomiting, abdominal cramps, constipation, weight loss,
  lethargy
Joint stiffness/contractures
Muscular atrophy
  Thrombophlebitis/pulmonary embolus
Hypostatic pneumonia
Hypostatic edema of lower extremities
Decubitus ulcers
Urinary retention, incontinence
Insomnia
Depression
Confusion
Problems in instrumental activities of daily living

jects who moved about early, but the rate of complications in experimental subjects was only 17% as compared to 46% for those in the "usual treatment" (bed rest for 10–15 days) control group. Steinberg (8) has shown that "immobilization carries a morbidity of its own, which can be modified or ameliorated by appropriate management." Browse (9) described in detail the physiologic effects of assuming the supine position and especially of prolonged bed rest. Spencer, Vallbona, and Carter summarized the findings of empirical research on physiologic effects of immobilization (10).

In a study of the recovery of elderly patients with hip fracture, one of the findings was that patients who had been immobilized (for whatever reason) prior to hip fracture were more likely than other patients to suffer acute confusion postoperatively (11). The hazards of immobility for the elderly can also be inferred both from clinical observations of old people (12–15) and from findings of studies of younger persons (16).

Table 1 lists some of the consequences of limitations in mobility. Symptoms or problems may occur after a short period or after lengthy immobility. Several of the symptoms may arise by multiple pathways. For example, weight loss may be associated with hypercalcemia or depression or both. Medical treatment of some of the symptoms may lead to even more serious complications (17). For example, treating someone who is not eating by nasogastric intubation predisposes that person to aspiration pneumonia; treating a confused person with drugs increases the likelihood of falls and thrombophlebitis. Each of the symptoms or problems tends to lead to further immobility.

Immobility that is not interrupted decreases the likelihood of future self-care and performance of instrumental tasks, and increases dependency and need for medical care. The initial limitations in mobility are generally disease or trauma related, but they may be superimposed on varying degrees of biological decline associated with primary aging. Despite a certain amount of decrement associated with normal aging, the serious consequences of limitations in mobility are not inevitable. Filner and Williams (18) note that physical immobility and mental confusion are the chief determinants of functional dependence, that descent into dependency is not inevitable, and that dependency can often be prevented, reversed, or reduced.

Although all potential consequences of mobility limitations in the elderly are important, the problem of falls and, in particular, hip fracture bears special attention. Hogue has reviewed the epidemiology (19) of injury in late life and showed that injury is a leading cause of death in the elderly, that more than half the deaths resulting from injury in persons 65 and older are caused by falls, and that beyond consideration of mortality, the disability, dysfunction, and need for health services that results from falls is far greater than that experienced by younger people.

Persons with mobility limitations are at higher risk for falls than others. The mobility limitations may arise from characteristics thought to be associated with normal aging in late life, including diminished postural control, gait changes, muscular weakness, and decreased reflexes. They may accompany pathologic conditions such as parkinsonism, stroke, arthritis, amputation, or foot problems, or they may be secondary to treatment with pharmacologic agents, especially psychotropic, diuretic, and antihypertensive drugs. Those who fall once are more likely to fall again. Furthermore, old people who fall are more likely than young people to sustain fractures, a consequence of osteoporosis. Only a small proportion of people who fall incur hip fractures (although the incidence of hip fracture increases markedly in the fourth decade for women and about 20 years later for men). Nonetheless, the cumulative lifetime risk of hip fracture or pelvic fracture is 42% for women and 19.5% for men (20). The annual incidence of hip fracture in the United States is 98/100,000, well over 200,000 each year (18). Melton and Riggs estimate that among elderly patients, "at least half of those who could walk before sustaining a hip fracture cannot walk subsequently" (21). The economic costs of hip fracture are also sobering: in 1977 dollars, the annual hospital treatment costs of hip fracture are estimated to be a billion dollars (22).

As the significance of mobility in the elderly is considered, the devastating interaction of falls and immobility must not be neglected. Those with mobility limitations are more likely to fall; those who fall are more likely to fall again; and those who are most frail are at highest risk for fracture. Fractures nearly always limit the mobility of older persons and place them at risk for subsequent decline in functional status with such bed-rest-related problems as confusion, not eating, incontinence, and skin breakdown.

The great significance of mobility and mobility limitations makes these high priority for care, for teaching, and for research in the TNH setting. Indeed, the case has been made that health care providers in institutional settings have "a strong ethical and perhaps legal obligation" to practice primary preventive strategies aimed at minimizing immobility (23).

MEASUREMENT

The measurement of mobility depends on one's understanding of the concept and on what aspects are to be measured. The measured aspects, in turn, depend on the role of the user and the purpose or function of the measurement. Kane and Kane (5) discuss five functions of measurement in long-term care: description of populations, screening, assessment, monitoring, and prediction. They also note that what is appropriate for decision-making for clinical care of individuals is not likely to be appropriate for program planning for groups (5).

Measurement of mobility also depends on whether the technology is available to obtain the required information. This section identifies some available sources of data relevant to considerations of mobility, points to sources of measures of mobility for those who wish to make their own assessments, and offers a few comments on the development or selection of measures.

Survey data collected by the National Center for Health Statistics can be used for making inferences about several factors related to mobility. What proportion (and number) of people over 65 walk with crutches or require wheelchairs to get around? What is the prevalence of arthritis, and how many days of restricted activity are associated? What are the leading causes of activity limitation (or contributory chronic conditions) for persons of all ages and for persons 65 and over? Are rates of disability and restricted activity increasing? How many adults need assistance in one or more basic physical activities? How many adults need help with walking or with getting in or out of bed or chair? How do those rates differ for persons 65 to 74, 75 to 84, or 85 years and over?

All of these questions can be answered by consulting the first five data sources in Table 2. However, those data represent only the noninstitutionalized civilian U.S. population, and thus they exclude persons residing in nursing homes at the time of the data collection. Such data sources are included here because the nursing home population comes from (and in some instances, returns to) the noninstitutionalized population.

The main source of large-scale survey data on nursing home residents comes from the two National Nursing Home Surveys, the more recent in 1977. Table 2 indicates some of the mobility-related information included. The survey data also include much more information about characteristics of residents and about residents discharged, as well as staff, facilities, and financial matters. Unfortunately, there are no data sets that allow us to compare the mobility of nursing home residents with the mobility of the noninstitutionalized population. Furthermore, in considering the characteristics of nursing home residents, it is important to remember that "nursing residents are not an homogeneous block but fall into two distinct categories.

TABLE 2. *Selected data sources relevant to mobility/immobility*

Source	Relevant measures
Use of special aids Vital and Health Statistics: Series 10, No. 135, E. R. Black. DHHS Publication No (PHS) 81-1563. Washington, DC. U.S. Government Printing Office, 1980. Household interviews in 1977	A special aid is a device used to compensate for defects resulting from disease, injury, impairment, or congenital malformation. Included are artificial limbs, braces, crutches, canes or walking sticks, special shoes, wheelchairs, walkers, and any other kind of aid for getting around
Prevalence of chronic skin and musculoskeletal conditions Vital and Health Statistics: Series 10, No. 124, G. S. Bonhom, DHEW Publication No (PHS) 79-1552. Washington, DC. U.S. Government Printing Office, 1978. Household interviews in 1976	Arthritis, rheumatism, osteomyelitis, and other bone diseases, displaced intervertebral disk, bunions, synovitis, tenosynovitis, and gout: prevalence, impact, and characteristics of impaired
Health characteristics of persons with chronic activity limitation Vital and Health Statistics: Series 10, No 137, B. A. Feller. DHHS Publication No (PHS) 82-1565. Washington, DC. U.S. Government Printing Office, 1981. Household interviews in 1979	Impact of chronic conditions or impairments on activity
Disability days: United States, 1980 Vital and Health Statistics: Series 10, No. 143, C. S. Wilder. DHHS Publication No (PHS) 83-1571. Washington, DC. U.S. Government Printing Office, 1983. Household inverviews	"Disability" is temporary or long-term reduction of a person's activity as a result of an acute or chronic condition. A "restricted activity day" is one in which a person cuts down on his or her usual activities for the whole of that day because of an illness or injury. For retired or elderly, usual activities might consist of almost no activity, but cutting down on even a small amount for as much as a day would constitute restricted activity. Persons who have permanently reduced their usual activities because of a chronic condition might not report any restricted activity days during a 2-week period. Therefore, absence of restricted activity days does not imply normal health
Americans needing help to function at home National Center for Health Statistics, B. Feller. Advance Data from Vital and Health Statistics, No 92. DHHS Publication No (PHS) 83-1250. Public Health Service. Hyattsville, MD, 1983. Household interviews	Numbers and rates of persons needing help with walking, ADL, and IADL by age and sex and the kind of help they need. Valuable for estimating needs for home care

TABLE 2. *(continued)*

Source	Relevant measures
National Nursing Home Survey National Center for Health Statistics, J. Van Nostrand. Series 13, No 43, DHEW Pub No (PHS) 79-1794. Public Health Service. Hyattsville, MD, 1979. Two-stage random sample of nursing homes in 1977	An ADL scale (based on the work of Katz) that includes mobility. Mobility is categorized as "walks independently," "walks with assistance," "chairfast," or "bedfast." Assessments were made on cross sections of residents and at the time of discharge. Chronic conditions and impairments, primary diagnosis, and special aids are among the many variables included

One group generally comes from a hospital and consists of patients convalescing from an acute illness. These 'short-stayers' get well or die in a fairly short period of time. The other group consists of those, usually elderly, often with mental problems, who are no longer able to live outside institutions. Such 'long-stayers' usually stay a long time, perhaps the rest of their lives (4, p. 363)." Comparing discharges and residents, Keeler, Kane and Solomon have shown marked differences between the short-stayers and long-stayers. For example, the short-stayers are much more likely to be married, to be male, to have fractures, to have cancer, and to be bedfast (4, p. 366). This sort of information suggests caution in the use of nursing home data and it raises interesting clinical and research questions.

Kane and Kane (5) have systematically reviewed measures of activities of daily living or physical functioning appropriate for use in long-term care. In addition, in 1983, the National Institute on Aging sponsored a conference on assessment technology, bringing together participants with a variety of experience and perspectives on functional assessment. It can be noted that the measures reviewed by the Kanes include assessment of such items as transfer, mobility, walking, bed activities, locomotion, propelling wheelchair, and physical condition of lower limbs. Nearly all are components of multidimensional measures, appropriate because of the intercorrelations of the components of functional status.

There is much on-going work in this area of measurement (1, 24–27). The linking of quality of nursing home care to outcome measures, a project of the Kanes at the Rand Corporation, is particularly interesting. Activities of daily living comprise one of six domains measured by their instrument. Their ADL measure builds on the Barthel–Granger scale (28), which includes four-point ratings, from total dependence to total independence, on grooming, using the toilet, washing, feeding, walking, and wheelchair mobility. Performance is emphasized over capacity, using the Performance Test of Activities of Daily Living of Kuriansky and Gurland (29). Partial credit is given for performance requiring assistance.

In addition to multidimensional measures that include mobility, more sharply focused measures of gait and balance are available (30–32; M. Tinetti, *unpublished*, 1983). Some require instrumentation, and one, the Tinetti Mobility Scale, requires systematic observation of gait (9 items) and balance (8 items) using a rating scale (M. Tinetti, *unpublished*, 1983). Of course, many clinicians assess gait and balance as part of a neurological examination without an instrument or rating scale (33).

Although the available instruments for measuring mobility may be less than entirely satisfactory, Kane and Kane note that new instruments should be at least as good as those we already have. Kaufert reports an empirical study which showed that four measurement problems affect the validity of measures of mobility and activities of daily living: "assessing the impact of aids, adaptations, and helpers; controlling for situational variation and motivational factors; controlling for the professional perspective of the rater; and controlling for the role expectations of the patient in the performance of certain functions" (34). It is probably unrealistic to expect an instrument to be equally effective for the clinical assessment of mobility and for research purposes. Kane and Kane offer helpful criteria for assessment instruments: one set for clinical assessment and one for research and evaluation purposes (5).

A CONCEPTUAL MODEL

There are a variety of approaches to mobility, but most of them have not been guided by theory. This lack of theoretical foundation makes it difficult for us to appreciate what we know, to consider how to use what we know, and to plan cumulative research. The conceptual model described below has potential for organizing information relevant to the mobility of older people in long-term care settings. Even though the model is rudimentary and requires much more specification, it has heuristic value for administration, for clinical practice, for teaching, and for research. The model (see Fig. 1), which is an ecological model for the enhancement of functional health, is a variant of the familiar ecological equation:

$$B = f(P, E, P \times E)$$

That is, behavior is a function of the person, the environment, and the interaction of the person and the environment. The model was adapted from Moos (35), was substantially influenced by Lawton (36), and builds on work by Lawton and Nahemow (37) and Hogue (38,39).

The model proposes that the competence of older people and the resources of the environment influence each other (see chapter by L. Pastalan for further information on aging and the environment). Individuals potentially select the environments they wish to enter, and environments choose new members they wish to admit. In addition, the level of competence of individuals can influence all aspects of the environment. Each of us has a

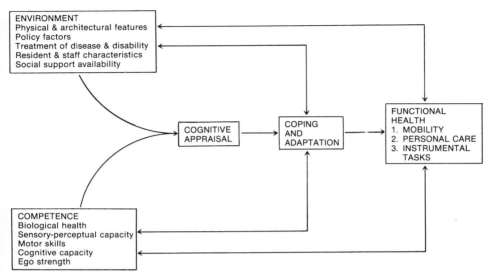

FIG. 1. An ecological model for the enhancement of mobility, personal care, and instrumental tasks in an institutional setting.

range of adaptive behavior that is influenced by personal abilities (competence) and by environmental press. Persons of high competence have a wide latitude of capacity to interact with the environment in ways that maximize adaptive behavior. On the other hand, persons with diminished competence may have maladaptive responses to relatively slight degrees of environmental press (39). For example, a frail elderly resident in a nursing home with parkinsonism (diminished motor skills) and impaired vision may slip on a puddle in a dimly lit hall and fall; a resident with better vision and gait will avoid the puddle and not fall. The first person has functioned outside her adaptive range, the second person within her range.

Lawton proposes that "lowered competence increases the proportion of behavioral variance that is associated with environmental, as compared to personal, factors" (36). Environmental factors and aspects of personal competence both influence cognitive appraisal or the way individuals perceive their environment. Cognitive appraisal, in turn, influences coping and adaptation, which ultimately influence functional health. Aspects of personal competence such as ego strength and environmental policies both can affect coping directly. Functional health is directly affected by biological health, by motor skills, and by the physical and architectural features of the environment. Functional health clearly has direct effects on biological health, and the functional health of individuals can have direct effects on the social climate and other features of the environment.

Depending on the disciplinary orientation and functional role of the user of the model, different variables can be expanded or developed. Furthermore, although the model is deliberately broad, there is no intention that any user study or apply all the classes of variables.

The environment in this model has five major domains of resources: physical and architectural features, policy factors, treatment of disease and disability, resident and staff characteristics, and availability of social support.

Physical and architectural features include features that aid residents in mobility and activities of daily living (prosthetic aids, orientational aids, safety features); physical features that add convenience and comfort and foster social and recreational activities; public and private space available to residents; physical features that make the setting more pleasant for staff; and physical integration of the facility with the surrounding community.

Policies can have important effects on elderly residents in nursing homes. Moos has noted that "some of the characteristics frequently observed among the elderly, such as feelings of depression and helplessness, may be attributable in part to the policies in such settings, especially the relative lack of environmental choice and control" (36, p. 80). Policies determine the balance that exists between individual freedom and institutional order and continuity.

Disease and disability treatment is closely related to the domain of policy. Critical considerations include the extent to which nursing and medical care are based on comprehensive functional assessment and on primary and secondary prevention of disability. What the clinical goals and preferred characteristics of residents are, the extent to which physical or chemical restraints are used, and whether prescribing patterns are sensitive to pharmacokinetics in the elderly are also important.

Resident and staff characteristics are included in the model because of research which has shown that people who have backgrounds and interests similar to those of the other people in their environment "tend to be more satisfied and secure and to function better in that environment" and because there is "evidence that a person's behavior and values may change over time to conform to those of the majority of the other people in a setting" (36). The activity level and functional health of residents as a group can influence those characteristics of individuals. Staffing levels, staff abilities, and stability are also part of what is sometimes called the suprapersonal environment.

Availability of social support, a class of variables sometimes called the personal environment, refers to one-to-one social relationships with family and friends, that is, the opportunities for social support.

Individual competence is defined in the model as the theoretical upper limit of capacity of the individual to function in the areas of biological health, sensation–perception, motor behavior, and cognition and ego strength.

Biological health refers to the absence of disease, to the condition of an individual portrayed by signs, symptoms, and laboratory tests of biological function, or to medical diagnoses. Biological health is different from functional health; functional health is a behavioral or performance outcome resulting from the interaction of personal and environmental factors. In other words, biological health and other aspects of personal competence are necessary but not sufficient for functional health. Recent fractures, moderate and severe cardiorespiratory disease, stroke, parkinsonism and other neurological disorders, articular and systemic rheumatic disorders, bone disease, and amputation all limit mobility. Because of the limited adaptive range of the elderly, acute illnesses that are considered minor in young people have the potential of limiting mobility among frail elderly persons and even leading to the downward spiral that can occur with bed rest. Clustering of illnesses, a common phenomenon among the frail elderly, has the potential for being particularly immobilizing.

Sensory–perceptual capacities include "the primary processes of vision, audition, olfaction, gustation, somesthesis, and kinesthesis as well as the more differentiated aspects of these senses such as depth perception, flicker fusion, or pain perception" (36).

Motor skills are clearly related to biological health and sensory–perceptual capacities, but they are of sufficient importance to the ability to use the environment and to functional health that the model shows a separate category for these skills. Neurological and muscular causes of impaired gait, either physiologic or pathologic, pain in the musculoskeletal system, and contracture of joints involved in ambulation all need to be investigated if a resident has a gait disorder.

Cognitive capacity refers to the presumed ability of the individual to comprehend, process, and cope with information from the environment.

Ego strength refers to another class of intraindividual factors that influence coping; these are relatively stable features such as self-concept and self-esteem.

The interaction variables in the model, cognitive appraisal and coping/adaptation, refer to the individual's perception of the environment as potentially harmful, beneficial, or irrelevant, the individual's perception of the range of available coping alternatives, and coping and adaptive responses. Quite a bit of promising research has been done on concepts in the interactive phase of the model, including perceived situational control, helplessness, and self-induced dependence (40–44).

Functional health is a set of behaviors that include mobility, personal care, and performance of instrumental tasks.

In discussing this model the emphasis has been on environmental factors over individual competence, not because they are important but because they may be amenable to changes not previously considered in relation to mobility, except in relation to falls, where the needs and opportunities for environmental interventions have been discussed (39).

It is our belief that this model has utility for administration, for clinical practice, and for teaching and research in several disciplines. It can help us keep in mind the "broad view," long-term goals, and the general relationships of factors that influence the functional health of residents. It can be used by interdisciplinary teams as a guide for making decisions on ethical issues, for thinking through assessment issues, for addressing staffing concerns from the standpoint of needs suggested by the model, and for appreciating residents' perspectives of their situation. For researchers, the model highlights broad areas in need of study. There are instruments available for operationalizing and measuring many of the variables in the model. For example, Moos and his associates have developed instruments to assess the physical and architectural features of residential settings (45), to assess the institutional policies of sheltered care settings (46), and to assess the suprapersonal environment (resident and staff characteristics) of nursing home settings (47). A variety of measures of social support are available (48); the Tinetti Mobility Scale is an example of an appropriate measure of physical skills (M. Tinetti, *unpublished*, 1983); and Hogue has developed an instrument, the FRAIL Scale (Falls Risk And Injury Likelihood Scale), that takes into account biological health and motor skills (C. C. Hogue, *unpublished*, 1982).

CONCLUSION

The downward spiral that can occur as a consequence of immobility is reversible. Even for those whose mobility is already impaired, the rate of further decline, the incidence of consequent impairment, may be minimized or decreased substantially through early detection and appropriate intervention. As the ecological model suggests, there is a need to consider comprehensive assessment of total persons in their environment, not merely their gait and balance. For example, correcting a problem of cardiac output or enhancing perceived social support could lead to increased mobility.

Furthermore, several research efforts are needed. Computerized bibliographies and inventories of research on mobility and related concepts would be useful to investigators needing access to empirical and theoretical literature, which is presently widely dispersed. Refinement of the measures of mobility is needed, as are descriptions of biological, psychological, and social processes that can enhance mobility and controlled studies to test the effectiveness of supportive interventions. The TNH is an ideal setting for such clinical research, and residents, staff, faculty, and students all stand to benefit from the synergy between research and clinical practice in long-term care.

REFERENCES

1. Linn MW, Linn BS: The rapid disability rating scale—2. *J Am Geriatr Soc* 1982;30:378–382.
2. National Center for Health Statistics: *The National Nursing Home Survey: 1977 Summary for the United States.* Vital and Health Statistics. Series 13, No. 43. DHEW publication No. (PHS) 79-1794, Public Health Service. Washington, DC, US Government Printing Office, 1979, p 136.
3. Leering C: A structural model for functional capacity in the aged. *J Am Geriatr Soc* 1979;27:314–316.
4. Keeler EB, Kane RL, Solomon DH: Short- and long-term residents of nursing homes. *Med Care* 1981;19:363–369.
5. Kane RA, Kane RL: *Assessing the Elderly.* Lexington, MA, Lexington Books, 1981.
6. Dietrick JE, Whedon GD, Shorr E: Effects of immobilization upon various metabolic and physiologic functions of normal men. *Am J Med* 1948;4:3–36.
7. Powers JH: The abuse of rest as a therapeutic measure in surgery. *JAMA* 1944;125:1079–1083.
8. Steinberg FV: *The Immobilized Patient.* New York, Plenum Press, 1980.
9. Browse NL: *The Physiology and Pathology of Bed Rest.* Springfield, IL, Charles C Thomas, 1965.
10. Spencer, WA, Vallbona C, Carter RE: Physiologic concepts of immobilization. *Arch Phys Med Rehab* 1965;46:89–100.
11. Williams MA, Holloway JR, Winn MC, et al: Nursing activities and acute confusional states in elderly hip-fractured patients. *Nurs Res* 1979;28:25–35.
12. Miller MB: Iatrogenic and nurisgenic effects of prolonged immobilization of the ill aged. *J Am Geriatr Soc* 1975;23:360–369.
13. Steinberg FU (ed): *Care of the Geriatric Patient.* St Louis, CV Mosby, 1983.
14. Libow LS, Sherman FT (eds): *The Core of Geriatric Medicine.* St Louis, CV Mosby, 1981.
15. Anderson WF, Caird FI, Kennedy RD, et al: *Gerontology and Geriatric Nursing.* New York, Arco, 1982.
16. Goldman R: Rest: Its use and abuse in the aged. *J Am Geriatr Soc* 1977;25:433–438.
17. Gillick MR, Serrell NA, Gillick LS: Adverse consequences of hospitalization in the elderly. *Soc Sci Med* 1982;16:1033–1038.
18. Filner B, Williams TE: Health promotion for the elderly. Reducing functional dependency, in Sommers AR, Fabian DR (eds): *The Geriatric Imperative: An Introduction to Gerontology and Clinical Geriatrics.* St Louis, CV Mosby, 1981, pp 127–168.
19. Hogue CC: Injury in late life: Epidemiology. *J Am Geriatr Soc* 1982;30:183–190.
20. Melton LJ, Riggs BL: Epidemiology of age-related fractures, in Avioli LV: *The Osteoporotic Syndrome.* New York, Grune & Stratton, 1983, pp. 45–72.
21. Lewinnek GE, Kelsey J, White AH, III, et al: The significance and a comparative analysis of the epidemiology of hip fractures. *Clin Orthoped* 1980;152:35–43.
22. Owen RA, Melton LJ III, et al: The national cost of acute care of hip fractures associated with osteoporosis. *Clin Orthoped* 1980'152:172–176.
23. Craig TJ: Ethical aspects of primary preventive measures among the institutionalized elderly. *J Am Geriatr Soc* 1982;30:175–176.
24. Cairl RE, Pfeiffer E, Keller, DM, et al: An evaluation of the reliability and validity of the Functional Assessment Inventory. *J Am Geriatr Soc* 1983;31:607–612.
25. Pfeffer RI, Kurosaki TT, Harrah CH, Jr, et al: Measurement of functional activities in older adults in the community. *J Gerontol* 1982;37:323–329.
26. Chappell NS: Measuring functional ability and chronic health conditions among the elderly: A research note on the adequacy of three instruments. *J Health Soc Behav* 1981;22:90–102.
27. Kane RL, Bell R, Riegler S, et al: Assessing the outcomes of nursing-home patients. *J Gerontol* 1983;38:385–393.
28. Granger CV, Greer DS: Functional status measurement and medical rehabilitation outcomes. *Arch Phys Med Rehabil* 1976;57:103–109.
29. Kuriansky J, Gurland B: Performance test of activities of daily living. *Int J Aging Hum Dev* 1976;7:343–352.

30. Nayak USL, Gabell A, Simmons MA, et al: Measurement of gait and balance in the elderly. *J Am Geriatr Soc* 1982;30:516–520.
31. Imms FJ, Edholm OG: The assessment of gait and mobility in the elderly. *Age Aging* 1979;8(Suppl):261–267.
32. Imms FJ, Edholm OG: Studies of gait and mobility in the elderly. *Age Aging* 1981;10:147–156.
33. Sabin TD: Biologic aspects of falls and mobility limitations in the elderly. *J Am Geriatr Soc* 1982;30:51–58.
34. Kaufert JM: Functional ability indices: Measurement problems in assessing their validity. *Arch Phys Med Rehab* 1983;64:260–267.
35. Moos RH: Specialized living environments for older people. A conceptual framework for evaluation. *J Soc Issues* 1980;36:75–94.
36. Lawton MP: Competence, environmental press, and the adaptation of older people, in: Lawton MP, Windley PG, Byerts TO (eds): *Aging and the Environment.* New York, Springer, 1982, pp 33–59.
37. Lawton MP, Nahemow L: Ecology and the aging process, in: Eisdorfer C, Lawton MP (eds): *The Psychology of Adult Development and Aging.* Washington, American Psychological Association, 1973, 619–674.
38. Hogue CC: Epidemiology of injury in older age, in: Haynes SG, Feinleib M (eds): *Epidemiology of Aging.* Bethesda, National Institutes of Health, 1980, pp 127–135.
39. Hogue CC: Injury in late life: Prevention. *J Am Geriatr Soc* 1982;30:276–280.
40. Seligman MEP: *Helplessness: On Depression, Development, and Death.* San Francisco, WH Freeman, 1975.
41. Langer EJ, Rodin J: The effects of choice and enhanced personal responsibility for the aged: A field experiment in an institutional setting. *J Pers Soc Psychol* 1976;34:191–198.
42. Schulz R: The effects of control and predictability on the psychological and physical well-being of the institutionalized aged. *J Pers Soc Psychol* 1976;33:563–573.
43. Chang BL: Perceived situational control of daily activities: A new tool. *Res Nurs Health* 1978;1:181–188.
44. Avorn J, Langer E: Induced disability in nursing home patients: A controlled trial. *J Am Geriatr Soc* 1981;30:397–400.
45. Moos RH, Lemke S: Assessing the physical and architectural features of sheltered care settings. *J Gerontol* 1980;35:571–583.
46. Lemake S, Moos RH: Assessing the institutional policies of sheltered care settings. *J Gerontol* 1980;35:96–107.
47. Lemke S, Moos RH: The suprapersonal environments of sheltered care settings. *J Gerontol* 1981;36:233–243.
48. Hogue CC: Social support, in Hall JE, Weaver BR (eds): *Distributive Nursing Practice,* 2nd ed. Philadelphia, Lippincott, 1984.

The Teaching Nursing Home, edited by Edward
L. Schneider et al. © 1985 The Beverly
Foundation. Raven Press, New York.

The Physical Environment and the Emerging Nature of the Extended-Care Model

Leon A. Pastalan

Department of Architecture, University of Michigan, Ann Arbor, Michigan 48109

Extended care or long-term care as an institutional response to health care needs has had a very short history. The modern concept of extended care goes back to 1965 with the passage of Medicaid and Medicare legislation. Medicaid and Medicare firmly established the medical nature of the extended-care concept, and passage of these acts was instrumental in helping to legitimize the extended-care facility as an integral part of the medical care delivery system. Just as the modern-day nursing home emerged from its past, it is reasonable to expect that its form will continue to evolve as societal needs and conditions change.

A major force for change in residential and extended care is the growing recognition that the traditional medical model is not sufficient in and of itself to respond to all of the needs of the persons receiving such care. The residential nature of extended care in the future will be given a new emphasis, since there is an increasing awareness that the person is only a patient for part of the time but is a resident all of the time and that a number of issues that currently are viewed as medical are, in reality, residential in nature.

Designing solutions for the physical environment cannot be done effectively without also considering the nature of the individual interacting with it. Each person has a past set of experiences and knowledge that he/she uses in interaction with the environment. Furthermore, even though basic human needs remain fairly constant across the life-span, the appropriate means of meeting these needs tend to vary with advancing human age. Consideration of such matters as familiarity with the environment, expectations about it, and the likelihood that both the individual and environment will be undergoing a process of change over time are important considerations. The heterogeneity of the elderly population cannot be forgotten. Those over 65 differ widely in terms of age, sex, social status, psychological well-being, health, and functional status. It must be recognized that the key factor is not aging per se but age-related sensory, cognitive, or physical deficits.

A PARADIGM MATCHING CAPACITY WITH DEMAND

A basic premise underlying the study of aging and environmental inter-action is the importance of matching the demands of the physical environ-ment with the competence level of the individual. The goal is to assist in-dividuals in helping to modify the environment so that it is maximally supportive. The concept of matching demand with competence ranges across the life-span continuum and includes a consideration of physical and developmental disabilities as well as different dwelling unit levels. In addi-tion to incorporating the changes that are generally, but not inevitably, experienced by all individuals as they develop from infancy to old age, this paradigm also incorporates those problems related to physical and devel-opmental disabilities experienced either temporarily or permanently by a subset of the total population. This approach avoids the narrow limitations that are usually present in dealing with the needs of special populations such as the elderly, the physically disabled, or the developmentally disad-vantaged. Furthermore, it obviates the necessity of trying to justify the im-portance of each problem group and places all of these groups within the context of normal expectations of the human condition.

What is proposed here is an approach that will enhance the relevance of architectural design by taking into account certain psychosocial and phys-iological facts of life. Although there are significant variations, it is generally true that an 80-year-old person cannot handle the same level of environ-mental complexity as a 25-year-old. There is a need to identify how the environment can be designed to compensate for age-related limitations and conditions. For example, sensory or cognitive deterioration may necessitate a different order of stimulus intensification and orchestration. One's posi-tion on the life-span continuum can be expected to affect the types and amount of spaces needed. The level of mastery in terms of competence *vis à vis* an environmental demand such as getting to a dining area can be integrated by design. Since nursing home residents spend most of their days within their rooms or immediate surroundings, serious thought must be given to what needs to be compensated for in the total environment because of these limitations.

Organizing Principles

The environment can be viewed as a language. The messages that the environment conveys have salience only to the extent that the message can be perceived, processed, and responded to meaningfully. If for some reason the message cannot be clearly perceived, then the response will tend to be incomplete or inappropriate. Because very elderly patients are likely to have suffered from sensory and health-related decrements both mental and physical, their ability to function optimally may be compromised. The following design concepts are an attempt to structure the environment so that this special population can function as independently as it possibly can.

Organized Space as Orientation

Organized space as orientation is a design concept that seeks to organize spaces for predictive value. The idea is that, in general, a space should have a singular and unambiguous definition and use. The concept has several important dimensions. In terms of orientation, the spaces are cued with landmarks that act as focal points for functionally different spaces: color-coded surfaces to signal functionally different spaces in terms of visual perception; textured surfaces for the tactile; a series of distinct smells for olfaction, etc. The purpose is to sensorily load the spaces so they may more effectively serve as points of reference.

Another dimension of this concept is to organize spaces around three distinct spatial sets: personal, social, and public. Spaces that denote private uses for sleeping, certain medical procedures, toilet activities, plus other activities such as reading, thinking, letter writing, or simple withdrawing from others to be or do things alone should be distinctly bounded. Spaces for social and public uses should be similarly treated. These spatial sets with distinct boundaries not only provide options for the different functions at any given time but also signal the appropriate uses of each set and provide a contextual relationship between and among these sets.

Organized Space as Mastery

Organized space as mastery is a concept with at least two important dimensions. The first has to do with designing spaces that assist individuals with reduced abilities to claim and defend such spaces as their own inviolate spheres. The goal is to make it as difficult as possible for staff or fellow patients who may be aggressive to assert a form of spatial deprivation among the resident population.

The other dimension has to do with scale and mastery. Scale in this case refers to size in terms of numbers (people) and size in terms of spatial dimensions. A major premise of this theory is that with advanced age and associated sensory and cognitive deficits, an individual's world shrinks so that over time one's ability or energy to master relationships with larger numbers of people and/or larger or more complex spaces tends to decrease. Thus, the amount of interaction a given space encourages in a particular setting and its spatial dimensions have a great deal to do with the type or category of resident status with which one is concerned.

The last statement emphasizes the utility of these design concepts in linking appropriate spatial arrangements with a given type of resident status.

As one moves across the continuum from independence to dependence, the more crucial the concepts become. The applicability of these concepts ranges from the smaller, personal level of the dwelling and/or nursing unit to the larger level of the entire facility.

EXAMPLES OF ENVIRONMENTAL INTERVENTIONS

Kane and Kane point out that among the most common problems encountered in long-term care situations are mental confusion, incontinence, falls, and immobility (1). Three of these problems (mental confusion, falls, and immobility) can and have benefited from the application of the above concepts. I shall use two examples from my work—the empathic model and preparation for relocation—for purposes of illustration.

Empathic Model

The empathic model is a technique that simulates age-related sensory losses. It is made up of an assortment of appliances that simulate the visual, auditory, and tactile sensitivity of a person in his/her late 70s or early 80s. Although the simulation is relatively crude, it does provide the first extension of personal experience to observations that can be repeated by others and verified. Over time, these observations can be validated and generalizations made about them (2).

Figures 1A and 2A illustrate how a person with intact sensory perception functions as compared to a person with age-related visual deficits (Figs. 1B and 2B) viewing the same environmental settings.

One architectural firm in Southfield, Michigan used the empathic model to aid in the design of a retirement community. All members of the firm on this project used the model extensively to develop personal empathy and to gather data. It was also used as a cross-validation tool in the programming and design phases. This direct experience with the model under a variety of conditions gave the design team a group cohesion during critical stages of the design process and a means of testing their conceptions during the progression from observations to programming to schematics to working drawings.

The resulting final design for the retirement community took into account the sensory deficits of elderly persons by improving sensory input with lighting, color, texture, and sound. Compensation for the reduced sensitivity of elderly residents to sensory stimuli was provided through redundant cuing of environmental messages.

An orderly hierarchy of personal, social, and public spatial zones was established. Spaces were cued with landmarks or focal points to facilitate orientation and were designed to have singular, unambiguous definition and use. Buildings were scaled and organized to compensate for hypothesized decreases in the elderly residents' ability to deal with large numbers of people and complex spaces.

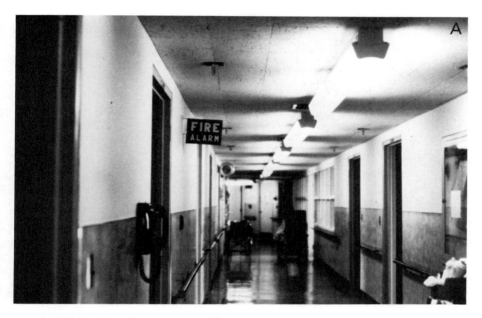

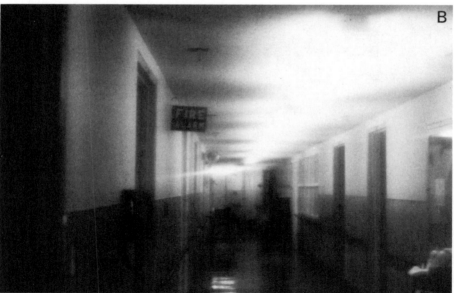

FIG. 1. Scene of a typical institutional corridor as seen (**A**) by a person with normal vision and (**B**) by a person with a visual deficit.

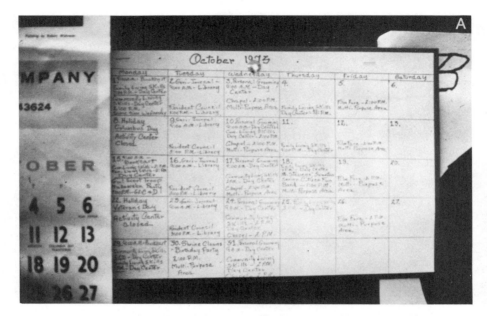

FIG. 2. Posted schedule of events as seen (**A**) by a person with normal vision and (**B**) by a person with a visual deficit.

A follow-up evaluation of the effectiveness of these environmental interventions indicated that mobility was increased as evidenced by an increase in appropriate social behavior. There were also fewer falls by the residents after they moved into the treated residential areas.

The model has proven to be a very powerful training tool for designers and others who work with physically vulnerable people, and it provides a link between researchers and designers. It has been used extensively with planning and design professionals, educators, social services personnel, housing managers, and community service personnel such as firefighters, police, and telephone operators who frequently deal with the elderly in emergency situations. Graduate students from a large number of disciplines have also worked with the model (3).

In addition to its use in training, this model has considerable potential for the field testing of design concepts. It also offers wide-ranging opportunities for research on the effects of visual impairment on the performance and well-being of both old and young people.

Preparation for Relocation

Forced relocation, which involves an involuntary move from one setting to another, has been a matter of concern for a long time. Two major questions emerge from the speculated negative effects of involuntary relocation of the elderly, particularly of frail, elderly patients in nursing homes. Do all older people under all conditions experience negative consequences following a move, or are certain types of individuals more susceptible to a move under certain conditions? What, if anything, can be done to facilitate adjustment to a new setting and reduce the potential "transplantation shock"?

Attempts to better understand how and why relocation affects elderly nursing home patients have revealed the importance of familiarizing them with the new setting prior to their move. Previous research has demonstrated that those patients who had participated in a preparation program had the lowest mortality rates (4). The heart of the preparation program was a series of purposeful site visits during which patients were familiarized with the spatial layout of important functional areas and with the social, medical, and other supportive services offered at the new facility. Hence, when the transfer is made, the patients will be adequately oriented in locational terms, i.e., they will know where their room is in relation to other important spaces in the facility They will have established this point of reference, and they will know the staff and be familiar with the various therapy and recreational programs. In sum, such patients will have a working knowledge of the new environment by the time they move in to stay.

Table 1 shows the relationship between the preparation for relocation and patient outcomes. Despite the life-saving value demonstrated by this ori-

TABLE 1. *Preparation for relocation: site visits and mortality by age, prognosis, and mental status*

Site visits	Died (%)	Survived (%)
Age		
≤65 Only one person died within this group (*N* = 54)		
66–80[a]		
No[b]	22 (19)	78 (69)
Yes[c]	5 (2)	95 (41)
81 +		
No	34 (52)	66 (99)
Yes	22 (8)	78 (28)
Prognosis		
Poor		
No	35 (41)	65 (76)
Yes	24 (04)	76 (17)
Fair[d]		
No	23 (25)	77 (86)
Yes	08 (03)	92 (34)
Excellent		
No	04 (01)	96 (22)
Yes	06 (02)	94 (30)
Mental status		
Confused[a]		
No	32 (58)	68 (126)
Yes	05 (02)	95 (38)
Alert		
No	15 (12)	85 (66)
Yes	14 (08)	86 (50)

[a] $p < 0.001$ by chi-square test.
[b] Patients did not visit site.
[c] Patients went on site visits.
[d] $p < 0.05$ by chi-square test.
From Pastalan et al. (4), with permission.

entation program, those patients of advanced age, poor prognosis, and confused mental status did less well than younger, healthier patients (4).

MENTAL CONFUSION AND THE PHYSICAL ENVIRONMENT

The purpose in citing the above examples is to emphasize that the physical environment does play an important role in the extended-care arena. There is another area in which the physical environment can play an even more important role. Mentally confused patients are rapidly becoming the most common type of patient found in an extended-care setting. How the physical environment can act to improve the quality of life of the mentally confused patient and improve the effectiveness and morale of the staff are addressed in the next part of this chapter.

Mental confusion among elderly nursing home patients has been dealt with in the literature primarily from a biomedical and/or psychosocial perspective. There has been very little in the literature about the degree to which confused behavior represents adjustments to a distressing environment as opposed to inherent cognitive incompetence.

Psychiatrists have long recognized that in practice no sharp line can be drawn among the elderly between so-called senile dementia (confusional states) and the cognitively normal. The one may merge imperceptibly with the other, and the diagnosis may be made on behavioral more than on other grounds. Broadly speaking, if the aged individual fits into the customary surroundings, he/she is usually considered to be "normal."

STAFF AND PATIENT PERSPECTIVES REGARDING MENTAL CONFUSION

From a patient perspective, cognitively intact patients and their families are disturbed by loud, incoherent talk, night wandering or night disturbance, as well as daytime wandering and disturbance, interference with other people's property, aggressive or violent behavior, and offensive eating, dress, or toilet habits. This disturbance is manifested by nonacceptance of the confused patient by the cognitively intact residents in such things as conversational patterns, communal activities, and friendship relations. In many cases, there is an overt defensiveness and rejection of the confused patient.

From a staff and programming perspective, the residential life of the confused patient is restricted. For instance, they are frequently given little choice as to what they will wear each day, little choice about bedtime or meal time, and are given few opportunities to help staff with small jobs. Additionally, recreational activities are highly monitored and limited, and little encouragement is given for self-care such as bathing. All in all, staff exhibits what many times may seem like overprotectiveness. It is possible that such tight supervision might reflect an overreaction to the alleged incapacities of the mentally confused person. Tight supervision or control is typically effected by physical constraints such as "geri" chairs, isolation, medication (drugs), physical force, ridicule, fear, and authority.

The above description depicts a situation in which the social and psychological fabric of the community is in a process of daily disintegration, and behavioral contagion is constantly in danger of veering out of control. The staff is in a perpetual state of suppressing the contagion with further restrictive measures at the same time that both confused and intact patients face a bewildering overload of stimulation and unpleasant surroundings. Clearly, bold new approaches are needed.

Optimum Stimulation Hypothesis

There is a literature in child development dealing with the *optimum stimulation hypothesis*, which has two specific predictions associated with it. The first is called the "preference" prediction, which states that organisms will prefer or approach an optimum level of stimulation. Optimum level is typically defined as a moderate degree of discrepancy between the organism's stimulus adaptation level and the complexity of the stimulus. The second is called the "enhancement" prediction, which states that a maximal level of functioning will be achieved if the individual is presented with stimulation optimally discrepant from the individual's own cognitive level or stimulus-processing ability (5). There are important similarities and differences in considering the applicability of the optimum stimulation hypothesis for the functional maintenance and growth of older adults, especially older adults with diminishing capacities. The optimum stimulation hypothesis has significant implications for extended care and should be evaluated among the elderly.

Levels of Stimulation

Let us start with the assumption that the individual functions optimally within a certain range of environmental conditions and, more particularly, of values of stimulation contained within the environment. We are referring here not only to properties of the environment, such as temperature and humidity, which exert a direct effect on physiological processes, but also to dimensions of the stimulus environment to which the individual responds primarily through the excitation of sensory receptor mechanisms, transmitting information to the higher neural centers. There are two important consequences of this assumption.

The first is that it is possible to view environmental stressors at the behavioral level as acting in a manner similar to physiological stressors, i.e., as exceeding the limits of tolerance for that individual. Second, just as physiological equilibria may be disturbed by deviations in either direction (e.g., extreme hot or extreme cold), so psychological stressors may likewise involve departures from some mode in the direction of either over- or understimulation. This is an important point, since in the past psychologists have been inclined to view the role of stimulation in the development and maintenance of behavior primarily from a "the-more-the-better" perspective. Both the animal research and the voluminous human literature on the effects of sensory deprivation have given dramatic evidence of the deleterious effects on behavior of marked reduction in the amount of stimulation present in an individual's environment. Very little attention, however, has been given to the effects of hyperstimulating conditions on behavior, and the possibility that such conditions may likewise exert adverse effects on behavior has not been seriously examined except for certain intensive variables of stimulation such as noise level or shock (6,7).

This is puzzling, since behavior theorists have increasingly invoked the concept of an optimum level of stimulation as essential to the maintenance of arousal and thus to maximally effective performance or to maximization of positive affect. Yet the limited evidence in support of such an optimization notion is based entirely on research on preference responses, ratings of liking, and similar measures. Extensions to possible impairment of performance or to deleterious effects on mental health have occasionally been suggested but rarely if ever have been put to an empirical test. The proposition that stress can result from either hyper- or hypostimulating conditions is consonant with the "sensoristasis" concept advanced by Schultz (8). In explicating this concept, Shultz draws an analogy to Canon's homeostasis concept and explicitly considers increases of stimulation beyond the optimal level as disturbing the internal balance and disrupting behavior. Further, he cites Lindsley's analysis of the role of the reticular formation, postulating similar effects of sensory restriction and sensory overload (9). Whereas the reference to Lindsley's model reinforces the plausibility of a comparable conception of hyper- and hypostimulation effects, it does not preclude the possibility—indeed, the strong likelihood—that the overt behavioral manifestations may be quite different in the two cases, just as bodily reactions to extreme heat and extreme cold take very different forms. It will therefore be essential to maintain the distinction between hyper- and hypostimulation in the search for possible similarities in the individual's general mode of response and adaptation to them (5).

MAIN VARIETIES OF HYPO- AND HYPERSTIMULATION

Three kinds of hypostimulation may be distinguished from Wolhwill's work: deprivation of sensory stimulation, of social interaction, and of movement (7).

Deprivation of Sensory Stimulation

Deprivation of sensory stimulation is the condition on which most of the experimental research has concentrated, inspired in large measure by the emphasis that Hebb has placed on a constant influx of stimulation as essential to the maintenance of behavior and by the dramatic effects of sensory deprivation that the pioneering work originating in the McGill laboratories under Hebb's auspices demonstrated. It typically involves the elimination of all potential sources of stimulus input across some or all sensory modalities.

Isolation (Deprivation of Social Interaction)

The stimulation provided by interaction and communication with other human beings is clearly of a special sort and deserves to be treated as separate from sensory deprivation. Most probably, the distinctive feature of social stimuli is the fact that they provide feedback to the individual's responses and perhaps, as a consequence, arouse an affect of a sort that the world of inanimate stimuli would be incapable of providing.

Confinement (Deprivation or Restriction of Movement)

Confinement represents yet a different form of hypostimulation; most likely, it owes its distinctiveness to the role of stimulation from the proprioceptors in maintaining posture and arousal. It is typically found in conjunction with either sensory or social deprivation or both, as in the case of a bed-bound patient in an extended-care facility who may be experiencing sensory deficits.

Sensory Overload

In sharp contrast to the topic of sensory deprivation, the effects of a hyperstimulating environment, that is, of very high levels of stimulation, on the individual have received virtually no attention on the part of psychologists except within the very restricted realm of the effects of noise, which can hardly be considered to represent the counterpart at the hyperstimulation pole of the sensory deprivation condition. Precisely what "overstimulation" may mean is more fully discussed below. In the meantime, the use of the prefixes "hyper-" and "over-" may be begging the question if anything more than a condition characterized by relatively large amounts of stimulus input is intended. Whether extreme amounts of stimulation will necessarily produce negative effects on behavior remains to be determined, of course. But the relevance of the problem for an understanding of the conditions of human existence in extended-care settings should be apparent.

One particular aspect of this concept must be noted here, since it relates to an important semantic distinction, that between sensory and information overload. This distinction concerns the question of whether the stimuli impinging on the individual do so merely in the sense of passive exposure or whether they contain information that require the individual to respond in a certain way. Therefore, it seems advisable to designate the upper end as "sensory overstimulation," given that the prefix "over-" is intended as merely descriptive, and to reserve the term "overload" to situations in which the individual must process information carried by the stimuli impinging on him/her.

It is useful to add one further category called "hyperdynamic." If restriction of movement can be considered "hypodynamic," then a condition reached by an inordinate amount of physical movement such as compulsive wandering can be considered hyperdynamic.

ADAPTATION LEVELS AND ENVIRONMENTAL INTERVENTION

Levels or zones of stimulation along particular dimensions that are maximally preferred, or otherwise optimal, should vary considerably from one person to the next depending on the adaptation level that has been established for that dimension. Behavioral adaptation to the environment is not a passive process but depends on a complex of interacting factors. For instance, the individual cannot respond continually to stimuli or aspects of his or her milieu of stimulation that are a constant feature of that environment with the intensity or magnitude of affective arousal he or she exhibits during the initial confrontation with that environment. It is essential that neutralization of affect occur, at least with respect to negatively experienced aspects of the stimulus environment over which the individual exerts little or no control.

Providing such control must start with the restructuring of the physical arrangements of the facility. One of the essential functions of this spatial reconfiguration must be to provide a basic element of control. From a staff perspective, such control will help to contain certain types of patient behavioral contagion such as wandering or loud, meaningless, and repetitive oration.

Control from a resident perspective would allow the individual to regulate the amount and kind of stimulation, a jurisdictional control over who penetrates his or her space, and a spatial arrangement that will facilitate privacy, sociability, and therapeutic activity (Fig. 3).

SPATIAL ORGANIZATION

The specific configuration of the spatial envelopes will vary from facility to facility and between floors or wings within a single facility. The design concepts cited above, namely, treating space as a language together with organizing space as a function of orientation and of mastery both in terms of jurisdictional control and of capacity levels, should serve as organizing principles.

Most extended-care facilities are based on the corridor concept (Fig. 4). Although the corridor provides a good movement system for linking rooms to the main circulation network, it represents in fact a street function and as such does not provide a context for neighboring or other forms of social interaction. This causes confusion and conflict in space use, since it is used not only as a through connecting link (public use) but also as a place to stop and chat with friends and neighbors (social use).

The psychological impact of the corridor arrangement is similar to that of leaving one's living room and stepping out to the street. What is needed is a spatial arrangement that buffers one's personal space from public space, that is, one that can provide a transition from personal activities to public activities and back again. This arrangement (as illustrated in Figs. 5 and 6) would also provide the resident with greater autonomy as well as providing staff with more assistance in the delivery of programs through greater access and control.

When the spatial zones that are required to meet the behavioral needs of the residents are applied to the next logical step, the relationship between units, the cluster layout satisfies the need for the semiprivate or semipublic

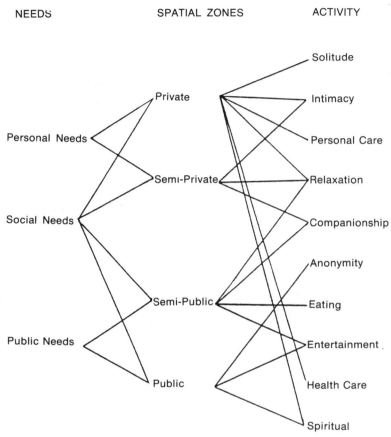

FIG. 3. Relationship of resident/patient needs, spatial zones, and activity. The spatial zones needed to satisfy personal needs are private and semiprivate. The behavioral response linked to a private space zone is solitude or the desire to withdraw from others and be alone. Intimacy means that one can opt to interact in privacy with members of one's family or close friends. Other kinds of behaviors within the private spatial zones are personal care such as toilet activities or bathing, relaxation such as television watching or reading, and health care, involving various medical or nursing procedures, which typically require physical privacy. As one follows the connecting lines from left to right, from needs to spatial zones to activity, the relationships become readily apparent. This chart can serve as a summary of the complex relationships that exist in conceptualizing appropriate support systems for any aging person as well as appropriate intervening support systems as a person continues to age.

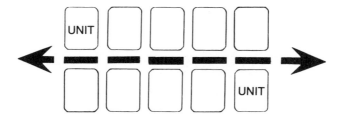

FIG. 4. Typical corridor arrangement.

zone between the individual unit and the corridor. By providing a common space accessible to all units in a cluster, a space is provided for social interaction, which may, over time, develop the cluster into a cohesive social unit.

Using the three spatial sets (personal, social, and public) in this way also provides an orientation function for the resident by virtue of the distinct uses and direct and proximate relationship to each other. By linking a group of clusters together, another common space accessible to each cluster can be provided to meet the needs of a larger group. Wherever possible this principle of clustering should be maintained if the concept of a hierarchy of spaces from private to public is to be followed. Figures 5 and 6 illustrate how the units may be clustered.

A congenial home-like atmosphere must be created and maintained to make extended-care patients feel they are living in a "home" and not an institution. The prerogatives of every-day life must be assured, such as privacy, personal autonomy, and opportunities for engaging in social interactions as well as disengaging from them.

Physical organization of space can assist in the function of control for both patient and staff. This assurance of control creates a number of opportunities. Once behavioral contagion no longer consumes as much valuable staff time and energy, staff will have more of themselves to give to the improvement of quality of patient life. On the other hand, residents

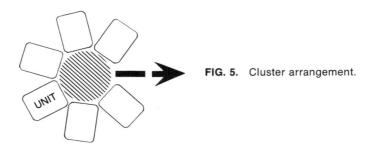

FIG. 5. Cluster arrangement.

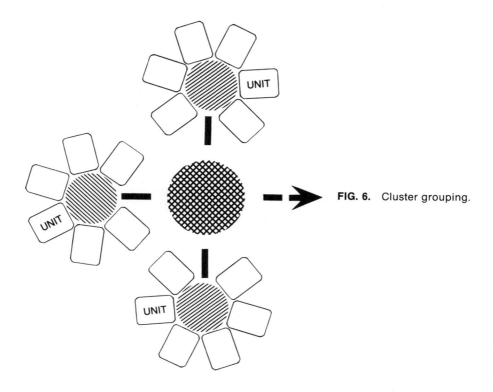

FIG. 6. Cluster grouping.

who have their capacities matched with appropriate environmental loads will be less demanding of staff for daily necessities of life and will presumably be more interested in matters beyond survival.

Once the spatial context is set, long-term testing of the optimum stimulation hypothesis in terms of the two dimensions associated with it, i.e., preference prediction and enhancement prediction, can be undertaken. Sorting out the environmental, managerial, and therapeutic factors as they interact with a very complex array of patient, staff, and organization characteristics requires a long-term commitment in terms of program and research activity.

REFERENCES

1. Kane RA, Kane RL: *Assessing the Elderly*. Lexington, MA, Lexington Books, 1981.
2. Pastalan LA: Environmental design and adaptation to the visual environment of the elderly, in Sekuler R, Kline D, Dismukes K (eds): *Aging and Human Visual Function*. New York, Alan R. Liss, 1982, pp 323–333.
3. Pastalan LA: Designing housing environments for the elderly. *J Architect Ed* 1977;31:11–13.
4. Pastalan LA, Davis L, Haberkorn S: *Pennsylvania Nursing Home Relocation Program: Interim Findings*. Ann Arbor, MI, University of Michigan Press, 1976.

5. Wachs TD: The optimal stimulation hypothesis and early development: Anybody got a match? in Uzgiris I, Hunt J (eds): *The Structuring of Experience.* New York, Plenum Press, 1978, pp 153–173.
6. Wohlwill J: Human adaptation to levels of environmental stimulation. *Hum Ecol* 1974;2:127–147.
7. Wohlwill J: The physical environment: A problem for a psychology of stimulation. *J Soc Issue* 1966;22:29–37.
8. Shultz DP: *Sensory Restriction: Effects on Behavior.* New York, Academic Press, 1965.
9. Lindsley OR: Geriatric behavior prosthetics, in Kastenbaum R (ed): *New Thoughts on Old Age.* New York, Springer, 1964, pp 147–184.

PART V
Research in the Teaching Nursing Home

The Teaching Nursing Home, edited by Edward
L. Schneider et al. © 1985 The Beverly
Foundation. Raven Press, New York.

Introduction

Matilda White Riley

*National Institute on Aging, Behavioral Sciences Research, National Institutes of Health,
Bethesda, Maryland 20205*

This section of the book examines the opportunities and the challenges of research that can be performed in a teaching nursing home (TNH) program. As more people survive to very old ages than ever before, research becomes essential as a guide to professional practice and public policy in optimizing care and treatment.

In these chapters, many kinds of research are discussed for which the TNH program serves as a useful laboratory. Research conducted inside the nursing home is considered on how to prevent or treat the diseases unique to the end stages of life, how to make the institutional surroundings more "home-like," and how to generate the respect that is due to long-lived human beings as well as to their caretakers. Research that extends beyond the nursing home also is considered on alternative systems of care for the ill and disabled elderly and on earlier stages of life before the end stages of disease have become entrenched. This research can build on a growing body of studies demonstrating that not all the ills of old age are inevitable—that, indeed, many are preventable, reversible, treatable, or capable of being so managed as to maintain functioning, alleviate pain, and enhance well-being.

Taken together, these chapters provide details of the sophisticated methodologies that can be adapted for research both inside the nursing home and beyond. Many pertinent research problems are defined and constructive approaches are proposed, such as the inability of confused patients to answer questions in an interview and special procedures for training interviewers, the possible contamination of comparison sample by experimental sample in a clinical trial and ways of avoiding such contamination, the need to allow unusually large amounts of time for studies of frail older people, the obstacles to recruiting and managing the multidisciplinary research teams often required for these studies, and the danger of overgeneralizing to the aged population as a whole from the most disabled and dependent segments.

Six research topics, together with the appropriate methodologies, are proposed for TNH programs:

1. Disease processes in old age.

2. The fit (or lack of fit) between the needs of old people and the care and support provided in institutions, community facilities, and their own homes.
3. The kinds of medical and social interventions that can improve functioning and well-being.
4. The means of integrating the nursing home with the range of other health care systems.
5. Public attitudes toward nursing home personnel and the effect of these attitudes on personnel morale and on patient outcomes.
6. Implications and consequences for older people and their families of alternative methods of financing long-term care.

In addition to these common themes and numerous special topics, there is frequent reference to research on the interacting biomedical, social, and psychological factors that affect health, functioning, and the need for long-term care.

In summary, these chapters develop in detail the remarkable opportunities as well as the problems of research in the TNH program, ranging from the call by Maddox for a broad research agenda for the future and by Ostfeld for an epidemiological outreach to Rowe's practical analysis of the cornerstones of geriatric research and Eisdorfer's concern with the disparity between systems of health care and the actual health needs of older people. Moreover, these chapters go beyond the research itself to discuss strategies for translating research findings into programs of action at the levels of both professional practice and public policy.

The Teaching Nursing Home, edited by Edward
L. Schneider et al. © 1985 The Beverly
Foundation. Raven Press, New York.

The Teaching Nursing Home and Beyond: Research Objectives for the 1980s

George L. Maddox

*Departments of Sociology and Psychiatry and Center for the Study of Aging and Human
Development, Duke University, Durham, North Carolina 27710*

Scientific research is necessarily a public enterprise. How this enterprise is planned and develops involves distinctly social, not just intellectual, components. Public review by peers in the scientific community of work proposed and done by individual scientists is universally recognized as essential and valuable. This chapter focuses on the National Institutes of Health (NIH) as a case in point for discussing how research objectives in aging are identified, reviewed, and implemented. Peer review is the strategy of choice both for certifying the criteria for theoretically and methodologically sound science and for selecting the best research proposals from the marketplace of ideas to advance scientific knowledge and the public interest. For many if not most scientists who propose and review research, the best policy for the development of science is to insure free competition of individuals in the marketplace of ideas. However, there are other problems in planning and implementing research. There are typically more good scientific proposals than resources to fund them. Further, good science does not insure that all identified socially important issues are equally likely to be addressed. Left to their own preferences, scientists tend to work on scientific puzzles they believe they can solve with available theory and methods. Who decides what is socially as well as scientifically most urgently important?

The NIH leadership inevitably exercises an executive function and effects, however cautiously and tentatively, the free operation of the marketplace of ideas. This is done by directing or suggesting to the scientific community a particular idea or problem for investigation that might otherwise have been neglected, directing research through contracts or set-asides, or allocating resources to centers and program projects dedicated to pursue a particular, complex problem systematically rather than to individual scientists. Such constraint is frequently viewed with ambivalence if not hostility by the scientific community, although there is a promise that individual projects in a program project are purportedly viewed on their merit and that the proportion of resources of an Institute devoted to program projects is relatively small. One would not expect a nationally funded program labeled "the teaching nursing home" (TNH) to be exempt from similar constraints.

The public aspect of the scientific enterprise necessarily insures that more than peer review of the quality of individual research proposals generated in the intellectual marketplace will be considered. Societies invest in scientific research with a reasonable expectation that identifiable social benefits will be delivered. The promise of science following the Second World War was perceived to be very high. Public expectations about the usefulness of investing in scientific research were concomitantly high. The love affair between science and society that followed has produced a number of offspring, but none more favored than the NIH. Although the favored status of NIH has insured its substantial freedom to pursue its own developmental course at its own pace on behalf of science and society, the NIH has not been immune to practical political considerations in setting its research agenda. As a case in point, neither NIH leadership nor the leadership of most scientific organizations in the early 1970s wanted a National Institute on Aging (NIA). Whereas the intellectual marketplace of ideas in the scientific community did not demand a National Institute on Aging, Congress demanded it (1). Thus, the NIA, created with objectives to pursue behavioral and social as well as biomedical research and to serve as the Federal focal point for research in aging, was not demanded by free competition in the intellectual marketplace.

Although there are different TNH models and sponsors (see the Introduction, E. L. Schneider, *this volume*), this chapter will focus on the NIA initiative, since NIA is the agency primarily responsible for furthering national research on gerontology and geriatrics related to long-term care issues (see N. List, M. Ory, and E. Hadley, *this volume*, for a detailed description of the NIA program).

Good sense as well as good science are involved in setting and implementing research agendas. The NIA TNH Program strikes this observer as an illustration of good sense probably complemented by the expectation of good science. Among NIH institutes, the NIA has an unusually explicit mandate to consider psychosocial, societal, and environmental as well as biomedical dimensions of health and well-being in its multidisciplinary research agenda. Selecting nursing homes as a major setting for long-term care research has obvious merits for a program of multidisciplinary research but is not without risks (2).

There is no question that nursing homes, socially visible and societally important as they are, have remained relatively foreign territory for the scientific research community. As Thomas Kuhn observed a long time ago, scientists have preferences for problems they perceive to be solvable. The utilization of nursing homes as attractive sites for basic and clinical research and training in aging would not be likely to occur spontaneously to most basic and clinical scientists and teachers. The neglect of nursing homes as research and teaching sites illustrates once again that the social importance of problems is not ordinarily a primary motivation in determining preferences for research and training topics and sites. The TNH as a strategy for research development in aging did not emanate from the scientific community; rather, NIA leadership promoted the strategy with the concurrence of its National Advisory Council.

Whether the TNH Program generates research producing new knowledge about chronic disease and its effective management in later life that would otherwise not have been produced remains to be seen. Whether the program produces models demonstrating the effective and beneficial movement of nursing homes into the mainstream of gerontological/geriatric research and teaching remains to be seen. There is no reasonable basis for dismissing these hopes and expectations *a priori*. On the contrary, there is a basis for optimism. This new program initiative has developed in a context in which peer review and relatively open competition in the intellectual marketplace and public review of outcomes have been preserved.

As of March 1984, five investments in TNH Program projects involving 22 specific research projects have been made. The funded research proposed and most highly valued in the peer review process provides an opportunity to describe what reputable scientists and their peers in aging believe to be some important research objectives for the 1980s. Summarizing these objectives will constitute our first task. The second task will be to assess this list of research objectives in relation to NIA's recently completed *A National Research Plan for Research in Aging* (3). The final task will be to provide a balanced view of research objectives in aging for the 1980s and of the contribution of the TNH Program to those objectives.

TEACHING NURSING HOME PROGRAM: OVERVIEW OF RESEARCH TOPICS

Within the context of a peer review strategy of selecting quality research in gerontology and geriatrics, the 22 proposals from five academic institutions and related long-term-care facilities illustrate the high-priority objectives generated in the intellectual marketplace and certified by peers (see chapter on NIA TNH program by N. List, M. Ory, and E. Hadley). The following pattern emerges:

1. Central nervous system functioning and pathology
   a. Dementia studies in the context of the TNH
   b. Cognitive and genetic aspects of SDAT
   c. Regional metabolism and blood flow in aging and dementia
   d. Vasopressin release in dementia
   e. Clinical and neuroendocrine measures of depression in SDAT

2. Urinary functioning and pathology
   a. Bladder function and incontinence in frail elderly
   b. Urinary tract infections in a geriatric population
3. Rehabilitation, interventions, and training effects
   a. Cognitive rehabilitation of stroke
   b. Modification of exercise capacity in the elderly
   c. Cardiopulmonary effects of training in an aging population
4. Sleep
   a. Sleep apnea in the elderly
   b. Aging, adiposity, and sleep-disordered breathing
   c. Neurobehavioral performance in aging and the role of sleep-disordered breathing
5. Pulmonary functioning and pathology
   a. Performance and control of the respiratory muscles
   b. Autonomic and airway reactivity
6. Behavioral sciences and epidemiology
   a. Predictors of functional dependency in the elderly
   b. Identification of persons at risk of institutional placement
7. Miscellaneous systems
   a. Osteoarthritis: synovial cell–cartilage interactions
   b. Aging, adiposity, physical fitness, and endocrine metabolic function
   c. Vitamin D nutrition in the institutionalized
   d. Falls in the elderly
   e. Syncope and blood pressure homeostasis in the elderly

Overinterpretation of this summary of topics at the beginning of the TNH Program as the research strategy for NIA in the 1980s is not invited or encouraged. It is admittedly a partial and particular view of gerontological and geriatric research objectives for the decade. It is, however, as definitive a view as we have of what our peers in scientific research believe to be among the important Federally specified objectives for the 1980s that can be pursued effectively in nursing homes. The importance attributed to central nervous system pathology and to urinary and sleep disturbances is hardly surprising given what we know about the incidence and prevalence of these conditions in older, institutionalized individuals. These conditions create problems of management that surely increase the risk of institutionalization and complicate the management of institutionalized patients. Although one might second-guess the investigators and our scientific peers about the relative importance and scientific merit of these projects in relation to projects not funded, intuitively, none of the funded projects seems irrelevant or trivial.

THE NIA RESEARCH PLAN AS A REFERENCE POINT

NIA's research plan for research in aging (3) provides as definitive a reference as we have with which to compare the research objectives derived from the TNH projects to the more comprehensive plan developed by the Institute. The published plan is the only comprehensive statement we have on research objectives in aging for the 1980s, and thus we may use the plan as a frame of reference for locating the TNH projects.

The subtitle of the research plan, "Toward an Independent Old Age," would not encourage one to think immediately of nursing homes as a strategic site for research. But the statement is explicit on this matter (3, p. 180). Under the heading "Special Opportunities," the following two paragraphs appear:

> Patients in nursing homes and similar long-term settings present special challenges and opportunities for further study and understanding of the disabilities, both functional and disease-based, which contribute to their need to be in such settings. Studies carried out in the nursing home setting to modify the environment, through adding variability and other stimuli and observing for possible benefits in patients' status, would have potential applicability to other social settings in which the environment is particularly relentlessly unchanging. Widespread interest in development of home support services, as an alternative to institutional care, makes this an excellent time for demonstration and evaluation projects of this type. The role of education in eliciting cooperation and compliance in therapeutic regimes, with inducement of the long-term care patient to participate actively and independently in therapeutic decisionmaking and treatment, is an area that now requires rigorous research.
>
> High-quality nursing homes are a special resource for teaching and research. They provide a distilled essence of disease and functional disability where the multiple pathology characteristic of old age can be demonstrated. Nowhere else can far-advanced, individual disease states be better observed and studied by students of the health professions. Such facilities are a valuable resource to help teach about advanced disease in old age and motivate students to recognize disease early and prevent its progression in the independent elderly.

The TNH research projects listed above would appear to provide an opportunity to observe "a distilled essence of disease and functional disability where the multiple pathology characteristic of old age can be demonstrated" (3, p. 180). The stated expectation that disease and disability, their course, and their management as observed in nursing homes can be used to compare the condition of older persons in other settings is less obviously accounted for in the referenced projects. However, it should be noted that in several projects in the first five funded program projects, noninstitutionalized elderly are targeted for comparative study. Even less obvious in the referenced, approved projects is interest in the nursing home as a social environment within which staff and patients interact or in the societal context in which nursing homes operate. Although the social allocation processes leading to institutionalization are included in some projects, nursing homes as a social institution are not a focus of attention.

The NIA research plan includes reports from subpanels on three major areas of research: basic mechanisms of aging, clinical manifestations of aging, and interactions between older people and society. One would intuitively expect the TNH projects to fall primarily in the second area, and this is, in fact, the case. All of the referenced projects fit into one or more of the 18 priority categories in the plan for clinical manifestations of aging (3, pp. 113–186). The research objectives in this section of the plan not apparently addressed by the funded TNH projects warrant noting without prejudice; they are:

1. Sensory functioning
2. Skin
3. Neoplastic disorders
4. Bioengineering supports
5. Ethics.

Thirteen of 18 of the research objectives listed under the "Clinical Manifestations of Aging" section of the NIA research plan are addressed by at least one of the TNH projects. Since it is unlikely that the TNH investigators developed their proposals with the current NIA research plan in hand, this observer views the outcome as a favorable commentary on the good sense of allowing an informed scientific community a great deal of freedom to generate its own priorities, constrained only by the general objectives that the research was obligated to pursue. Whether, in their totality, the funded TNH projects should be faulted for their concentration on one or another research objective or their neglect of others can be debated and probably should be.

There is little behavioral and social scientific research in the funded projects. The kinds of strong research groups that generate successful program projects do not, by definition, insure a balanced mix of biomedical, behavioral, and social scientific projects. My guess is that some excellent program projects may have had weak behavioral and social scientific projects. And, conversely, some strong behavioral and social scientific projects were embedded in weak program projects. Short of directing the scientific community to produce a certain balance of projects in different substantive areas, multidisciplinary balance is not very probable. In any case, achieving a desirable balance is not easy.

THE TEACHING NURSING HOMES AND BEYOND

The TNH Program is not NIA's research strategy on aging. The program is a tactical move to generate socially useful as well as scientifically sound research and to stimulate a relationship between academic institutions and nursing homes.

Development of Nursing Homes as a Site for Aging Research and Research Training

The TNH Program constitutes, as Campbell might observe, a quasi-experiment in allocation of scientific resources (4). One might hope if not expect NIA to be curious about the effectiveness and efficiency of its investment and to monitor outcomes with some care. Will the TNH Program produce notable good science in reasonable quantity? Who will be taught what? Will careers in aging be focused in a distinctive way? Will the interaction between academic institutions be changed distinctively in the institutions involved and in other institutions not involved directly in the program? Cumulatively, do the funded program projects present the kind of disciplinary mix and balance required to provide the scientific information we need about effective management in long-term care settings and the role of nursing homes in the continuum of long-term care?

These are ponderous and difficult questions. But they are answerable, or at least they appear to be so. As a principal investigator of many research and training grants, this observer has been asked to provide answers to such questions regularly. In the case of the TNH Program, to which substantial sums are being dedicated, formal and systematic review of the outcomes of this investment in TNHs seems warranted. A primary recommendation to NIA and to basic and clinical scientists with career interests in aging is to take a scientific view of the effects of allocating scientific resources in a distinctive way. It will be interesting to see whether the scientific community will generate in the context of this special program, or in the context of other NIA programs, research projects that address a broad range of behavioral and social scientific issues not currently observed among the funded projects.

Attention is called here to the instructive exchange among Ahronheim (2), Schneider (5), and Posner et al. (6) regarding the potential and limitations of the TNH Program. Briefly, Ahronheim expressed four concerns:

1. The great majority of older persons are not in nursing homes, and nursing home patients, many with end-stage chronic diseases, are not an adequate basis for generalizing about aging or age-related disease.
2. The assumption that exposure to very sick, impaired elderly patients will generate positive attitudes toward older patients on the part of scientists and clinicians is dubious.
3. Experimentation with institutionalized, frail elderly may not be a good idea scientifically, much less ethically.
4. Important as the physician is, the physician has not been and is not likely to be the primary professional caregiver in nursing homes. And, one might add, important as nursing homes are, most long-term care is provided elsewhere.

Schneider (5) countered by arguing that the TNH Program is *a* research program, not *the* research program of NIA. "Recognizing the importance of multiple sites for long-term care," he noted, "NIA encourages biomedical, social, and behavioral research in a variety of home, community, and institutional settings." Posner et al. (6) indicate that the Philadelphia group takes a broad view of the mission of their TNH Project.

Broadening the Research Agenda in Aging

This focused exchange among Ahronheim, Schneider, and Posner et al. is instructive in several specific ways in broadening our thinking about and planning of research in aging for the 1980s. An opportunity was provided for NIA to reiterate that its TNH Program is a timely and important but limited tactical move, not its total strategy for research in aging. The NIA total research plan, of which the TNH Program is only a part, is a matter of record. However, some important issues of substance and methodology were raised.

Research on the Attitudes and Behavior of Scientists and Clinicians

The challenge to NIA's assumption that exposure of academic faculty and students may be beneficial both in producing and cementing a productive relationship between academic institutions and long-term care institutions and in promoting new knowledge, new skills, and positive attitudes among participants warrants further critical discussion. This assumption is more properly a hypothesis that NIA and its awardees should make a systematic effort to test.

Ethical Issues in Research

The challenge that doing research on severely impaired institutional populations raises both ethical and scientific questions also warrants attention (see C. K. Cassel, *this volume*). The total NIA research plan identifies ethical issues associated with the use of patients in research and alternative care experiments as germane to its interests and as a research objective for the 1980s. Scholarly review of such ethical issues in TNH research is not found explicitly among the 22 projects approved to date. Possibly a project focused on ethical issues is not appropriate for any single program project and would be more appropriately commissioned by NIA as a resource for all the TNH projects. In any case, a project addressing ethical issues would seem to be wise.

Methodological Issues

A scientific as well as ethical issue is also raised by the use of severely disabled, institutionalized patients. One of the classical methodological issues in medical sociology and epidemiology is the problem posed by generalizations from treated cases to larger populations from which the treated cases are drawn. The challenge by Ahronheim poses the problem in terms of misleading program participants to believe that observations based on an institutionalized population and on the disease processes exhibited there are broadly generalizable, reinforcing a stereotypically negative view of later life.

There are several concomitant scientific concerns. For example, the natural histories of disease processes and the precise effects of interventions in these processes are frequently neither well documented nor well understood. Are generalizations about these processes based on observations of selected treated samples applicable even to institutionalized patients much less to older adults generally, and are they scientifically justifiable? A great deal of caution would be in order here. Attention should be given at the minimum to comparisons across program project sites and to comparisons between project sites and other long-term care facilities. The process of allocating people to treatment sites is complex and has a distinctive social component. And the match between the characteristics of individuals and the characteristics of treatment sites is known to have an effect on behavior, health, and well-being (7).

Further, whereas Ahronheim's challenge questions the ethics of scientific studies of institutionalized elderly patients, this observer would be more concerned about whether TNH residents are scientifically suitable subjects for the research and experimentation proposed. It seems highly probable that investigators in the TNH projects will, in fact, be driven to broaden the subject pool to include more than nursing home residents not only for the purposes of comparison but also because many available TNH residents will be found to be too impaired for many research purposes. How the TNH investigators deal with issues of sampling and generalization of findings will be followed with considerable interest.

Psychosocial and Societal Issues

Behavioral and social scientists may be somewhat reassured by NIA's declaration of its commitment to study the psychosocial and societal aspects of aging processes and the experience of aging in the TNH Program and in the Institute's other programs. The psychosocial aspects of aging and the experience of aging are not totally missed in the funded projects of the TNH Program, but neither do they appear to be central. Apparently little or no attention is directed toward long-term care institutions as the immediate social environments (the milieus) of behavior in later life. There is a substantial body of research in the tradition of social and psychological ecology that documents the importance of person/environment congruence for understanding health and behavior in various settings (7–9). Institutional—more broadly, environmental—settings constitute treatment effects that warrant research in their own right. Individuals are not adequately characterized by their International Classification of Diseases (ICD) alone; they bring to treatment settings a variety of personal and social characteristics, including knowledge, coping strategies, and social supports, that affect functional capacity and capacity for rehabilitation. Special living (or treatment) settings are not all alike either. These settings are organized socially in different ways reflected in the number, training, program resources, and

care philosophies of staff. Explicit scientific curiosity and systematic research on long-term care environments as treatment settings or as organizations in a societal context are not evident in the funded TNH projects.
This is a loss that would not be corrected by having such research done in
other settings.

These considerations would lead this observer to make a strong recommendation that NIA include in its TNH Program—or as an adjunct to it—
a comparative study of long-term care organizations as special living settings.
Schneider's statement on the TNH Program (5) indicates NIA's possible
interest in the topic. What is needed is the implementation of appropriate
social psychological and social scientific research projects. Whether the
TNH Program is the best mechanism for promoting such research is a separate issue. The research itself needs to be done.

This recommendation leads to a still broader recommendation, which is
at least partially germane to NIA's broad research mandate and is partly
anticipated by several of the funded TNH projects. Special living settings
such as long-term care institutions represent the social construction of care
systems and social processes of allocating both residents and resources to
these special settings. If congruence of personal and environmental characteristics is as important as limited current research suggests, then a major
research objective of the 1980s would be to develop and apply reliable, valid
procedures for characterizing personal and milieu settings in order to assess
the implication of person/milieu congruence or incongruence. An extension
of such research would focus not only on the risk of institutionalization but
also on the social processes involved in allocating specific individuals to
specific care settings and the consequences of these assignments (6). Further, the potential of experimenting with the effects of environmental interventions on behavior, health, and well-being of nursing home residents
is appropriately a matter for research (7–9).

Societal allocation of resources in ways that structure, intentionally or
incidentally, the care system in distinctive ways also warrants attention. The
issue of the characteristics and consequences of alternative care systems
has in the past decade been the business of the Health Care Financing
Administration (HCFA) and National Center for Health Services Research
(NCHSR) in the Department of Health and Human Services (HHS). But
NIA has an obvious interest in these issues, at least at the level of remaining
informed, and, as appropriate, stimulating and articulating health care and
health services research supported by other Federal agencies with the interests of NIA. At a minimum, NIA has an incentive to insure that its TNH
Program is not an implicit endorsement of accepting the status quo in the
organization and financing of long-term care.

A recent summary volume on perspectives of long-term care provided by
research and demonstrations from HCFA (10) indicates how far we have
come in the past decade—and how far we have yet to go—in understanding

the demography and epidemiology of aging populations and the efficiency and effectiveness of alternative organization and financing of systems of care appropriate for these populations. Several conclusions suggested by this volume seem inescapable. The NIA's TNH Program will be severely and inappropriately truncated if it does not eventually include an integral or a supplemental research interest in the nursing home as an organizational construct reflecting processes of social allocation of people and resources in the United States. The participants in TNH programs will remain significantly uneducated if they do not understand the societal processes that produce and sustain, for better or worse, nursing homes as central to national health care policy.

Teaching in the TNH Program

One final question about why the TNH is a useful point of departure for discussing research objectives for the 1980s involves asking "Who is supposed to be taught what?" A narrow answer is that physicians are to be taught about chronic disease and its management in later life. We must also decide, however, whether it is equally relevant to teach physicians about the distinctive roles of other health care professionals and other health care professionals about the distinctive roles of physicians? It is equally relevant to teach health care professionals about scientific research on social processes of allocating people and resources to health care institutions and the consequences of these allocations? Is it relevant for health care professionals to understand the basic public policy issues raised by our society's larger commitment to the use of nursing homes? This observer concludes that the answer to these questions is affirmative.

It may be premature to insist on answers to these broad questions, to assume we know the answers, to assume that any satisfactory answer exists, or to assume that the TNH Program alone bears the responsibility for the answering. The NIA, however, has an obligation to answer and to plan its research on aging for the 1980s accordingly. An opportunity to do this lies in the development of a broad research agenda for NIA in the 1980s that includes the TNH Program and perhaps more than this Program currently promises.

SUMMARY AND CONCLUSIONS

The federally sponsored TNH Program has developed in the context of NIA's peer review procedures, which encourage initiatives from the intellectual marketplace, and in the context of a broader explicit comprehensive research plan. This is a sound and reassuring procedure to help insure that a particular programmatic tactic such as the TNH Program is perceived as a tactic, not as the total research strategy of NIA. Peer review will help insure that the currently funded TNH projects are not only the best available of their type but also are related to the Institute's total research objectives.

The following are recommendations for research in the 1980s that relate to possible extensions and elaborations of the TNH Program or possibly to supplemental programs for NIA or other agencies in cooperation with NIA.

First, the TNH Program is an experiment in the allocation of research and training resources. This experiment should be evaluated systematically in terms of its stated objectives to increase the interaction of academic and care institutions, to contribute to knowledge about disease processes, and to change the attitudes of health care personnel in beneficial ways.

Second, a TNH is not only a potential model for investigating disease processes and care management but also a focal point for investigating both how society allocates people and resources in care systems and the comparative efficiency and effectiveness of alternative care systems. This broader objective is important for research relevant for any aging society in this decade.

Third, research on the clinical manifestation of disease processes in particular populations in special settings must be related comparatively to the study of these processes in other settings to assess generalizability and must be studied over time.

Fourth, one of the very fertile areas of research, which is by definition multidisciplinary, is exploration and application of methodologies appropriate for characterizing both individual and social contexts and the effects of interactions between these characteristics. Nursing homes are appropriate settings for addressing this question, but comparative research in a broader range of special living environments and in communities where most older adults live out their lives is obviously necessary.

Fifth, an exciting development in current theories of aging is an empirical basis for exploring an old maxim of experimental and clinical sciences: to understand something, try to change it. Although we do not know the limits of our capacity to change aging processes and the experience of aging, the mutability of these processes and experiences is clearly part of scientific thinking currently. The issue is not just the potential contribution for rehabilitation in the interest of a more independent and productive old age. The issue now has been broadened to explore the potential of psychosocial interventions designed to document how perceived personal control and personal effectiveness can be enhanced and how the mobilization of social supports might buffer the impact of challenging life events. In the broadest sense, research on alternative structuring of care systems acknowledges that special living environments are, in effect, modifiable treatment environments.

In understanding aging and the experience of aging, understanding personal and social systems is as important as understanding biological systems. The NIA leadership understands this and is committed to the implications of understanding this in its comprehensive research plans for the decade.

This is why NIA has a comprehensive research plan within which its TNH Program may be kept in perspective and why the leadership of the funded TNH projects are well advised to take a broad view of their research mandate.

ACKNOWLEDGMENT

Preparation of this chapter was supported in part by a grant from the Sandoz Foundation (U.S.).

REFERENCES

1. Lockett BA: *Aging, Politics, and Research: Setting the Federal Agenda for Research on Aging.* New York, Springer, 1983.
2. Ahronheim JC: Pitfalls of the teaching nursing home. *N Engl J Med* 1983;308:335–336.
3. National Institute on Aging: *Toward an Independent Old Age: A National Plan for Research on Aging. Report of the National Research on Aging Planning Panel.* Washington, D.C., US Department of Health and Human Services, 1983.
4. Campbell D: Reforms as Experiments. *Am Psychol* 1969;2(4):409–429.
5. Schneider EL: Teaching nursing homes. *N Engl J Med* 1983;308:336–337.
6. Posner J, Kaye D, Miller B, et al: The Teaching Nursing Home. *N Engl J Med* 1983;308:1604–1605.
7. Moos R: Specialized living environments for older people: A conceptual framework for evaluation. *J Soc Issues* 1980;36:75–94.
8. Schulz R, Hanusa B: Experimental social gerontology: A social psychological perspective. *J Soc Issues* 1980;36:30–46.
9. Rodin J: Behavioral medicine: Behavioral effects of self-control training in aging. *Int Rev Appl Psychol.* 1983;32:153–180.
10. Vogel R, Palmer H: *Long-term Care: Perspectives from Research and Demonstrations.* Washington, D.C., Health Care Financing Administration, Department of Health and Human Services, 1982.

The Teaching Nursing Home, edited by Edward
L. Schneider et al. © 1985 The Beverly
Foundation. Raven Press, New York.

The Teaching Nursing Home:
Research Strategies and Issues

Adrian M. Ostfeld

*Yale University School of Medicine, Department of Epidemiology and Public Health, New
Haven, Connecticut 06510*

Research on the interrelated health and social problems of the elderly is
beginning to move from the descriptive to the analytic phase. This discussion of the strengths and weaknesses of the teaching nursing home (TNH)
as a setting for research and the kinds of research the TNH best facilitates
is in keeping with the reality that many activities besides research must go
on in a nursing home.

Most research on the physical and mental health of older people and on
the biomedical and psychosocial factors determining health has been done
in teaching hospitals, mental institutions, outpatient departments or their
equivalent, and on populations in the community. The teaching hospital
and the research center offer the opportunity for exquisite monitoring of
physiological and biochemical functioning, for new, daring, and risky therapeutic measures, and for linking biopsy and autopsy data with antemortem
findings. The TNH cannot easily do any of these things. The community
study can provide data on morbidity and mortality change, reasons for the
change, the effect on health of exposure to life crises such as bereavement,
retirement, or housing change and can delineate behavioral and biological
risk factors for a variety of illnesses and fatal events. The TNH can do none
of these things.

Where then does the TNH fit in? What can it provide that other research
settings cannot? Studies in hospitals must usually be completed in a short
time and are often very expensive, and long-term follow-up is difficult. Studies in the community may illuminate why some people go to institutions
and others do not but will not reveal what happens in those institutions.
To know what goes on in the TNH, we must study the TNH itself. Moreover,
hospitals and communities are such exceedingly complex and often rapidly
changing physical and social environments that research related to them is
very difficult.

The chief advantage of the TNH as a setting for research is that it is a
relatively slowly changing, geographically compact social and physical sys-

tem of moderate size and complexity offering access to the problems of a very ill and disabled group. The patient population is relatively stable: turnover is slow compared to hospitals, and the stay is usually months or years. These factors create the opportunity for careful planning, allow multiple and repeated measures of the desired variables, and permit a relatively long follow-up period. For the nursing home patient, the problems of coming to the research center or hospital do not exist. The TNH patients do not have to contend with inadequate transportation, fear of crime, wintry weather, and slippery streets. One cannot keep a patient in an acute-care hospital for months for repeated medical observations. Nor can one see a community population daily or weekly for the same purpose. The TNH patient presents clear advantages for studies in which daily or weekly contact with researchers is needed.

In the TNH, the population available for study is known and categorized. Participation rates and dropout rates are easily monitored. There is no need to go door to door looking for participants as in community studies; no need to check the hospital admission diagnostic list every day to see who might be a study participant. The relatively high rates of illness and disability are tragic for the patients and their families, but they provide a high concentration of both research opportunities and participants.

A major advantage of the nursing home is that it provides an excellent opportunity for a wide variety of controlled clinical trials, far more than evaluations of new drugs. Many kinds of trials are feasible. Consider the hypothesis that training the more alert and active TNH patients to help the more disabled patients with meals, by social attention, and by assisting the staff with provision of care will improve morale, patient–patient and patient–staff communication, patient mobility and activity, eating habits, and adherence to prescribed regimens. A "treated" group and a comparison group in different parts of the TNH are created, and the judgments about benefit are made by investigators ignorant of the composition of the two groups and with no vested interest in the outcome. Similarly, one could set up special programs of training for nursing home staff and evaluate the effectiveness of the training on quality of care and behavior of patients and staff. The nursing home could become a center for training of the family or close friends of patients to provide the needs of the patient so that transfer back to the home could be facilitated.

There is, of course, an opportunity to carry out placebo-controlled double-blind studies of new medications for dementia or treatment of bed sores, and to evaluate bioengineering devices that improve urinary incontinence, mobility, self-care, and feeding.

There are other opportunities besides such clinical trials. One can study the relationship among health, patient care, and visitation. Visits to each TNH resident could be quantified with respect to number of visits, relationship of visitor to patient, length of visit, the communication between visitor and visitee, and the behavior of both. These data could be correlated with measures of morale, mobility, food intake, adherence to medical regimens, and episodes of symptoms and illness and lead to prospective studies of the relationship between visits and multiple patient outcomes.

There is a need to sharpen our measures of quality of care, especially of long-term care, and to improve the evaluation of care. The opportunity for methodologic research resides in many nursing homes.

There is the opportunity to study the last moments of life. When that time comes, what proportion of the moribund are awake? Comatose? In pain? Comfortable? What proportion have family and friends at the bedside? What do people say at the last moment of life?

Consider the limitations and problems of research in the TNH. Any single institution may have a patient population that is nonrepresentative of any larger group. The nursing home may have disproportionate numbers of patients of one religion, one social class, one ethnic group, or atypical physical or administrative features. It would be hazardous to generalize from a single institution to all others in a community or in a state. Replication of results in other institutions is the best evidence that generalization is warranted.

The TNH is likely to be better staffed and funded and more innovative than the nonteaching nursing home. These circumstances create an atmosphere of hope and optimism and may have nonspecific beneficial effects on patients and staff. In such an atmosphere, success of any measure may be more easily achieved than in a more poorly staffed cautious institution. It is important to avoid generalizing from one kind of nursing home to another and to replicate the successes of TNH in more characteristic institutions.

Much of the research done with institutionalized elders has been short term. But short-term success does not necessarily predict long-term benefit. It is important to plan longer studies when the effects of long-term interventions are to be evaluated.

A mechanism is needed for disseminating information about research that has not confirmed its hypotheses and programs that have failed. Such results are ordinarily not published, but they need to be, perhaps in much abbreviated form. Identifying failure can be very important to planning research.

Histories of prior hospitalizations, physician's visits, medications, or symptoms are not clearly and accurately recalled by most people after the passage of a few months to a year. Problems in recall are likely to be worse in nursing home patients or their elderly family members and friends. This means either that research protocols heavily dependent on past medical history should be avoided or that historical data be buttressed with hospital and physician's records. The latter sources are not without their difficulties.

A major issue in TNH research is the number of participants required for research or the sample size. The issues determining sample size in a hypothetical experiment in which both a new treatment and a placebo are administered to all participants, to be compared in their effectiveness on some measure of disability, may differ from those in a parallel design in which the participants receive only a new treatment or a placebo.

The first exercise is to decide at which level to set the probability that the difference in outcome of the treatment and placebo is statistically significant. The smaller one sets the probability that the results could have occurred by chance, the higher the number of participants needed.

Second, if there is a real difference, what assurance is there that the experiment will produce a statistically significant outcome. In other words, what power is required in the experiment. The higher the power desired, the larger the group that must be recruited.

Third, the expected difference in effectiveness between treatment and placebo will have a marked effect on sample size. Obviously, the greater the difference, the smaller the numbers required.

A couple of examples will clarify these issues. If the significance level and power of the experiment are at conventional levels of 0.05 and 0.80, and if the treatment is expected to benefit two-thirds of the participants and the nonspecific effects of the trial and placebo to help one-fourth of the participants, then about 30 participants in each group will be quite satisfactory. On the other hand, if some new treatment improves 10% of participants and the treatment or placebo with which it is compared helps 5%, then 400 subjects in each group may not be enough. If the treatment has differential beneficial effects by gender, then even larger numbers are needed to determine effectiveness in men and women. There must be a large difference in outcome of two treatments if the numbers usually available in the TNH are to be large enough for the study.

A relatively small and enclosed institution like a TNH poses other problems for research, problems that arise out of the communication and physical compactness of the TNH. For example, in the Multiple Risk Factor Intervention Trial (MRFIT) funded by the National Heart, Lung and Blood Institute, one group of men at high risk of coronary heart disease was to undertake a series of interventions on behavior to reduce their risk of heart disease. The comparison group, who were not deliberately encouraged to reduce their risk of heart disease, began to do the same things the treated group did. They began to stop smoking, start exercising, change diet, and get their high blood pressure treated. The comparison group refused to remain a comparison group, and the outcome of the trial was confounded.

Similarly, a nursing home group, seeing that people in the same institution are involved in certain potentially beneficial activities, may begin these activities themselves. The benefit of the intervention measures will become difficult to determine. It will require care and ingenuity to avoid such problems.

It may be difficult to carry out more than one or two studies in a TNH at the same time. Staff may confuse protocols or feel excessively burdened, and one study may contaminate the other.

Although the TNH is one site, there are broader opportunities for study. Teaching nursing homes are located in communities, and nursing home patients have family and friends who are not institutionalized. The nursing home is only one mode of providing care for the ill and disabled elderly. These relationships provide opportunities for comparing the nursing home with congregate elderly housing, with the home, or with the elderly day-care center as a site for activity and for treatment of the less severely ill and disabled. Not only effectiveness of treatment but costs and the burdens to family could be compared. The TNH may develop cooperative arrangements with retirement communities, housing projects for the elderly, day-care centers, and congregate housing in which a smooth continuum of residence based on health and ability could be explored. An elderly person could move back and forth from one setting to another depending on the status of his/her physical and mental health and the support available from the family and the community. Creation of such organizational frameworks would require careful study and evaluation at every step of the way.

There are a few essential principles to keep in mind when planning research. First, research starts with a question. The question may be, "If we make this change in our procedure will it help the patients?" Or, "I wonder why patients on this new medication lose their appetite?" Or, "How can we prevent patients from becoming disoriented at night?" To proceed, frame the research interests in the form of single-sentence questions and then work to specify exactly what is to be done, step by step, to answer the questions. The next step is to consult a researcher who is experienced and quantitatively oriented. This consultant may be an epidemiologist or bio-statistician, but there are other kinds of investigators who can do the job. Write down research protocol, develop a schedule of work and a budget, and seek the funds to do the work. Needless to say, all this is easier to describe than to carry out. But it is not formidably hard either. Curiosity about something coupled with methodical planning are two important qualifications for a researcher.

GENERAL REFERENCES

1. Phillips JL Jr: *Statistical Thinking*, 2nd ed. San Francisco, WH Freeman, 1982.
2. Nutt PC: *Evaluation Concepts and Methods: Shaping Policy for the Health Administrator*. New York, SP Medical and Scientific Books, 1981.
3. Miller DC: *Handbook of Research Design and Social Measurement*, ed 2. New York, David McKay, 1970.
4. Mausner J, Bahn A: *Epidemiology: An Introductory Text*. Philadelphia, WB Saunders, 1974.
5. Multiple Risk Factor Intervention Trial Research Group: Risk factor changes and mortality results. *JAMA* 1982;248:1465–1469.

Factors Facilitating and Impeding Research in the Teaching Nursing Home Setting

John W. Rowe

*Division of Gerontology, Joint Department of Medicine, Beth Israel and Brigham and
Women's Hospitals, Boston, Massachusetts 02215*

There are numerous factors or characteristics of a teaching nursing home
(TNH) that might be seen as facilitating the conduct of research as well as
some that represent perils or pitfalls to the development of a robust research
program. This chapter is mainly based on experience in developing a research-oriented TNH program consisting of a consortium of the Hebrew
Rehabilitation Center for Aged, the Beth Israel Hospital, the Harvard Medical School, and the Boston University School of Nursing.

There are several major facilitators to the development of research in a
TNH, several major impediments, and a number of important characteristics that, if they are present, are major facilitators and, if they are absent,
can represent very substantial barriers.

The most important facilitators are the funds made available by the National Institute on Aging (NIA) for the TNH Program. Many of the TNH
programs that have recently appeared would not have been developed as
quickly or as well if the NIA had not allocated funds for the support of these
activities. Another important driving force for the development of the TNH
is the very substantial and well-recognized need for research on disorders
that represent prominent causes of morbidity and mortality in institutionalized chronically ill elderly. A third major facilitator is the positive effect
that the establishment of academic programs can have on the quality of
care in the long-term care setting.

A final major facilitator is the nonacademic interests of hospitals and
medical centers in long-term care. Over the past year, prospective reimbursement plans have been enacted that provide acute-care hospitals with
an economic incentive to limit the length of stay of elderly patients. In
response to this incentive, many institutions have sought to develop meaningful relationships with long-term care centers. In many cases, these relationships include total or partial ownership of long-term care facilities by

acute-care hospitals. There is also growing recognition of the need for the expertise and resources of acute-care hospitals to be brought to bear on the problems of long-term care. These factors provide an excellent base for the development of TNH programs.

It is critical for planners of TNH programs to recognize the importance of these facilitators and to utilize them to their maximum advantage as catalysts for developing a strong commitment on the part of all members of the consortium. It is especially important that individuals at medical schools and teaching hospitals, where the impetus for the development of a TNH often develops first, to recognize that they must share these resources rather than hoard them and coerce the long-term care facility into submission. Specifically, it is important that financial resources as well as prestige be shared as effectively as possible. For instance, if a long-term care facility has adequate experience in grants management, one might consider having the long-term care facility serve as the grantee for the TNH application, and an investigator based at the medical school and teaching hospital as the principal investigator. This provides all major members of the consortium with adequate amounts of control and prestige and prevents isolation of the TNH as an institution that is being used for, but not participating in, the benefits of the TNH program.

There are two major barriers to development of TNHs. The first is the general lack of well-developed academic programs in geriatrics. There is a lack of investigators with interest and experience in geriatric research and of investigators capable of conducting research in a long-term care setting. A second factor potentially inhibiting progress is a lack of experience on the part of administrators, patients, and staff of nursing homes in the conduct and administration of research programs in the long-term care setting. There is a widespread concern, if not in some cases a fear, that elderly impaired individuals will be experimented on unnecessarily with little gain. Long-term care facilities as well as patients and their families often voice this concern as their major objection to the development of TNH programs.

Both of these major impediments can be successfully overcome. The lack of expertise on the part of the research faculty can be addressed not only by the recruitment of new faculty but more quickly and less expensively through the involvement of present faculty in research programs based in long-term care. The inducements here are not only the resources that might be made available via a TNH grant but also the very substantial number of important and exciting research questions that have not yet been examined. Many investigators who have not worked in geriatrics have a bias against aging or geriatric research and simply have not yet fully grasped the major importance of questions that they could effectively answer. Uncertainty on the part of long-term care facilities, their patients, and their family members regarding the goals and safety of clinical research can rather easily be addressed in a systematic educational program, which should be a forerunner, as well as an important ongoing component, of any TNH program.

There are a number of major characteristics that, if present, can have a beneficial effect on facilitating research in the TNH setting and, if absent, represent important impediments that need to be addressed before the program is developed. Too frequently, efforts are made to develop a broad-based large TNH program without these cornerstones in place. Such programs, although they may appear theoretically sound, have an ominous prognosis.

Preexisting academic programs in geriatric medicine and nursing are important components of the proper substrate for a TNH. These programs provide a focus for schools and hospitals as they develop a partnership with a nursing home. Schools without current programs in geriatrics might view the NIA's TNH grant as an opportunity to acquire the requisite resources to initiate such a program. This approach is generally unworkable unless substantial additional university-based resources are also simultaneously available. Funds in the NIA TNH program are not adequate to support the TNH itself and also establish academic programs in schools of medicine and nursing and teaching hospitals. Key faculty in geriatrics are unlikely to have adequate time to develop these programs in parallel. Schools that wish to develop programs in geriatrics that include a TNH in their efforts are better advised to adopt long-term plans that place TNH development in a later phase.

A preexisting program in geriatrics has several obvious potential strengths to bring to the TNH effort. If a program in aging has a research component, then experienced investigators are available to assist in the design and conduct of the TNH research. At the very least, there should be one experienced gerontological investigator so that the principles of geriatric research will be recognized as projects are developed. One cannot simply take a group of investigators who have an interest in or skills relevant to studies in the elderly and transplant them to a nursing home, hoping for the best. Special considerations that are important here relate not only to knowledge of the theoretical aspects of aging research, such as the importance of cohort effects, the importance of separating age and disease effects, and consideration of psychosocial factors when studying biomedical areas, but also practical aspects of clinical gerontological research.

Some practical considerations include:

1. The importance of developing a thorough, efficient, noninvasive screening procedure for all potential research subjects.
2. The importance of recognizing the substantial resources in terms of personnel and time required to perform clinical research in the elderly when compared to young adults. This factor cannot be overemphasized. Most clinical investigators are experienced in research on healthy

young adults with normal physical examinations who can read and understand informed consent forms, remember instructions, have few if any possibly confounding biomedical problems, are able to get dressed and undressed quickly, can fill out forms and questionnaires easily, have excellent veins, can void on request, often when lying supine if necessary, and are willing to undergo studies on successive days and to stay in clinical research centers for days to weeks. These individuals adapt well to changes in diet, and their daily schedules generally comply well with protocols requiring collection of blood, urine, or stool and rarely suffer adverse effects of physiologic studies. Elderly residents of long-term care facilities are more difficult to study than these healthy young volunteers. They require very detailed screening and a major time investment on the part of the investigator. One of the most important components of an efficient productive clinical research program in geriatrics is expert nursing personnel who are familiar with and committed to studies in the elderly and who can provide the warm, nurturing, and sensitive research atmosphere required.

3. The importance of prior research experience in the long-term care setting. Either ongoing projects or short pilot studies are required before a research program can be planned in a TNH. Such experiences provide the following benefits:

a. The administrators and boards of directors of long-term care facilities become experienced with researchers and research, thus eroding a major barrier to research—their concern for its impact on patient care.

b. Research staff and administrators develop expertise with the acquisition of informed consent from potential study subjects in the long-term care study. This requires a collaborative effort on the part of administrators, nurses, social workers, researchers, and primary care physicians. Families will often need to be involved in discussions of informed consent but not always. Long-term care facilities planning to be the site of substantial research should develop their own institutional review board.

c. Individual components of the long-term care facility gain an understanding of the impact of research on their personnel and programs. This is most important in the nursing sphere. It is not uncommon for clinical investigators to be naive regarding the impact of their research on the long-term care nursing staff. They often fail to realize that nurses are generally overworked and have no research experience. Researchers may expect nursing staff to obtain blood pressures, pulses, and weights on patients, administer mental status examinations, and perform functional assessments. They expect nurses to administer study medications and observe patients carefully for any adverse effects and often assist in the conduct of physiologic studies. This approach is often counterproductive and not only results in inconsistent data but often polarizes nursing staff against the research program, thus crippling the entire TNH effort.

   d. The interdisciplinary research team gains knowledge of the medical record system in the long-term care facility. Too frequently, researchers assume that nursing home records are equivalent to the records in acute-care hospitals and are unaware that much of the data they require may not be readily available.

   e. The overriding issue of respondent burden comes clearly into focus as several pilot studies are initiated simultaneously in a nursing home. Researchers become aware that in many cases they each wish to study the same individuals. This can sometimes be effectively addressed by careful planning and initial collection of data on patients who are relevant to more than one study. Frequently, investigators find that inadequate numbers of subjects will be available for their studies. If they are not to overburden individual patients, additional sources of subjects need to be identified prior to the initiation of the research plan.

   f. Investigators become aware that, unlike healthy young volunteers, frail institutionalized elders often become sick, sometimes requiring hospitalization, or die; and long-term studies (i.e., those requiring serial observations over a month or longer) will require more subjects initially than the investigators might expect from their experience with healthier subjects.

The following suggestions are made to individuals planning research activities in the context of an NIA TNH program:

1. Establish pilot research programs—this is mandatory.
2. Include major input from all consortium members in all stages of planning.
3. Address the issue of informed consent early and in detail.
4. Approach the effort as an institutional rather than a programmatic collaboration, i.e., involve boards of trustees, advisory committees, deans, etc.
5. Proceed at a pace consistent with the development of mutual trust.
6. Hold meetings with patients, families, nursing staff, and primary care physicians in the long-term-care setting to discuss the general and specific goals of the program.
7. Include long-term-care facility nursing staff in the planning process.
8. Develop educational programs that benefit the long-term-care facility patients and staff as part of the initial teaching nursing home effort.
9. Involve long-term-care facility nursing and medical staff in all research programs when possible.

10. Minimize the transfer of patients from the long-term care facility to other research sites.
11. Share the wealth and the public relations benefits in order to facilitate TNH development.

There is no intent to present a pessimistic picture. Although clinical gerontological research certainly is not easy, it can be exceptionally satisfying. No area of clinical research has been more neglected or presents greater current challenges. No setting seems more appropriate for needed research than the nursing homes in which frail, multiply impaired elders reside.

The Teaching Nursing Home, edited by Edward
L. Schneider et al. © 1985 The Beverly
Foundation. Raven Press, New York.

Implications of Research for Public Policy

Carl Eisdorfer

Montefiore Medical Center, Albert Einstein College of Medicine, Bronx, New York 10467

There is a serious disparity between our present system for providing health care and the actual health needs of the elderly. Cost containment has become the dominant theme of those who make health policy, although appropriateness, quality, and outcome are scanty, at best.

Our health care system is founded on powerful cultural beliefs that give highest status and support to the diagnosis, treatment, and cure of acute diseases and to relevant research. At the same time, we accord relatively low priority to the functional evaluation of chronically impaired individuals and to the care of chronic health problems. Of course, it is these lower-valued chronic problems that are most prevalent among the elderly.

Any system of care reflects and reinforces current beliefs concerning what is valued and how to accomplish valued ends. Americans are technophiles; we are fascinated with and proud of our scientific achievements (1). We hold in high esteem the miracles of modern medicine and the science and technology that make many of these miracles possible. Accordingly, we have adopted strategies involving everything from training to financing mechanisms that encourage the use of high technology in diagnosis and treatment.

Clearly, the present organization and financing of health services reinforces the long-held belief that hospitals constitute the best settings for care. Unfortunately, we simply do not have a data base to show policymakers the benefits of alternative caring strategies.

As demographic and fiscal imperatives of this era have drawn attention to the nation's older citizens, we have become aware of the incongruity between our traditional beliefs and strategies of care and the needs of these consumers. With increasing life expectancy, these needs are predominantly long term, involving multiple illnesses and crossing the border between health and nonhealth functional needs, and they are often not amenable to traditional strategies of disease diagnosis, treatment, and cure. The goal of long-term care can be to restore full function. More often, however, it includes the slowing of decline, helping a patient or family to adapt to a given level of disability, reducing pain, improving social and psychological maintenance, or providing a humane environment for dying.

For the functionally disabled, the care needed is not primarily medical in nature, nor does it require sophisticated equipment. Usually a combination of physical care, supportive services, and personal appliances can help. Family members, nurses, social workers, psychologists, rehabilitation therapists, and others may be employed as principal caregivers.

The goal of the service provided is to compensate for functional loss rather than to effect a nonexistent cure. Often, simple personal appliances can be a crucial variable in functioning, but such technology is rarely accorded the priority in development or financing that reflects its potential benefits. Improved hearing aids, wheelchairs, walkers, or household appliances simply have not captured the medical imagination as have computerized tomographic scans, digital angiograms, or positron emission tomographic scanning devices.

Research increasingly demonstrates that with a proper financial investment and service structure, quality care can be delivered effectively in noninstitutional settings. In general, older people would prefer to be cared for at home whenever possible, and personal technology along with human service supports may help to achieve this goal for many. Indeed, the nursing home as a rather impoverished version of the hospital arguably sustaining the wrong approach to caring may be something to eliminate in its present form in favor of a system of long-term caring better suited to those in need.

Why, then, support the nursing home model through such programs as the teaching nursing home (TNH)?

A good many professionals have devoted much of the past few decades to the recommendation that we reexamine our pattern of health care delivery. Instead of maintaining an almost exclusive focus on hospital and long-term institutional care, perhaps policy should be oriented to insure noninstitutional, community-based long-term caring services and finances distributed accordingly. Indeed, this idea is not new; the phrase "alternatives to long-term care" is so often used by government policymakers that it may replace "In God we trust" on our currency.

From a public policy perspective, then, does it make sense to invest substantial time and effort in strengthening the nursing home, elevating it to the Aesculapian heights of the academic (medical) model? This seems a particularly wry note, since it is precisely the academic medical model that has been criticized for serving the elderly so poorly, and this program would appear to risk reinforcing the worst component of nursing home care, namely, the nursing home as a minihospital.

This concern that we are perpetuating those very institutional models from which we need to move away is valid, and we ignore it at our peril. However, the TNH as a concept need not reinforce old and inappropriate strategies of care.

Others have made the point that institutional settings devoted to long-term caring are a necessary resource in our society. Even the most optimistic must admit, however grudgingly, that nursing homes play a crucial role in the provision of care for many elderly, and, for the foreseeable future, a larger number of elderly will require ongoing supportive care, probably in just such institutions. That is reason enough to address the problem of how to improve nursing homes.

The TNH, if understood as an experiment in long-term caring rather than as an evolved institution, offers possibilities for study of geriatric disease, new types of treatment, and new models of service delivery that will lead us in the direction we would like to go, that is, toward a more comprehensive, flexible continuum of health services designed specifically for the needs of large numbers of elderly and delivered in the least restrictive settings possible. The TNH offers the opportunity to conduct long-neglected clinical research and professional training that will enable us to improve our understanding and care of many of the disabilities and diseases associated with age.

Such advances are, on the face of it, needed and desirable. But research at the TNH could have a more broadly based mission than just clinical disease investigation. The TNH also gives us the opportunity to test new ways of organizing and financing service delivery, training and retraining staff, setting up a therapeutic milieu, developing positive interactive relationships with other service providers, and addressing the ethical issues that arise in the care of the elderly, to identify just a few examples of what is needed. Research into these areas would take us beyond the existing relatively stereotypical academic medical models and would begin to provide us with the appropriate data base for policymaking. This chapter examines a number of potential research areas.

CLINICAL RESEARCH

A strong program of clinical research in long-term care has never been undertaken in this country. Perhaps, at least to some extent, we can attribute our national policy against long-term care to the dearth of relevant research concerning treatment potential and the clinical course of the older patient. During the decade of the middle 1960s to the middle 1970s, we experienced a growth of long-term care institutions. Then, for the sake of simplicity and reimbursement strategy, the range of long-term care institutional types was reduced. A strategy of reevaluating patient needs and the alternatives within long-term care awaits careful study and analysis, the implication of which is powerful. In New York State, 7.5% of hospital bed days are for patients awaiting nursing home placement.

The TNH provides an excellent environment for addressing this clinical research. Subjects are accessible and centralized; monitoring of environmental, treatment, and other research variables is simplified. The role of families as the basic support system and an understanding of social alternatives and family needs to sustain patients could be investigated with a view toward developing interventions that may have far-ranging policy implications.

Although the elderly population residing in nursing homes is not representative of older persons as a whole, studies of the health problems of the nursing home group can have a beneficial impact on the noninstitutionalized aged population as well as on acute hospital care. The nursing home group differs mainly in demographic characteristics: age, gender, and the presence of a family network to provide help on an informal basis.

The health problems experienced by the nursing home and non-nursing home groups are similar. It has been estimated that although only 5% of older persons live in institutions at any one time, for each aged nursing home resident, there is at least one equally disabled elderly person living in the community (2). Thus, both institutionalized and noninstitutionalized elderly stand to gain from research conducted into chronic disease and disability in the nursing home.

Many concerned professionals have spoken of the need for research on chronic diseases that has been virtually ignored until recently (3).

Understudied but common causes of institutionalization among the elderly include the irreversible dementias, depression, loss of bladder and bowel control, osteoporosis, diabetes, and osteoarthritis. Decubiti, gangrene, falls, sleep disorders, wandering, and problems in feeding all demand attention.

Our traditional focus on acute care has diverted our attention from the persistent chronic problems that the long-term care clinician encounters frequently. These management problems are also the difficulties that are of great concern to patients and their support systems and are as deserving of medical study as the more exotic diseases that seem to draw so much attention.

The TNH could and should open up clinical research opportunities into the use of various technologies that help patients to adapt to chronic disability. For example, the TNH could examine the adaptational and financial value of medical prostheses, including computer-based self-stimulation, particularly for those who are cognitively impaired.

Studies of prevention and of the management of patients with incontinence, decubiti, contractures, feeding problems, or nocturnal wandering have the potential not only of helping us to improve the care of older people but of reducing the cost of care for such patients.

RECONCEPTUALIZING THE NURSING HOME

Beyond providing a fertile setting for clinical research, the TNH offers us the opportunity to test new ways of conceptualizing the nursing home and its delivery of care (4). The TNH provides the context for taking beyond the discussion stage many of those ideas that have been under discussion for years.

The patient entering the long-term care facility usually has social and adaptational difficulties as well as chronic medical problems (1). Yet our nursing homes, modeled after hospitals, tend to neglect these important needs. Undue attention to physical disorders sometimes precludes the recognition that the nursing home is a home and not a hospital and that the patients really are residents.

One important aspect of shifting the nursing home from its present focus involves changing the quality of the relationships between staff and residents. Patients in greater control behave more like real people and are likely, therefore, to do better in caring for their own needs.

The TNH offers a context for developing models of care designed to meet the needs of the whole person, not just those parts requiring medical treatment. In the context of the TNH, we can examine the question of whether we ought to resocialize the nursing home and change the nature of the environment from its present emphasis on health and disease to an adaptational and functionally oriented setting.

Architectural changes might be included. The integration of health and social services, the design of more home-like and comfortable physical environments, and the rebalancing of power relationships among staff and between staff and residents need to be studied and could affect both staffing and reimbursement patterns.

Brody and others have identified the fact that nursing homes presently are serving two distinct resident populations (5). One group has temporary convalescent needs; members of this group generally stay in skilled nursing facilities for relatively short periods (usually 90 days or less). Brody called this short-term long-term care (STLTC). The second group, in long-term long-term care (LTLTC), have significantly longer stays and are less likely to be discharged to their homes.

With the advent of DRG regulations, it is likely that the need for short-term long-term care services will increase. As hospitals respond to incentives to reduce length of stay, they are likely to discharge older patients who still have convalescent needs and require some temporary form of institutional care.

The TNH could play an important role in identifying ways to restructure services to bring them more into line with the needs of the two different types of nursing home residents. A possibility is to modify the nursing home into two components, one becoming a chronic disease hospital with a rehabilitation focus and the other offering functionally oriented support programs.

A well-staffed rehabilitation facility acting in lieu of a hospital could significantly influence certain health care costs, as the high-technology capital investment in these facilities could be minimized.

In the LTLTC setting, physicians could be replaced by nurse practitioners, physician's assistants, and psychosocial workers who could probably care adequately for a substantial portion of the needs of targeted and well-examined groups. This alternative orientation could give us a chance to do much more aggressive studies of the effect of rehabilitation on patient management and to focus on a series of issues that challenge and overwhelm the family or the individual and result in institutionalization.

A multilevel long-term care facility could distinguish problems requiring intense care from those that demand less attention. In the less intense cases, the nursing home could limit its role to that of a primarily day or night caring agency acting in collaboration with the patient's family. Reductions in the costs of care and in stress on the family could be important by-products.

A related concept for the TNH is the use of nursing home beds for alternate supportive services. Examples include respite care, which allows families to take a breather from caring for elderly relatives, day or night care, and the use of nursing home beds for diagnostic purposes or for family training. In this context, families would have the opportunity to learn how to better manage the care of frail, aging relatives.

None of these ideas is new, but the TNH could make an important contribution by translating them into successful, evaluated program models. As part of this effort, the TNH would need to experiment with alternate methods for financing these services, since insurance coverage for them is presently limited (5). The development of innovative private–public insurance or other financing strategies is a key public policy issue worth investigation.

Models for providing respite night care and other forms of long-term care—and for providing this care in an affordable manner—would significantly improve our ability to support family caregivers. We are not sufficiently aware that the family is this country's major source of care for the elderly. It is worth investing substantial time and effort to find ways to protect this precious, and at times fragile, resource. At the same time, the aged without family are at higher risk for nursing home placement. Alternate living styles such as that of the Philadelphia Geriatrics Center need to be examined and a range of policy issues from funding to zoning regulations pursued.

THE NURSING HOME AS A MINI-MENTAL HOSPITAL

One of the key policy concerns of the TNH ought to be research into the mental health care of the aged. Careful evaluation of nursing home patients, with particular attention to their psychiatric needs, would explode several myths. One of these is that the profound advances in psychiatry credited with reducing the number of psychiatrically ill people who require care in state hospitals has benefited the elderly. Indeed, data support the notion that most of the beds that have been closed in state psychiatric facilities have reopened as nursing home beds, but without the benefits of mental health professionals. Medicare and Medicaid reimbursement incentives have encouraged the diversion of patients from state hospitals to long-term care facilities with no requirement for provision of mental health services.

It has been shown that the post-1960 decrease in the number of individuals in state hospitals has been met with an equivalent rise in the number of nursing home patients (6). Thus, for elderly individuals, deinstitutionalization has merely meant reinstitutionalization in a facility less well equipped to meet their psychiatric needs.

Data emphasize the urgency for attending to the mental health needs of the institutionalized elderly. A 1976 study found that about three-quarters of the nursing home residents were either formally diagnosed with a psychiatric disorder or were "*de facto* psychiatrically impaired." Projecting this finding to a national level suggests that there may be more than three-quarters of a million nursing home residents who have psychiatric problems but have little or no contact with psychiatrists (6).

This is a major public policy issue involving Medicaid financing and Federal–state relationships. Here the patients—and particularly the LTLTC patients—have become the victims. This use of Medicaid dollars has also had its impact on the broader spectrum of Medicaid-eligible persons of all ages.

Critical tasks for the TNH include: improving diagnosis of psychiatric illness among older patients, particularly in functional terms; clinical research into appropriate use of psychotropic drugs and their side effects; and alternate psychosocial strategies. Many experts suspect that psychotropic drugs are being used as a less expensive strategy in lieu of other, perhaps better, therapies. Under present policy, reimbursement is more readily forthcoming for nonpsychiatric physicians' employment of psychotropic drugs than for a range of other approaches designed to improve function.

The TNH presents a most important opportunity to study a range of innovative techniques such as cognitive retraining and to reduce reliance on sedating or restraining medication.

LINKING THE NURSING HOME WITH OTHER HEALTH CARE PROVIDERS

At the moment, the nursing home is often operated apart from the array of supportive and caring systems that exist in the community to serve the elderly. The TNH could play a significant role in linking the nursing home not only with the family but with a range of provider organizations within the health and human services systems.

Elaine Brody (*this volume*), among others, has dispelled the myths that families abandon their elders or dump them in institutions. We know that, for the most part, institutions are used as a last resort, either when an elderly person has no family or when the care needs of the elderly person extend beyond the physical or psychological capabilities of the family.

The TNH is capable of addressing many important questions about the family. For example: How can the nursing home build a collaborative relationship with the family? What are appropriate financial arrangements that balance the fiscal needs but do not force pauperization of the spouse or children?

Just as the TNH can find ways for families and nursing homes to reinforce each other's efforts, the TNH can help to move the nursing home toward the health and social service systems from which it presently is somewhat isolated. Preferred provider arrangements, the nursing home as a component of a vertically integrated hospital, and other such arrangements require close examination. The positive and negative implications of each should be assessed, and implications of DRGs for the hospital–nursing home relationship are also of immediate interest. Similarly, models for improved relationships between nursing homes and social agencies should be developed.

TRAINING AND DEVELOPMENT

In addition to the need for more medical, nursing, and other professional training in dealing with aged and chronically impaired persons is the need to substantially increase our investment in the education of nurse's aides. Nurse's aides are the people who provide the bulk of care to the elderly residents of nursing homes and yet are the least well-trained and probably have least job satisfaction. Although a great deal of attention has been given to this issue, little has actually been accomplished in terms of upgrading training.

Since we have kept nurse's aides at the lowest economic and educational levels, it is not surprising that the general quality of care given is low and that staff turnover rates are high where other employment opportunities exist. If we truly wish to improve the quality of care in our long-term care institutions, it is imperative that we equip those with the most "hands-on" responsibility with proper skills and education for the job. Additionally, we need to find ways to attract and keep personnel once they are trained. The TNH is perfectly suited to the tasks of evaluating the socioeconomics of improving the quality of staff and developing new training models.

The nursing home as a work setting must be explored. The recent report by Eisdorfer (7) has identified potentially serious problems among the RN and LPN staffs of several nursing homes. Whether these problems are secondary to adverse selection or to job-related stress, the implication for patient care is extraordinary and should be a basis for careful scrutiny and possible changes in the system.

FINANCING CARE

The TNH must address the issue of making long-term care affordable. Despite enormous expenditures for health care, we are not meeting existing needs; yet, we are pauperizing families in the process.

Rhetoric notwithstanding, there is every indication that we are already rationing both acute and long-term health care in many parts of this country. The TNH could offer an appropriate setting for developing alternate models of long-term care financing and service delivery that will enable us to extend scarce resources to those who need them.

We need to correct the major imbalances in our existing health care financing programs for the elderly. Our present system focuses on acute care when the need is primarily for chronic care management; it dichotomizes health and social services when an integrated service package is what most people need. The result is the eventual medical indigency of even middle- and upper-middle-class patients who require institutional care. Middle-class elderly who are ineligible for Medicaid on admission to a nursing home find themselves rapidly impoverished by the exorbitant costs of care (2). The process of spending down to Medicaid eligibility levels requires the older patient or spouse to exhaust virtually all assets including lifetime savings and home.

In short, older patients must divest themselves of the very resources that would enable them to return home following a period of institutionalization. The pauperization of the elderly is a devastating problem; it deserves high priority on our investigative and policy agendas.

TRANSLATING RESEARCH INTO POLICY

One of the greatest impediments to formulating policy on long-term care in this country is the lack of a solid data base about the long-term care of the elderly and the value of the services provided to them. An example that currently illustrates this point is the Congressional debate on the expansion of home health care services for the elderly. The number of General Accounting Office and Congressional Budget Office reports on the pros and cons of expanding home care are endless. Yet Congressional leaders still do not have good data to determine whether home care reduces the number of days of nursing home care, decreases hospital use, or reduces total health care costs. Quality-of-care issues abound, and we risk setting up a series of new problems by coming up with simple solutions without appropriate feedback from committed and well-recognized providers.

For example, to insure quality of care in some areas we insist that a skilled nursing facility do daily temperature checks as part of skilled nursing. Since a substantial portion of the SNF population may have Alzheimer's disease or a related dementia without other physical problems, this has resulted in daily rectal temperatures of disoriented persons who often resist mightily this intrusion on their being and require several people to hold them down. It is not surprising, therefore, that the debate just lingers on.

In conclusion, a few points can be made about strategies for increasing the likelihood that research findings will affect policy decisions. First, data are essential. Second, we should not expect that policy decisions will always be made from a sound data base.

The documented history of the creation of the National Institute of Aging (8) gives ample testimony to the nature of the political process influencing policy. The recent upsurge of interest in Alzheimer's disease in Washington and throughout the United States is hardly the result of any report by the Center for Disease Control on the outbreaks of a new Alzheimer's disease epidemic. A major route to policy formulation is to have individuals or groups of people exert their political influence in the correct place at the correct time. The advances in polio research under the Roosevelt administration, in cancer funding under Nixon, and in mental retardation during the Kennedy era need no further elaboration.

There is another good way to affect public policy: a successful demonstration project, strategically placed, has enormous power. Consider, for example, the community-based long-term care model at On Lok in San Francisco. The Health Care Financing Administration reportedly decided about 2 years ago not to extend On Lok's waiver, which was essential to their financial survival. Yet this relatively small demonstration program had United States senators virtually competing with each other on the Senate floor in their effort to override the Administration's decision—not because of any political clout but because of the program's considerable success in taking care of the long-term health needs of the frail elderly Chinese–Americans in the San Francisco area. Finally, anyone who ever attended a Congressional hearing is struck by the power of the afflicted to promote their cause.

Perhaps the TNH has the greatest likelihood of affecting policy if it produces a few excellent demonstration projects and focuses on the impact of improved care on individual patients and their families. The TNH has the potential of identifying new and successful models for organizing, financing, and delivering long-term care services. However, only if the models work and work demonstrably well should they have a chance of influencing national policy.

REFERENCES

1. Eisdorfer C: Care of the aged: The barriers of traditions. *Ann Intern Med* 1981;94:256–260.
2. Avorn J: Beyond the bedside: The social context of geriatric practice, in Rowe J, Besdine R (eds): *Health and Disease in Old Age*. Boston, Little, Brown, 1982, pp. 25–37.
3. Besdine R: The data base of geriatric medicine, in Rowe J, Besdine R (eds): *Health and Disease in Old Age*. Boston, Little, Brown, 1982, pp 1–13.
4. Schneider E: Teaching nursing homes. *N Engl J Med* 1983;308:336–337.

5. Brody S: Health services: Need and utilization, in Brody S, Persily N (eds): *Hospitals and the Aged*. Rockville, MD, Aspen Systems, 1984, pp. 39, 106.
6. Gelfand D: *The Aging Network*. New York, Springer, 1984.
7. Eisdorfer S: Differential impact of educational programs on nurses working in a long-term care setting [Dissertation]. Seattle, University of Washington, 1983.
8. Lockett BA: *Aging, Politics and Research: Setting the Federal Agenda for Research on Aging*. New York, Springer, 1983.

PART VI
The Teaching Nursing Home as a Focus for Training

The Teaching Nursing Home, edited by Edward
L. Schneider et al. © 1985 The Beverly
Foundation. Raven Press, New York.

Introduction

Leslie S. Libow

*Department of Geriatrics and Adult Development, The Mount Sinai Medical Center, New
York, New York 10027*

In the earliest model academic nursing home program, teaching was the
mechanism by which we attempted to insure improved patient care and
improved quality physician training (1,2). By contrast, the Teaching Nursing
Home (TNH) Program of the National Institute on Aging (NIA) is funded
with a major emphasis on research, with the hope that teaching will occur
under the umbrella of research (3,4). Indeed, this hope seems realistic, and
the early advances seem promising.

Students, medical faculty, visitors, and patients all fear the nursing home.
The connotation is decline, death, and general disarray. Yet the nursing
home must become central to all health care systems. We can expect to see
remarkable changes in the nursing home by developing teaching programs
with their accompanying improved quality of atmosphere, skill, and attitude
(5,6). These changes will not be accomplished if the nursing home is treated
as a museum. For example, students should not be brought to the nursing
home for courses in physical diagnosis that focus on the "interesting murmur" rather than on the human beings involved in their struggle for survival
and quality of life.

Appropriate clinical care of the frail elderly, institutionalized or not, cannot be carried out by one practitioner, whether it be physician, nurse, or
social worker. A team of skilled clinicians is necessary to deal with the multiplicity of simultaneous medical, social, psychological, and environmental
problems. This team should be integrated into the health care system that
is developed and built around the nursing home. The team, of course,
cannot be defined as a series of individuals of various disciplines sitting in
the same room once per week. Rather, it must be a well-designed and then
redesigned instrument, put through a variety of trials before it is effective,
and then applied where appropriate.

Training in the nursing home will affect health care approaches for those
of all ages. Nursing home medicine is a less technological and less costly
approach to those with a variety of severe illnesses. The clinical trainee
learns that not every sepsis requires intravenous medication, not every pneumonia requires hospitalization, not every stroke must be seen by a neurol-

307

ogist, and not every myocardial infarction requires a cardiac care unit. By increasing clinical skills, diminishing dependency on laboratory and technology, and improving judgment and common sense, the physician will be able to extrapolate this skill not only to the elderly in the community but to young and middle-aged patients in community and hospital.

REFERENCES

1. Libow LS: A fellowship in geriatric medicine. *J Am Geriatr Soc* 1972;20:580–584.
2. Libow LS: A geriatric medical residency program: A four-year experience. *Ann Intern Med* 1976;85:641–647.
3. Butler RN: The teaching nursing home. *JAMA* 1981;245:1435–1437.
4. Schneider EL: Teaching nursing homes. *N Engl J Med* 1983;308:336–337.
5. Duthie EA, Priefer B, Gambert SR: The teaching nursing home. *JAMA* 1982;247:2787–2788.
6. Fisk AA: Comprehensive health care for the elderly. *JAMA* 1983;249:230–236.

The Teaching Nursing Home, edited by Edward
L. Schneider et al. © 1985 The Beverly
Foundation. Raven Press, New York.

Medical Student and Postgraduate Physician Training in the Nursing Home

Richard W. Besdine

*Hebrew Rehabilitation Center for Aged and Department of Medicine, Division on Aging,
Harvard Medical School, Boston, Massachusetts 02131*

Although the elderly are disproportionate consumers of American health resources, they continue, with few exceptions, to be ignored in the mainstream of American medical education. A recent report from the Institute of Medicine documents the deficiency of and need for training in geriatrics. The data base of geriatrics includes a cohesive but multidisciplinary body of knowledge, which is at best fragmented and incomplete in most current curricula. The data base includes:

1. Clinical geriatrics with its multiple subsets.
2. Normative aspects of biological and physiological aging (gerontology) and their interactions with disease.
3. The relationship of various life stages to psychologic and physiologic accompaniments of illness.
4. The transdisciplinary structure and cooperation required for teaching in clinical care relating to elderly patients.
5. The principles and specific details of the health care delivery system and modifications that likely would generate improved care for the elderly.

The goal of geriatric program development is not the creation of a cadre of clinical specialists who would take over the care of people reaching age 65 from the professionals who brought them to 65. Such an effort would be intolerable philosophically and operationally in America. The present goal is to produce small numbers of academic physicians committed to the study of aging who would develop and implement geriatric curricula. These efforts would provide the exposure and education for all health professional students, who will be spending increasing proportions of their professional lives caring for elderly patients.

There is a serious shortage of clinically skilled, academically oriented geriatricians and gerontologists in America. Although more than 75 of the

126 American medical schools responded affirmatively to an Institute of Medicine questionnaire about aging programs in their institutions, the great majority still seek leaders for their nascent programs. Few candidates with adequate academic experience are available simply because there have been few or no academic training programs in aging. Although many patients in acute hospitals are elderly (one-third or more at any time), general or medical subspecialty postgraduate training programs do not include specific didactic or clinical experiences for trainees addressing the special focus and data base of geriatrics. Training in long-term care institutions and exposure to the continuum of care, which are essential for successful maintenance of elderly patients, are absent in the postgraduate education of physicians who are candidates for academic positions in medical schools and teaching hospitals. Effective curriculum development in aging must await effective faculty development.

The logical first step in generating teachers of geriatric medicine is to attract good candidates from general medicine and provide them with post-residency fellowship training in geriatrics. These new geriatricians must be provided with the knowledge base and attitudes to equip them for careers in patient care and teaching exclusively focused on aged individuals, especially those frail elders at highest risk for functional decline and thus institutionalization. During training, fellows must also acquire competence in the evaluation and production of new knowledge in an area relevant to geriatric care to remain academically credible and competitive. Clinical training must provide the fellow with exposure to the multivariate continuum of care required to successfully meet the varied needs of frail elderly. The training must, in addition, be truly interdisciplinary, providing the fellow with a comprehensive understanding of the function and contribution of the numerous disciplines, in addition to medicine, required for successful management of vulnerable multiply impaired elderly. Such appreciation requires that the fellow be part of an interdisciplinary patient care team that includes, at a minimum, the primary care disciplines of nursing and social work, along with medicine.

Currently, most educational efforts in geriatrics are focused within health professional schools and their affiliated institutions, the majority being acute-care hospitals. In spite of the dominance of older patients in acute-care hospital beds, the acute-care hospital encourages a distorted view of the ill old person. The educational and attitudinal goals of geriatric training are best accomplished in a variety of settings, and the acute-care hospital bed is probably the most common but least typical setting to study disease and behavior in old age. The community, its supporting organizations, and long-term care institutions are the realistic settings in which health impairments, functional disability, and treatment responses can best be studied. But examination of current teaching sites and practices in undergraduate, postgraduate, and continuing health provider education reveals a monotonously recurring mismatch between the loci of training and the spectrum of care sites for the elderly (home, community support systems, and nursing homes).

Although long-term care simply means caring for someone over a long period of time, it has traditionally meant nursing home care; nursing homes have not been institutions with attractions for the academic teaching, research, or service community in any health profession. In spite of the relatively small numbers of elders in nursing homes, the distilled disease essence of the most frail elderly individuals is easily and reliably available for study in the nursing home. And for each frail elderly nursing home resident, there are at least two disabled home-dwelling elderly who qualify for institutional care and differ from the nursing home group primarily in having a family network capable of providing the informal supports that allow continued community dwelling. Thus, the study and learning of health care for the most frail resource-consuming segment of the elderly population (15–20%) can most easily be accomplished in the nursing home setting. That other sites are suitable and necessary is not disputed, but the major clinical geriatric teaching resource, as yet largely untapped in America, is the nursing home.

A set of major interrelated problems confronts long-term care institutions in late 20th century America. Knowledge concerning the management of frail elderly individuals must be both increased and translated into adequate, coordinated, continuing interdisciplinary health care. The production of the teachers and investigators who will introduce geriatrics into the mainstream of medical education is a first priority. The clinical education they receive and research they pursue must be focused on the nursing home, where, for the most part, an enormous untapped clinical and investigative need exists. The long-term care institution is also the appropriate hub of general health professional education in geriatrics as well as the site for training of specialist educators and investigators. The goals that, when achieved, will solve the problem of inadequate expertise in care of nursing home residents are as follows:

1. To produce new health professional educator/investigators committed to geriatrics who will assume responsibility for teaching principles of geriatric medicine to all students.
2. To provide for health professionals the data base of geriatrics by clinical example in the nursing home setting.
3. To train health professionals from the different clinical disciplines in the same setting using interdisciplinary teams.
4. To improve and reverse negative ageist attitudes among health professionals themselves.
5. To teach the principles and demonstrate the gratifications of long-term care.

Long-term care is the essence of geriatrics and of much contemporary medicine, with professional success and gratification derived from restoring and preserving maximum function and improving life in the face of chronic or recurrent disease, in contrast with the widespread myth that cure is the only goal of modern medical intervention.

Unlike acute hospitals, nursing homes, although they provide health care to many heavy consumers of health resources, have rarely developed ties to health professional schools. The absence of such relationships has meant, first, that professional students have rarely had experience in nursing homes and, second, that nursing homes have been deprived both of the experience of having students around and of the influence of academic faculty on health care delivery. Unfortunately, unfamiliarity and occasionally suspicion characterize interactions between professional students and nursing homes. Furthermore, students, the academic medical community, and society in general often regard the nursing home as a profit-motivated, poor-quality care-delivering institution to be avoided if at all possible. Thus, a major attitudinal barrier may exist between students and the nursing home.

Another barrier to development of professional education in long-term care settings is the shortage of qualified faculty, not simply faculty in geriatrics but, more important, faculty in geriatrics who have adequate knowledge and experience in long-term care.

A fourth barrier is the absence of evaluation standards for any program in geriatrics providing education for health professional students and graduates.

Last and most important among the barriers to all progress in care of the elderly is the specter of ageism. Negative attitudes about debilitated, incontinent, demented elderly who are concentrated in nursing homes will be an ever present impediment to training programs focused in these institutions. Nevertheless, with sensitive faculty and careful curriculum development, this barrier can be overcome as well.

The existence of good quality nursing homes is a special resource, providing a distilled essence of disease and functional disability for study in elderly residents in an optimistic setting of care delivery. Nowhere else can individuals with advanced disease states be observed and studied by students, often allowing the teaching of the entire natural history of a single disorder. The same diseases that are beginning to be functionally troublesome for the community-dwelling individual are often present with the full spectrum of pathology in the institutionalized patient. The existence of far advanced disease in some nursing home residents should not be disturbing to students provided adequate explanation of the processes is sensitively given beforehand. It is useful to remind students that debilitated individuals are volunteering to help teach about advanced disease in old age so that as future physicians the students will recognize disease early and prevent its progression in the independent elderly.

The nursing home presents a unique opportunity to teach "Comprehensive Functional Assessment in the Elderly" (CFAITE) as the cornerstone of geriatric health care. Impairment of the ability to function independently at home is the final common pathway of the broad array of diseases encountered frequently with increasing age. Functional impairment is the decreased ability to meet one's own needs, including the functions allowing mobility, cognition, eating, using the toilet, dressing, hygiene, shopping, cooking, and managing money. Unlike young persons, when elderly individuals become ill, the first sign of new or recrudescent chronic disease is rarely a single specific symptomatic complaint that helps to localize the organ system or tissue in which the disease occurs. Rather, old patients usually announce active illness with one or more nonspecific disabilities, which rapidly produce functional impairment.

The crucial implication for health care and life quality maintenance in old age is that deterioration of functional independence is a reliable marker of active, usually inadequately managed, disease. These diseases producing functional impairment in old people often are treatable and improvable, but detection is essential. Success of health maintenance or early intervention strategies in geriatrics requires a sensitive and accurate ability to assess functional status initially and over time in vulnerable elders wherever they are found. Thus, CFAITE emerges as a crucial capability for our health care system. The nursing home, given its high concentration of frail elders, is the best setting in which to teach CFAITE.

One crucial principle of geriatric medicine best taught in the nursing home using CFAITE is the lack of correlation between functional impairment and disease burden. Because prevalence of disease and functional loss increase with age, it is commonly assumed by most health professionals that the number of conditions identified on the problem list of an elderly individual determines the severity of functional loss. On the contrary, many independent old people have astonishingly long and impressive problem lists. It is also assumed that the specific type of functional loss is determined by the locus of the disease, so that problems with mobility originate in arthritis or stroke, problems of confusion originate in brain disease, problems with incontinence in bladder or kidney disease, weight loss in gastrointestinal pathology, and so on.

This principle of medicine, generally valid in young and middle-aged persons, is not valid in the elderly. Rather, as discussed, certain organ systems responsible for crucial functions permitting independence are vulnerable to the influence of disease in any organ system. Additionally, the severity of disease as measured by objective laboratory tests does not necessarily determine the presence or severity of functional impairment. For example, asymptomatic complete heart block may be discovered on a routine electrocardiogram, or startling but symptomless elevation of blood urea nitrogen on multiphasic screening in an independent elderly person. In situations of an impressive laboratory abnormality with minimal or no obvious functional impairment in an old person, objective CFAITE may provide the courage to withhold treatment for the symptomless aberration, especially if the treatment, such as a pacemaker or dialysis, carries with it substantial risk, discomfort, or expense. There is a clear educational mandate to equip health professionals with both the skill and awareness to perform CFAITE to permit maximum continuing independence and to permit prompt detection of decline, possibly indicating need for treatment.

The lessons taught by these noncorrelations between function and diagnosis are crucial for good care of elders. First, functional impairment must be assessed and quantified independent of the problem list in the problem-oriented medical record. Second, although an impairment of function may seem to correlate with a single organ system, the existence of that functional impairment does not necessarily imply disease in the parent organ system, nor does it justify attribution of the impairment to a disease identified in that organ system. For example, an old woman with urinary incontinence may, on exhaustive evaluation, be found to have a normal urinary tract and be incontinent because her diuretic medication fills her bladder faster than she can walk to a distant toilet and urinate. Even if a bladder infection were documented, treatment of the infection may not improve her incontinence. Only the restoration of continence by successful treatment of the infection allows attribution of incontinence to infection.

The central importance of functional impairment to the elderly person underscores the need for CFAITE. Health professionals may focus their concern on objective parameters of disease such as physical findings, blood chemistry values, X-ray results, and electrocardiogram. For the elderly person, these values are unimportant compared with the impact on life quality of the functional impairment. Therapeutic goals must be measured for the elderly individual by the quantification and then reduction of the burden of functional loss. The educational uses of CFAITE emerge here again for professionals caring for the elderly in allowing gratification for the provider and satisfaction for the patient by targeting and relieving the worst symptoms.

The educational objective for health professionals caring for vulnerable elders is to acquire skills and readiness to use CFAITE in parallel with classic disease-oriented evaluation techniques. A listing of all functional impairments, assembled side by side with the problem list, will facilitate careful comparison of diagnosis with lost function. Within the list of functional losses and their severity, items on the problem list can be identified as most likely etiologic of the most troublesome functional impairments for the elderly individual. By addressing problems using this functionally oriented priority system, the health provider is likely to satisfy the patient/client and, by seeing important gains in independence measured by continuing CFAITE, reap personal satisfaction as well. Additionally, if interventions produce no benefit, they can be confidently abandoned and new priorities addressed.

Most nursing homes care for some independently functional individuals who are institutionalized not because they need the full complement of nursing home services but because what they do need is not available in their own communities. These persons, besides providing relief from the discouraging aspects of severely impaired nursing home residents, also provide an appropriate focus for demonstrating how and why old people get into institutions.

In order to teach long-term care of the elderly effectively in the nursing home, three considerations must be addressed: faculty to do the teaching, curriculum to be taught, and credibility of the nursing home as an educational site. All the faculty teaching in the nursing home need not have the same scientific credentials demanded of full-time academics. But some primary care responsibility for the nursing home patients by the faculty is essential so that in the teaching process students can see clinician–educators deriving professional gratification from treating elderly patients. Academic credibility is important, and care of the elderly should never be considered a second-class activity: disinterested academics fulfilling a teaching obligation in a nursing home with patients they do not know would have a potentially disastrous impact on student attitudes. The protective caring shown by most professionals functioning in a primary care role is attractive to students and enhances learning.

Curriculum content for the nursing home educational experience needs to be chosen carefully. Departure from the high-technology intensive-care unit atmosphere of the teaching hospital is a welcome relief for most students and is consistent with the therapeutic goals of nursing home care. Emphasis on practioner–patient relationships, with direct student precepting by faculty, allows the bedside teaching that is less and less available in the acute-care hospital. In the teaching of geriatrics, a *potpourri* curriculum of sequential subspecialty medicine applied to old patients should be avoided. Adequate documentation of the data base for geriatrics exists and should be consulted in curriculum design. Two major attitudinal objectives of geriatric teaching for students are to learn that:

1. Curing is a relatively rare event in modern medicine, and successful caring for elderly patients over the long term of chronic or recurring illness is a source of gratification.
2. Sick old people are sick because they are sick, not because they are old. Functional loss occurring in old age is usually caused by disease, not aging; disease is usually improvable if not curable.

Making the nursing home a credible educational site has attitudinal and substantive components. The institution must be adequately prepared to receive students. Staff anxiety about being criticized in their professional performance or about having patients "used as guinea pigs" must be directly confronted. Students need to be told both what to expect and what their roles will be at the institution. Adequate facilities must be available to make the students' experience pleasant, and student impact on the functioning of the institution must be considered in scheduling sessions. All nursing home staff must understand why students are there. An introductory presentation of the problems and goals of long-term institutional care will help students realize the burden that nursing homes undertake when caring for elderly residents. Most important, students and the nursing home will each profit from the presence of a skillful faculty committed to medical education and successful long-term institutional care.

There is no disagreement that ambulatory and even well elderly should interact with medical students to provide a realistic view of successful aging in an independent setting, but the core of clinical geriatrics is taught best with moderately to severely impaired nursing home residents. Although the frail elderly, in and out of nursing homes, may comprise only one-fifth of the population over 65 years of age, they will, as major consumers of health resources, occupy a disproportionately large share of physician practice time, and, therefore, emphasis on their problems and health care is appropriate in health professional training. As appropriate information conduits and trainees in their own right, fellows in geriatrics and advanced residents in medicine and primary care should teach and learn along with faculty and students in the nursing home and other less intensive clinical long-term care sites.

The response of the Hebrew Rehabilitation Center for Aged (HRCA) to problems of geriatric education and medical care has been an innovative coordinated long-term effort culminating in a current program that has made the institution the hub of an integrated university-wide clinical and research postdoctoral fellowship training program in geriatric medicine. All eight primary care physicians of the medical staff provide, in varying amount, faculty supervision in clinical and investigative activities of the fellows. Two graduates of the program have joined the medical staff and spend a majority of their clinical professional time delivering care to frail aged nursing home residents. One has undertaken and completed a research project studying the value of periodic laboratory screening in nursing home dwellers. Another graduate has been appointed to an academic position spanning medical school, acute-care hospital, and nursing home, which will be his primary base for teaching and research. In studying syncope at the HRCA, he has uncovered a unique phenomenon of postprandial hypotension, which is currently under further investigation.

Each year, 35 to 40 second-year medical students are taught part of their physical diagnosis course at HRCA by its medical staff and the geriatric fellows, and special geriatric sessions are provided for those students as well. First-year medical students are introduced to functionally intact elderly residents and discuss issues in aging with an interdisciplinary staff group from the institution. Third- and fourth-year students from the related and numerous other medical schools take clinical didactic electives and preceptorships in geriatrics at HRCA. Medical house staff at the second and third postgraduate-year levels from several of the medical school's acute teaching hospitals take a 1-month elective course in geriatrics at HRCA throughout the year. Currently, several clinical research projects germane to geriatrics are being carried out at the nursing home by fellows and medical staff, largely under the aegis of an NIA TNH award.

This broad array of multilevel educational activities and research projects at one long-term care facility summate to provide a true academic or teaching nursing home. Identification of some key elements allowing the synthesis of this program may permit other institutions to consider undertaking related projects. The first initiative at HRCA was the recruitment and hiring of an academically oriented clinician in geriatrics, partly supporting some of his specialized geriatric training and underwriting his full-time salary. The encouragement to develop strong medical school linkages and a fellowship beyond the walls of the institution was essential. The director of the fellowship program spends part time supervising fellows and delivering primary care at the nursing home but also spends substantial time teaching at the medical school and acute-care hospital connected to the nursing home. Partial salary support for fellows primarily training at the institution came soon after the fellowship program began. Administrative approval and encouragement for broad support of the fellows and their faculty was crucial in securing the cooperation of institutional staff.

Fellows in geriatric medicine are recruited for a 2-year program at the completion of residency training, usually in internal medicine. After a comprehensive orientation, fellows spend 1 year three-quarters time delivering interdisciplinary team primary care to one nursing unit of institution residents under the supervision of a faculty member on the medical staff. All fellows also attend weekly tutorials in geropsychiatry. Specialty clinics are held frequently at the institution in dentistry, podiatry, ophthalmology, neurology, gynecology, general surgery, audiology, psychiatry, dermatology, and radiology. Fellows are taught in these settings, usually focusing on their patients. A weekly didactic conference at which a fellow discusses an important clinical topic in geriatrics is held at the institution and attended by medical staff, fellows, and other professionals from the entire academic community who are interested in aging. Fellows serve in their units as physician representatives in staff conferences and family meetings.

The benefits to the nursing home of such academic relationships are numerous. First, the nursing home and its residents benefit from the medical care provided by the physicians who are receiving training in the institution. Not only does this relieve the shortage of physicians willing to provide care for nursing home residents, but it also provides physicians lacking specific geriatric training with exposure to newer diagnostic thera-peutic strategies in care of elderly individuals. Second, these clinical phy-sicians have an opportunity to share in the medical educational process. Third, new physicians completing training are more likely to work in the nursing home setting when the medical director or staff positions need to be filled. Fourth, the interaction of motivated, enthusiastic medical trainees with a broad range of professionals working in the nursing home gives the staff a sense of pride in participation in the teaching programs. Fifth, in-terdisciplinary training, in which professionals from different disciplines learn and work together, enhances the care given to the elderly and helps all involved staff to better understand the roles and capabilities of their colleagues. Sixth, the presence of clinical training and research focused on better care of the elderly enhances the community image of the nursing home and aids in staff recruitment. Seventh, the increased movement of professionals between nursing home and acute-care hospital improves the care given to nursing home residents when they are hospitalized. Eighth, the presence of educational and investigative programs aids the nursing home in attempts to obtain outside funding for further innovative projects.

The comprehensive program described is large and complex, but com-ponents are identifiable that can be developed by smaller institutions with-out established medical school and teaching hospital connections. Increas-ing numbers of medical schools, teaching hospitals, and Veterans Administration facilities are developing training programs in geriatric med-icine. All need to identify long-term care institutions that can provide place-ments for fellows, house staff, and students who must learn geriatrics. Abun-dant evidence indicates that the nursing home is the ideal site for geriatric training. The task is to make such training available.

GENERAL REFERENCES

1. Akpom CA, Mayer S: A survey of geriatric education in US medical schools. *J Med Ed* 1978;53(1):66–68.
2. Butler RN: Testimony before the US Senate Special Committee on Aging. Medicine and Aging: An Assessment of Opportunities and Neglect, 1976.
3. Institute of Medicine: *The Elderly and Functional Dependence.* Washington, DC; National Academy of Sciences, 1977.
4. Somers AR: Geriatric care in the United Kingdom: An American perspective. *Ann Intern Med* 1976;84:466–476.
5. Institute of Medicine: *Aging and Medical Education.* Washington, DC; National Academy of Sciences, 1978.
6. Besdine RW: The data base of geriatric medicine, in Rowe JW, Besdine RW (eds): *Health and Disease in Old Age.* Boston, Little, Brown, 1982, pp 1–14.
7. American College of Physicians: *Conference Proceedings: Changing Needs of Nursing Home Care.* Philadelphia, American College of Physicians, 1980.
8. Besdine RW: Educational utility of comprehensive functional assessment in the elderly. *J Am Geriatr Soc* 1983;31:651–656.
9. Butler RN: The teaching nursing home. *JAMA* 1981;245:1435–1437.

The Teaching Nursing Home, edited by Edward
L. Schneider et al. © 1985 The Beverly
Foundation. Raven Press, New York.

Nursing Students and Postgraduate Nursing Training in Nursing Homes

Thelma J. Wells

University of Michigan School of Nursing, Ann Arbor, Michigan 48109-2007

Nursing is a term with several meanings, creating confusion in any discussion but particularly in one focused on long-term care. It is important to distinguish these meanings at the outset. In generic usage, nursing refers to caring or nurturing activities such as what a parent does for a child or a gardener for a plant. Based on this general sense, certain institutions in the community are called nursing homes to denote their purpose of providing care and nurture to their inhabitants. These institutions, in common with the health care industry as a whole, designate job titles that often use the generic term "nurse" or "nursing." In specific usage, nursing is a proper noun referring to the profession of a Registered Nurse, that is, an individual who has completed a particular course of study and has passed a particular licensing examination. Nursing as a profession functions under individual state practice acts regulated by Boards of Nursing.

It is most unfortunate that the generic term "nursing" is so widely used in the health care industry where the context of its use connotes professional practice. The subsequent lack of clarity does not benefit health care delivery and, surely, is unhelpful to the consumer. The resulting confusion is unnecessary, since the health care industry has been able to avoid a generic use of the term "doctoring" and has spared society the muddle of doctoring homes and doctoring aides. Perhaps with time and in the interest of fundamental fairness, the health care system can restrict its generic terminology when it reflects participating professions.

Nursing in this chapter always refers to the specific meaning as a profession unless otherwise noted. However, if the nursing profession is understood simply as all those holding a Registered Nurse License, further specificity is needed. Currently there are three quite differing types of preparatory education, the satisfactory completion of any of which entitles one to take the Registered Nurse Licensing Examination. These programs are all at the postsecondary education level. The oldest is the diploma nursing program, organized in American hospitals since 1872 (1). These programs are 2 to 3 years in length and over the last several decades have been closing. For example, between 1971 and 1980, the number of such programs declined by almost 50%, with those remaining contributing a steadily decreasing percentage of basic nursing education graduates, e.g., only 17% of graduates in the academic year 1980–1981 (2). The youngest nursing education program is the associate degree, organized in community colleges since 1952 (1) These programs are 2 years in length and have steadily grown in number. Such programs contribute about half of the graduates from basic nursing programs (2). The third preparatory nursing program is the baccalaureate degree, organized in colleges or universities since 1909 (1). These programs are 4 years in length, have been increasing in number, and produce about one-third of basic nursing education graduates (2).

It is clear that basic nursing education is in transition. Consistent with the recommendations of every national study of nursing since 1923, nursing is moving toward a collegiate system of education (3). The American Nurses' Association in 1965 advocated that all nursing education be in institutions of higher learning and resolved in 1978 that there should be only two entries into practice by 1985. The two nursing practice categories proposed were the professional nurse, prepared at the baccalaureate level, and a second type of nurse, not as yet distinguished by name, prepared at the associate degree level (4). Although implementation of these proposals has been slower than planned, it must be acknowledged that significant progress is evident despite resistance from those challenged by the professional development of nursing. The reality of both this progress and the clear intent of the nursing profession prescribes that the term nursing student in this chapter mean an individual in a baccalaureate nursing program, the entry point into the nursing profession. Postgraduate nursing education will mean that achieved after the baccalaureate level, that is, the Master's and Doctoral degrees. Thus, the educational institution of focus is the university/college school of nursing. It is essential to gain a clearer perspective of such schools and nursing homes, beginning with an overview of university/college schools of nursing and proceeding to gerontological nursing in such settings and to nursing homes in general before examining teaching nursing home (TNH) concepts.

SCHOOLS OF NURSING

Nursing education has put a priority on preparing nurse faculty at the doctoral level. From 1959–1960 to 1980–1981, the number of doctoral programs located in nursing schools with majors in nursing or a related field such as public health increased from two to 22 (2). Recruitment for graduates of these programs as well as for nurses with doctorates in other fields was intense, but by 1980 only 14% of baccalaureate and higher-degree nursing program faculty were doctorally prepared (2). Although this does represent significant gains compared to 6% in 1970, most doctoral faculty in schools of nursing engage primarily in teaching or administrative activity.

A study of the majority of nurses with doctorates in 1979–1980 found that the mean percentage of time spent in research activities was only 12% (5).

Although university/college schools of nursing have improved their faculties' preparation, an imperative need for more doctoral faculty remains. Styles notes a consensus among schools of nursing that their first purpose is "to generate knowledge through research" (6). Given the economic constraints on centers for higher education, nursing is being held to account. If nursing does not meet its primary purpose in universities, generating knowledge through faculty and student research, it will be unlikely to justify either its claims as a profession or its place in academic centers. Both by belief and necessity, discussions of nursing must center on research implications. Recognizing this, it is useful to explore the development of gerontological nursing in general and as it relates to these settings.

GERONTOLOGICAL NURSING

Gerontological nursing can be traced to ancient times when those occupying nurturing roles in the family or broader society provided care to frail, ill old people. But it is commonly agreed that the modern origin of the field extends from the 1935 Social Security Act and the resultant development of boarding homes for older people, many of which were owned and/or managed by registered nurses (7). A review of recent history reveals a characteristic specialty growth pattern in gerontological nursing as forces of increased knowledge, technological advances, and a concerned public have created a particular area of nursing (8).

In 1966, the American Nurses' Association established a Division of Geriatric Nursing Practice. Ten years later, the division title was changed to Gerontological Nursing Practice, reflecting a belief that nursing responsibility extended beyond the illness–institutionalized connotation of the term geriatric (9). The division has pursued an active leadership role. It has determined standards of practice, which were published in 1970 and revised in 1976 (10). It has defined the scope of gerontological nursing practice and articulated the dynamic role of such practitioners in a series of publications: A Statement on the Scope of Gerontological Nursing Practice (9), A Challenge for Change, The Role of Gerontological Nursing (11), Gerontological Nursing: The Positive Difference in Health Care for Older Adults (12).

Within this not quite 20-year-old nursing specialty, progress is evident. In 1982, Wells identified significant advances specific to gerontological nursing: an increase in basic textbooks and related topic books by nurses, an increase in primary nursing journals, an increase in relevant content in general nursing journals, an increase in the number of studies conducted by nurses utilizing samples of older people, a continued increase in academic programs, an increase in multidisciplinary practice/research programs facilitated by Federal and private sources, the development of private funding directed to nursing, and increased evidence of positive, innovative practice (13).

University schools of nursing have played an essential role in the development of gerontological nursing because, in nursing, specialization occurs at the Master's degree level. The first such program to prepare nurses as clinical specialists in gerontological nursing was developed by Virginia Stone at Duke University School of Nursing in 1966 (8). Although it is difficult to acquire an accurate count or description of existing specialty graduate programs, an American Nurses Association 1980 document lists 23 schools that offer a Master's degree with specialization in gerontological nursing. Recently, Brower surveyed 51 graduate programs identified as having a major or minor focus in gerontological nursing and found that 28 had a functioning major leading to a Master's degree (14). However, the data revealed that overall student enrollment was small, with continuing recruitment difficulties evident.

Among the 22 doctoral programs in nursing, five (Case Western Reserve University, University of Colorado, University of Illinois, University of Michigan, University of Wisconsin) offer a focus in gerontological nursing, and several others are planning to provide relevant emphasis in their overall programs (15). Of concern is the need for nursing faculty with either doctorates or postdoctoral work in gerontology/gerontological nursing to provide leadership and a research base for graduate level study. A 1980 American Nurses Association survey of all doctorally prepared nurses revealed only 18 (0.8%) with such gerontology/gerontological emphasis (16). With the rapid expansion of gerontological nursing, there is clearly a leadership crisis.

As gerontological nursing developed at the graduate level, interest at the undergraduate level enlarged. Four major surveys of gerontological content in all three levels of basic nursing programs were reported between 1953 and 1977 (8). A review of these surveys shows that although an increasing number of schools were providing specialized courses usually required in this content, only 14% of all preparatory programs had such offerings in 1975. The majority of schools stated that they incorporated principles of gerontological nursing into some aspect of course work. Although there are no published surveys exclusive to the university/college nursing programs, Tollett and Adamson explored four baccalaureate faculty and student groups to determine opinions about placement of geriatric and gerontology content in curricula (17). They found high and consistent agreement that such content was needed and should be required. Interestingly, they also included for comparison the opinions of a registered nurse group who were practitioners in a variety of settings. This latter group agreed with the faculty and student belief as to the need for a requirement in gerontological nursing but differed strongly in regard to curriculum placement. Faculty thought such content should be integrated throughout a curriculum, but the registered nurse practice group stressed the need for specific course offerings.

The issue of whether to integrate or separate gerontological nursing content at the undergraduate level may really be a discussion of staff resources. To provide exclusive content in a specific course suggests both considerable knowledge of that content as well as related differentiation skills. True integration of specialty content across a variety of courses requires high-level knowledge and skill in many faculty members. With a small supply of Master's and Doctoral gerontological nursing specialists, it is unlikely that many programs can offer either a specific course or true content integration. The suspicion holds that most gerontological nursing content at the undergraduate level is superficial and inadequate.

Although the lack of faculty prepared in gerontological nursing is the major problem, Gress reviewed nursing literature and identified seven compounding issues evident in university/college schools of nursing: lack of acceptance of gerontological nursing as a specialty, negative faculty attitudes toward the old, lack of clinical emphasis with older people, lack of gerontological nursing research, negative student attitudes toward the old, early curriculum work that questioned the value of content in gerontological nursing, and conflicting demands on limited school resources (18). Further barriers to development of gerontological nursing at the undergraduate level include the historic and continuing focus on acute care, the dominance of older nursing specialty areas, lack of licensing requirements in the specialty, lack of license examination questions in the specialty, and the complexities of effecting curriculum change in general.

It is essential to note that there is great breadth to gerontological nursing practice. Knowledge about healthy aging is important across the life span. Health and/or illness care of older people is provided in a range of community services as well as numerous institutional settings such as acute-care hospitals, Veterans Administration Medical Centers, chronic-care hospitals, and nursing homes. Although the focus of this chapter is the nursing home setting, the broader background of gerontological nursing should be kept in mind.

NURSING HOMES

Before discussing university/college schools of nursing experience with nursing homes as clinical sites, it is useful to examine briefly relevant features of nursing homes in general. As noted earlier, the term nursing in the title nursing home is in the generic rather than professional sense. In fact, as of 1977–1978, only 5% of the registered nurse work force were employed in such settings, and of these, only 12% had a baccalaureate or higher degree (19). A review of the 1977 National Nursing Home Survey data reveals that the predominant care providers are aides, representing 76% of full-time and 62% of part-time staff (20). Only 10% of full-time and 21% of part-time employees are Registered Nurses, with Licensed Practical Nurses making up the rest of the complement. With the entry point for nursing defined at the baccalaureate degree level in this chapter, analysis of the 1977 National Nursing Home Survey data discloses only 1.6% of all nursing home staff to have this or higher qualification. Applying this percentage to the 1,402,400 nursing home beds in 1977 yields a ratio of one professional nurse either full time or part time per 134 nursing home beds. Given this less than minuscule level of professional nursing in nursing homes, the misnomer of the latter is evident.

Staffing levels in nursing homes as specified by health codes are not derived from known staff competencies related to expected patient outcomes. Set staffing requirements derive from what is minimally acceptable as determined by a grossly empirical guess. Williams, estimating all levels of nursing personnel needed in his long-term care institution, concluded that his current 3.2 nursing personnel per patient was 50% below need (21). The need for more workers in long-term care is easily understood from a review of two large nursing home surveys that included patient dependency needs. These studies found that assistance was needed for the following percentage of patients in each activity: 89% to 94% bathing, 72% dressing, 34% to 50% eating, 55% to 68% use of toilet, and 70% in mobility (20,22). Since reimbursement is based on what patients cannot do, hiring untrained minimum-wage workers and assigning large work loads yields a custodial but profitable outcome. The few Registered Nurses involved serve primarily in administrative roles rather than as direct care providers. Typically, their salaries, like those of all levels of their staff, are lower than for similar roles in any other part of the health care system.

In addition to staffing issues, long-term care facilities range widely in terms of structural design and basic equipment. Although health codes have made considerable progress in this area, the work environment in nursing homes is still a critical problem. Space for patient dining, activity, and rehabilitative work areas is limited. Space for staff education such as classrooms and conference rooms is almost nonexistent. Equipment to facilitate patient care is often substandard or scarce for even such standard items as chairs or towels.

Nursing homes have a poor image as attested by a variety of book titles: *Too Old Too Sick Too Bad, Nursing Homes in America* (23), *Unloving Care, The Nursing Home Tragedy* (24), and *Old, Alone, and Neglected: Care of the Institutionalized Aged in Scotland and the United States* (25). Evidence presented in these books verifies the negative image.

There is an isolation to nursing homes. Few qualified health professionals practice there; those who provide periodic service or consultation do not stay long. Since patient care needs are complex, and custodial care is the main service, staff can easily feel overwhelmed. The atmosphere is often one of depression and deprivation.

Nursing is well aware of this negative background to nursing homes. Nevertheless, several baccalaureate programs have reported using a nursing home as the initial clinical learning site for students (26–30). Reasons given for selecting a long-term care rather than an acute-care setting are varied but include the following: stable patient population, slower work pace, desire to motivate students to work with the elderly, patient care needs being holistic and thus suitable to a nursing model, patient need for numerous nursing skills, which provides practice opportunity, and patient familiarity with technical procedures, which allows the student to focus most on skill attainment. Although the five reporting programs placed the nursing home experience in the first semester, duration was incompletely reported. It appears that some programs use the nursing home as one of several initial sites, rotating all students through them with very different time frames depending on the program, e.g., 18 hr (26) or 10 days (27). Other programs select a subset of students for a full semester of nursing home placement, e.g., 25% of the class on a 1 day a week basis (30) or all students placed in such a site for all of their initial clinical experience, e.g., 4 hr per week (28).

The great variance in student nursing home placement among these few reports is consistent with clinical site usage patterns in university/college basic nursing programs. Graham and Gleit surveyed a stratified random sample of deans in National League for Nursing (NLN)-accredited baccalaureate nursing programs and found a pattern of moderate use of a large variety of clinical sites rather than an extensive use of a single site (31). The educational bias seems to be for a breadth rather than depth exposure for basic-level students. It seems likely that this pattern will continue with only a limited time potential for nursing home experience at the basic nursing education level.

In gerontological nursing specific note is made of the need to emphasize well elderly experiences in addition to exposing the student to a continuum of care (7,32–36). Brower challenges the early placement of beginning nursing students in nursing homes because such students lack knowledge of normal aging and have not acquired sufficient performance skills or decision-making ability to function with the complex needs of ill, old, long-term patients (37). Her concern that nursing home experiences can be used to perpetuate myths and misconceptions of the elderly is especially relevant in regard to her observation that no basic nursing program has reported using such sites for senior-year leadership experience.

Indeed, evaluation of nursing homes as initial clinical sites is limited. Although learning objectives are reported as met, several papers relate dissatisfactions. Barrett and Metz found resistance in all students selected for the nursing home site placement and mixed reactions after the experience, although comparison between those and initial acute site placement students showed no difference in skill performance in the subsequent year (29). O'Driscoll and Wister report that more than half of their students who all experienced nursing home placement felt that it was not appropriate for their learning needs (27). Given the negative background of nursing homes, the persistent disinterest in gerontological nursing by basic nursing students (17,32,38,39), and the limited potential time for clinical site use of nursing homes, nursing education programs must be very selective and carefully plan the experiences of undergraduate students in nursing homes.

At the graduate level the literature contains little information about nursing homes as a practice site. However, informal discussions indicate that all graduate programs utilize nursing homes, although the extent of such use varies. A helpful measure of such involvement is the research outcome. Although there is no index of gerontological nursing research, a review of the monthly *Journal of Gerontological Nursing* for 1983 indicates that of 11 research reports by nurses, a third had utilized traditional nursing homes as the study site (40–43). Of special importance is the appropriateness of site selection to explore the clinical problems addressed, e.g., falls (40) or range of motion exercise (42). It is evident that a small body of nursing research is being generated from nursing home sites.

THE OPTIMUM RELATIONSHIP

The context of a special agreement that might occur between a university school of nursing and a nursing home should be considered. This special agreement is not the relatively simple clinical placement or affiliation contract, though it might grow from such. It is a thoughtful commitment between education and practice. It should not be considered in terms of what is typical but rather what should be optimum in terms of personnel, site, and goals.

Personnel

From the school of nursing standpoint it is essential that at least one doctorally prepared tenured faculty member with a strong background in gerontological nursing and both research and administrative strengths be involved for a major portion of her/his academic appointment. The faculty side of a nursing home relationship can simply not survive if vested exclusively in junior academic titles or clinical appointments. Neither can it survive if only fractional time is allocated to the highly qualified leader described, because the multiple demands on such a limited resource combined with the extensive problems to be resolved require a maximal effort. From the nursing home standpoint, it is essential that the nursing director have specialty preparation in gerontological nursing, i.e., a Master's degree with a concentration in gerontological nursing. All supervisory and head nurse levels must be filled with Registered Nurses, some of whom have baccalaureate in nursing degrees. Apart from the impact to patient care that such a prepared nursing home staff could engender, it is critical that practice and academic sides share a common communication and belief system.

In addition to these basic sides of the relationship certain personnel need to have formalized commitments that bridge the interests. Some recognition may take the form of maximum interest but minimal action such as unfunded adjunct appointments on the alternate side for administrative posts that serve important communication functions. However, there must be some truly joint appointments in which split or partial funding is provided by both sides. Such appointments could be a mixture of direct patient care and education roles such as a Master's-prepared clinical nurse specialist–instructor. However, schools of nursing must use great caution that such joint roles become neither *de facto* clinical tracks nor traumatic traps for naive junior faculty who would be better advised to continue their studies and pursue research.

Implicit in the personnel requirements is a common commitment between the schools of nursing leadership as represented by the Dean and Executive Committee and the nursing home owner and/or board of trustees. The optimum relationship between a school of nursing and a nursing home must be concrete, carefully formalized, and meant to be long lasting. It seems likely that such an intense relationship is also exclusive, making utilization of the site by other nursing programs less probable and certainly a matter of mutual discussion and agreement.

Personnel considerations extend beyond nursing roles in the optimum nursing home–school of nursing relationships. The complex needs of elderly long-term care clients require the skills of a multidisciplinary team. The nursing home medical director should take an active role in establishing and facilitating quality medical care. The Social Service Department should be under the direction of a qualified social worker. There should be a qualified physical therapist on staff and an activities program directed by an occupational or recreational therapist. A volunteer service should be functioning and an interface with the community evident. There are equally important personnel considerations within the school of nursing. Certainly, there should be an established department or unit of gerontological nursing. There should be a cadre of funded nurse researchers and a functioning doctoral program. Evidence of multidisciplinary research and collaboration with other university schools is relevant. In short, leadership in both institutions should be qualified and, thus, most likely to thrive in interaction.

Site

An optimum nursing home site from a university school of nursing perspective is within a half-hour's travel time and can be reached by frequent public service transportation or has adequate, secure parking space for private cars or vans. The size should be at least in the 100- to 199-bed range to allow for sufficient patient variance. The facility must be properly licensed and be rated by external inspectors as a good-to-excellent home. The building(s) should be in good repair and maintenance with an agreeable decor.

Adequate space should be provided for patient dining and recreational areas as well as special services such as hair care and a personal items shop. There should be an accessible clinic room with an examination table, weight scale, sink, basic physical examination supplies, and simple laboratory facilities equipped to examine urine. There must be office space available to interview patients privately and a larger room area to provide for patient group sessions. Educational space should be, at minimum, a large conference or classroom with a blackboard and projection screen. Additional school of nursing space needs include lockers for students, an office for school of nursing faculty providing leadership at the site, and some storage area for ongoing educational research materials.

The optimum nursing home site is well furnished with appropriate, functioning equipment that provides for flexible care needs. That is, there are a range of varied chair and commode designs, bathing facilities that extend from showers to hydraulic lift baths, and a stock of varied patient assistive devices.

The nursing home would do well to consider some features of the university school of nursing. The availability, quality, and access to a gerontology/gerontological nursing library, audio–visual materials, consultants, and conferences should be explored. Opportunities may be possible for academic study in relevant content areas and/or collaborative research projects.

Goals

In the optimum nursing home–school of nursing relationship, the central goal, quality care to patients, should not differ. Although the home's focus is primarily service and the school's focus primarily teaching, a mutual research interest should be appreciated by both.

Common goals and agreed philosophies are fundamental to any collaborative venture. Thus, it is essential to note that the majority of nursing homes are businesses run for profit, whereas university schools of nursing are nonprofit organizations. It seems logical that there might be inherent conflict between such groups. At the heart of the controversy about nursing homes is the economic issue with the concern that profit is made through reduction in patient care. It is extremely important that this issue be discussed early in any exploratory collaboration between a proprietary nursing home and a school of nursing. This is not to negate the optimum potential but to indicate that special concerns may be raised in the alliance of profit and nonprofit institutions.

Of course, goal variance can occur between nonprofit institutions too. Vladeck notes some useful monetary factors to evaluate in nursing homes, which may reflect underlying philosophies and potentially serious relationship difficulties: (a) tight working capital yielding limited stock inventories, recurrent shortages, and fluctuating care standards; (b) a disproportionately high share of revenue to capital financing rather than to patient direct benefits; and (c) perpetual administrative instability as ownership and/or the financial structure frequently change (25). Nursing schools would be wise to check these specific points.

Personnel, site, and goals desirable for an optimum relationship between a university school of nursing and a nursing home are extensive and impressive. There are those who will review the preceding and conclude that if such qualified components could be found they would be too good to need each other. This expression usually continues with the thought that university schools of nursing should develop a relationship with a typical nursing home, one that can rise from mediocrity through the infusion of academic blood. Such thinking has the wrong perspective.

Styles (6), acknowledging that the central concern for university schools of nursing is the relationship of education to practice, offers a series of questions and challenges for nursing, three of which are particularly germane to this discussion:

1. Whom does the professional school serve?
2. How are students socialized into the values and norms of the profession?
3. What is the actual/ideal effect of academia on reform in the profession? (7)

It might be useful to consider briefly at least some partial answers to Styles' questions. Professional schools do not serve the nursing home industry. Nursing schools serve societal needs; such service extends beyond manpower issues and rests in a research imperative. Students are socialized into the values and norms of the nursing profession to a great degree by contact with appropriate nursing role models. The typical nursing home may not have such models because it does not pay an adequate salary or attempt to recruit qualified professional nurses. And there will be no academic nursing effect on nursing homes until adequate numbers of prepared professional nurses are employed in such settings.

The naivete revealed in suggesting a special collaboration between less than exemplary nursing homes and outstanding schools of nursing is worrisome. The issues are more extensive than selecting an appropriate clinical site for students. The issues extend to balancing faculty practice and research responsibilities, reimbursement, legal constraints, expansion of nursing skills, and faculty governance. The issue is survival of nursing schools in university settings and the healthy growth of nursing research. Hence, the extension of university nursing schools into any arena must be carefully considered as the desirable qualities listed in the optimum relationship discussion attest. Of course, only a few university schools of nursing and nursing homes meet these qualities now, but with wise growth and committed planning other optimum relationships will develop.

There is little question that the proposed optimum situation is costly; the concern is "who will pay?" Pawlson, writing of medical education in nursing homes, identifies the need for a stable source of funding to support patient care, teaching, and research activities (44). He notes that private foundations, biomedical research grants, state governments, and professional service revenues have been supportive of medical education in such settings. But apart from the Robert Wood Johnson Foundation, nursing education has had no support for nursing home site utilization. It is critical that nursing funding issues be pursued in terms of both Federal or state initiatives and third-party payment.

Potential

The optimum nursing home–university school of nursing relationship rests on the premise that the minimum (minimum standards, minimum staffing, minimum professional nursing) has brought little change to the complex nursing problems of long-term care patients. Thus, a reduction in any part of the optimum weakens the merit of the endeavor as well as its consequence. This point is extremely important to nursing because outcomes attributed solely to nursing care are difficult to define (45). Haussmann et al., in a study of key variables thought to affect quality of care in 19 hospitals, found that although nursing action did relate to patient outcomes, this was significantly influenced by organizational variables in the patient care unit (46). Such variables included the following: for positive effect, increased Registered Nurse hours per patient day and a primary nursing structure; for negative effect, increased bed size and occupancy and increased numbers of nonprofessional staff. The optimum model will facilitate positve context variables and permit systematic exploration and evaluation of direct nursing care.

Research in gerontological nursing is increasing in quality and quantity (15,47–49). Nonetheless, clinical care abounds with opinions, admonitions, beliefs, ideas, and suggestions but few established facts or principles. Little is known about effective nursing interventions for the pervasive and complicated patient problems in long-term care such as urinary incontinence, wandering behavior, and multiple dependencies in activities of daily living. The foremost potential of the optimum university school of nursing–nursing home relationship is a quality nursing research program directed toward clinical questions with appropriate development of specific methodologies and relevant instruments.

A model setting could help resolve some of the issues related to gerontological nursing education. At the basic preparation level attention needs to be directed to appropriate learner objectives in long-term institutional care and to the placement of such experience in an overall program that includes well elderly practice experience. At the Master's level a core component in long-term institutional care is essential with a need to identify and test expected competencies. Nursing home educational opportunities for doctoral students focused in gerontological nursing need to be identified and evaluated. The possibilities are numerous to develop, plan, and test educational objectives in long-term care.

A needed outcome of educational development in such sites would be the production of relevant, quality teaching materials taking the form of varied core curriculum modules, specialized textbooks, and audio–visual productions. But perhaps the most exciting education potential is the opportunity for students to observe and work with positive faculty role models who can demonstrate the interrelationship of research and practice in a nursing home. It would be most valuable to monitor and evaluate this process for both immediate and long-term learner outcomes.

The impact of a model site on nursing practice as a whole would occur through many potential publications and presentations. It is likely that such sites would sponsor professional conferences, sharing findings and experiences, to challenge and to be challenged. Leadership has always resided in quality; the opportunity for quality to flourish in the optimum relationship envisioned would ensure meaningful outcomes for practice.

The potential of a model site to demonstrate the optimum relationship between a university school of nursing and a nursing home is so important that such consideration must not be made in either a sincerely enthusiastic but overly simplistic "bandwagon" manner or in a cleverly calculated but grossly underestimated "go for the dollars" mentality. A model site should be a precious and uncommon thing, carefully nurtured and responsibly supported. Looked to for leadership, it bears no less a responsibility than revolutionizing long-term nursing care.

REFERENCES

1. Kalish P, Kalish B: *The Advance of American Nursing*. Boston, Little, Brown, 1978, pp 86, 337–338, 593.
2. National League for Nursing: *NLN Nursing Data Book 1982*. New York, National League for Nursing, 1983, pp 6, 50, 79, 83.
3. Lysaught J: *Action in Affirmation, Toward an Unambiguous Profession of Nursing*. New York, McGraw-Hill, 1981, pp 98, 110.
4. American Nurses' Association: Resolutions. *Am Nurs* 1978;10(9):9–10.
5. Brimmer P, Skoner M, Pender N, et al: Nurses with doctoral degrees: Education and employment characteristics. *Res Nurs Health* 1983;6:157–165.
6. Styles M: *On Nursing, Toward a New Endowment*. St Louis, CV Mosby, 1982, pp 157–158, 173.
7. Davis B: The gerontological nursing specialty. *J Gerontol Nurs* 1983;9(10):527–532.
8. Wells T: Nursing committed to the elderly, in Reinhardt A, Quinn M (eds): *Current Practice in Gerontological Nursing*. St Louis, CV Mosby, 1979, pp 187–196.
9. American Nurses' Association: *A Statement on the Scope of Gerontological Nursing Practice*. Kansas City, American Nurses' Association, 1981, p 2.
10. American Nurses' Association: *Standards, Gerontological Nursing Practice*. Kansas City, American Nurses' Association, 1976.
11. American Nurses' Association: *A Challenge for Change, The Role of Gerontological Nursing*. Kansas City, American Nurses' Association, 1982.

12. American Nurses' Association: *Gerontological Nursing: The Positive Difference in Health Care for Older Adults.* Kansas City, American Nurses' Association, 1980.

13. Wells T: What does commitment to gerontological nursing really mean? *J Gerontol Nurs* 1982;8(8):434–437.

14. Brower HT: Graduate education in gerontological nursing. *Nurs Health Care* 1984 (in press).

15. Martinson I: Gerontological Nursing. A Statement to the National Advisory Council on Aging. October, 1980, pp 18–19. (*Unpublished document.*)

16. American Nurses' Association: *Directory of Nurses with Doctoral Degrees, 1980.* Kansas City, American Nurses' Association, 1980.

17. Tollett S, Adamson C: The need for gerontologic content within nursing curricula. *J Gerontol Nurs* 1982;8(10):576–580.

18. Gress, L: Governance and gerontological nursing in schools of nursing. *J Gerontol Nurs* 1979;5(6):44–48.

19. American Nurses' Association: *Facts About Nursing 1980–81.* New York, American Journal of Nursing Co, 1981, pp 11, 14.

20. US Department of Health and Human Services: *Employees in Nursing Homes in the United States: 1977 National Nursing Home Survey.* Hyattsville, MD, Office of Health Research, Statistics, and Technology, 1981, pp 2, 14.

21. Williams TF: Staffing problems in long-term care. *Med Care* [Suppl] 1976;14(5):85–93.

22. US Office of Nursing Home Affairs: *Long-term Care Facility Improvement Study, Introductory Report.* Bethesda, The Office, 1975, pp 22–25.

23. Moss FE, Halamandaris VJ: *Too Old Too Sick Too Bad.* Germantown, MD, Aspen Systems, 1977.

24. Vladeck BC: *Unloving Care, the Nursing Home Tragedy.* New York, Basic Books, 1980.

25. Kayser-Jones J: *Old, Alone, and Neglected: Care of the Institutionalized Aged in Scotland and the United States.* Berkeley, CA, University of California Press, 1981.

26. Wilhite M, Johnson D: Changes in nursing students' stereotypic attitudes toward old people. *Nurs Res* 1976;25(6):430–432.

27. O'Driscoll R, Wister E: Preparing nurse graduates for gerontology, a cooperative venture. *Nurs Clin North Am* 1979;14(4):653–664.

28. LaMancusa M, Robberson L: Nursing home for the initial clinical experience. *J Nurs Ed* 1981;20(2):4–8.

29. Barrett J, Metz E: An SNF for BSN students. *Ger Nurs* 1981;2(2):119–121.

30. Neil R, Casey T, Kennedy M: Nursing homes for initial clinical experience: Some specific advantages. *Nurs Health Care* 1982;3:319–323.

31. Graham B, Gleit C: Clinical sites used in baccalaureate programs. *Nurs Out* 1981;29:291–294.

32. Hart L, Freel M, Crowell C: Changing attitudes toward the aged and interest in caring for the aged. *J Gerontol Nurs* 1976;2(4):10–16.

33. Chamberland G, Rawls B, Powell C, et al: Improving students' attitudes toward aging. *J Gerontol Nurs* 1978;4(1):44–45.

34. Tobiason S, Knudsen F, Stengel J, et al: Positive attitudes toward aging: The aged teach the young. *J Gerontol Nurs* 1979;5(3):18–23.

35. Seigel H: Baccalaureate education and gerontology. *J Nurs Ed* 1979;18(7):4–6.

36. Strumpf N, Mezey M: A developmental approach to the teaching of aging. *Nurs Out* 1980;28:730–734.

37. Brower HT: The nursing curriculum for long-term institutional care, National League for Nursing: *Creating a Career Choice for Nurses: Long-term Care.* New York, National League for Nursing, 1983, pp 45–64.

38. Delora JR, Moses DV: Specialty preference and characteristics of nursing students in baccalaureate programs. *Nurs Res* 1969;18(2):137–144.

39. Gunter LM: Students' attitudes toward geriatric nursing. *Nurs Out* 1971;19(7):466–469.

40. Louis M: Falls and their causes. *J Gerontol Nurs* 1983;9(3):143–149,156.

41. Colling J, Park D: Home, safe home. *J Gerontol Nurs* 1983;9(3):175–179,192.

42. Clough DH, Maurin JT: ROM verses NRX. *J Gerontol Nurs* 1983;9(5):278–286.

43. Bahr SR: Sleep-wake patterns in the aged. *J Gerontol Nurs* 1983;9(10):534–537,540–541.

44. Pawlson LG: Education in nursing homes. *J Am Geriatr Soc* 1982;30(9):600–602.

45. Bloch D: Evaluation of nursing care in terms of process and outcomes: Issues in research and quality assurance. *Nurs Res* 1975;24(4):256–263.
46. Haussmann RK, Hegyuary S, Newman J: *Monitoring Quality of Nursing Care. Part II: Assessment and Study of Correlates*. Bethesda, USDHEW, 1976, pp 2,46.
47. Gunter L, Miller J: Toward a nursing gerontology. *Nurs Res* 1977;26(3):208–221.
48. Brimmer P: Past present and future in gerontological nursing research. *J Gerontol Nurs* 1979;5(6):27–34.
49. Kayser-Jones JS: Gerontological nursing revisited. *J Gerontol Nurs* 1981;7(4):217–223.

The Teaching Nursing Home, edited by Edward
L. Schneider et al. © 1985 The Beverly
Foundation. Raven Press, New York.

The Teaching Nursing Home as a Model for Interdisciplinary Team Training

Tom Hickey

Health Gerontology Program, School of Public Health, University of Michigan, Ann Arbor, Michigan 48109

During the past 10 to 15 years, we have seen the development of various options and programs that meet the long-term care needs of older people in their homes and in health care institutions. A current priority is to strengthen the linkages that exist between care options as evidenced by the rapid growth of assessment technology and the evolution of closer ties among hospitals, nursing homes, and home-care programs. An unstated assumption in this process is the necessity for involving different types of health care providers in the responsibility for long-term care. This chapter reexamines geriatric care and training priorities from the broad interdisciplinary perspective necessary to effect strong linkages in the long-term health care system. The following questions are addressed: what should be the various roles of different types of professional caregivers in the nursing home, how do ancillary and supportive health personnel fit it, and where does the model of a university-based teaching hospital best apply to the nursing home?

HISTORICAL ANTECEDENTS OF NURSING HOME TRAINING

In looking retrospectively at training deficiencies and staffing inadequacies in nursing homes, it is too simplistic to place the blame on physicians or even on the regulatory structure. The history of long-term care institutions in this country is rooted in a paternalistic philosophy that goes beyond the roles played by doctors or fiscal policies. This same paternalistic philosophy characterizes most of our societal institutions. Dependency at any age has been defined as deviancy from societal norms, whether referring to physical handicaps, mental retardation, criminal behavior, or chronic disability. When the care of such "deviants" exceeds the limitations of the family, responsibility has shifted to society at large. In all such examples of

335

dependency/deviancy, society's typical response has been to provide the protective isolation of a well-secured institution that abrogates the rights and wishes of the individual in favor of an impersonal, paternal caretaker.

The paternalistic philosophy that underlies societal caretaking assumes both responsibility and informed consent in determining its duties. Moreover, the focus of care in institutions is on problems rather than people. Whether nursing homes, mental hospitals, foster homes, or prisons, institutions have shared a similar approach in discharging responsibilities and duties. Given the historical roots and societal models, it is not surprising to find nursing homes that view the problem delegated to them by society as one of protective maintenance. In long-term caretaking, distinctions between medical and rehabilitative care, and between institutional capacity and personal care needs often become blurred. Thus, the institutional antecedents of current problems in improving long-term nursing home care are quite evident.

This past history provides several implications for staffing and training. By assuming that the major problem for institutions in long-term caretaking is that of 24-hr custodial maintenance, cost-effective staffing strategies have necessitated delegating day-to-day care to the least trained caretakers. Professionals have been involved largely in institutional and staff management rather than in patient care per se. As a consequence, the preparation of professionals and subsequent in-service training have dealt with role responsibilities that are defined horizontally. Physicians are trained to treat curable problems and to delegate to others the maintenance of chronic disabilities. Nurses, in turn, are trained to help others administer routine medical and nursing procedures and to supervise their performance. There are parallels in the training of other health professionals whose roles have evolved largely into that of a consultant.

The training of aides and ancillary nursing home staff is generally ignored for obvious reasons. Personnel turnover rates are too high, reaching as much as 200% annually in some nursing homes, making staff training not cost-effective for most institutions. Of course, high turnover is often planned as a "management" technique or, at minimum, is strongly influenced by low wages and job dissatisfaction, resulting in a vicious cycle. Morale might well improve along with job tenure if ancillary staff could derive more satisfaction in and be better rewarded for their work roles and task performance.

Where vertical staff training does take place, it is typically focused on technology, procedure, and regulations. Simultaneous training at all levels is usually directed at topics such as fire safety, meal preparations, cleanliness, and hygiene procedures. It can easily be argued that such training programs are not accurately "team training." Rather, they are directed at ensuring that all staff conform to good management procedures—largely for the benefit of the institution's cost containment goals and daily schedules rather than to improve patient care and personal needs.

However, very little training takes place, with the exception of minimal competency requirements for nurse aides. Regulations that have mandated minimal training standards have ended up defining limits or maximum standards. The regulations requiring "staff development training" are so loosely worded that they cover almost anything, including staff meetings.

NURSING HOMES AS GERIATRIC TRAINING CENTERS

Given this somewhat bleak history of training in nursing homes, it is difficult to identify good models or prototypes for developing an interdisciplinary teaching nursing home (TNH). The teaching hospital is perhaps the best example we have. However, it is not really an effective model for a TNH, since interdisciplinary training is noticeably absent from hospitals as well. Thus, at best, merging the teaching hospital with the long-term care facility represents only a viable starting point for interdisciplinary geriatric training.

A recent report by Breitenbucher and Schultz (1) describes a program in which teaching in an academic medical center was extended to several nursing homes in its immediate geographic region. Based in Minneapolis–St. Paul, the program focused on the training benefits for resident physicians as well as on the increase in the medical center's base of referral for acute problems. This program was intended to improve overall patient care. To the extent that patients received more attention as a result of the presence of doctors in the nursing homes and easier access to specialists at the medical center, geriatric care was improved. However, there appeared to be little interdisciplinary training or crossover between health care professionals. The authors noted that up to 90% of costs were recovered. The gap in cost recovery appeared to be at the level of the nurse practitioner, who was viewed, somewhat ironically, as essential to maintaining the day-to-day linkages between the medical center and the long-term care facilities. An important question here is whether the cost-effectiveness of such a program might be enhanced through increased emphasis on team training and the roles of other health professionals in maintaining a quality health care program. Some psychiatric hospitals, for example, assign a "primary therapist" to each patient on the basis of most appropriate need.

Although the Minnesota program and similar ones elsewhere have taken important steps toward improving patient care in long-term care settings, the concept of team care seems little advanced. To improve the interdisciplinary care of geriatric patients, fundamental changes must take place in both the concept and context of health care. Hospital-based models first must be modified to account for fundamental differences between acute and extended care. The needs of patients and the roles of physicians must be defined differently. Physicians cannot be viewed as "healers" in the traditional sense. Similarly, patients' needs cannot be defined solely in medical terms.

Long-term care, by definition, is longer, necessitating a continuing and recurrent monitoring of change. Ongoing assessment of geriatric patients in this context requires input from various individuals in addition to the doctor, and it encompasses a broader range of service and cost options beyond institutional care. Implicit in the definition of long-term care is the need to bring together diverse professional skills in the consideration of multiple treatment options. Thus, for a nursing home to become truly interdisciplinary in care, its institutional orientation must change. In this regard, the acute hospital model is limited by focus and tradition. The paternalism inherent in physician-dominated acute care tends to limit the scope of the teaching hospital model and is similarly constricting when applied to the long-term care and staff-training needs of a nursing home.

However, in attempting to design an innovative TNH, care must be taken not to throw out the proverbial "baby with the bath water." The linkage between acute-care hospitals and extended-care facilities remains critically important to success in meeting the needs of geriatric patients. Therefore, linking teaching hospitals with TNHs is important both for training purposes and for cost-effective continuity of care. The teaching model for both may be closely parallel or in tandem; however, the treatment context and goals must differ. An important difference in the nursing home is the relationship that patients have with professionals. A traditional view often held by older persons is that there is a dyadic relationship of patient to doctor, with other health professionals of minimal importance to either the patient or the physician. Such a perspective is often reinforced in the patient by his or her physician. Updated a bit, this view includes relationships between patients and several medical specialists (i.e., more than one doctor) but rarely the nurse practitioner or social worker.

For interdisciplinary care to be effective, patients must relate to many professionals beyond their physicians. To establish such a relationship, physicians can function neither as controllers of care nor as distant managers of long-term geriatric care. Similarly, other health professionals cannot serve merely as managers or consultants. The leadership role of physicians in the medical care of acute problems continues to be important. However, in the transition from acute to extended care, the institutional philosophies and care models must change—and visibly so to patients, health professionals, and physicians alike.

Despite the unsuccessful efforts to establish an interdisciplinary team-care approach for geriatric patients, the nursing home continues to have considerable potential for interdisciplinary training for at least three reasons. First, the context of care in nursing homes is different from that in the acute-care setting, regardless of the historical similarities as institutions. Second, physicians appear much less eager to dominate the care and treatment plans despite their traditional role. And, third, the various professionals necessary for maintaining team care are already working in nursing homes, albeit in managerial and consultant capacities, which need to be greatly expanded. The heart of the issue lies within this last point: interdisciplinary team teaching is essential for changing the roles and behaviors of health professionals—including doctors—to work effectively for the benefit of the long-term care of geriatric patients.

Interdisciplinary training for team care is only one-half of the equation. For health care professionals and nursing homes to initiate team care, the cost of such care must be included in planning and implementation. The need for team care and the assumption that it is less cost-intensive than the more traditional physician-dominated mode of care has wide acceptance. However, to match reimbursement with team care requires further empirical demonstration.

DESIGNING TEAM TRAINING FOR TEACHING NURSING HOMES

Where team training and care have been reported in the literature, little documentation of the generalizable ingredients for either success or failure is provided. Thus, most treatises that promote team care and interdisciplinary training tend to describe comprehensive program goals rather than practical priorities. Given the poor history of nursing home staff training and the obstacles to team efforts, a look at what is likely to work is desirable, rather than beginning with an ideal model.

Laying the Groundwork

There are a number of practical priorities to consider when implementing the concept of interdisciplinary team care. The fact that others have difficulty generalizing from their team experiences suggests the importance of the dynamics of a group and the charisma of its leader. Although discussion of group dynamics is beyond the scope of this chapter, the importance of the group process should not be minimized. Prior to initiating a team model for either clinical training or geriatric care, potential team members may need to know how a group operates and how to function in it individually. Similarly, the assumption and/or delegation of leadership and the distribution of responsibility may need to be taught as generic skills prior to focusing on interdisciplinary geriatric care. For emphasis here, it is important to restate the obvious: assembling a group of health care professionals and nursing home personnel under the new label "geriatric team" does not lead automatically to interdisciplinary team care.

A related practical issue to be confronted at the outset is the selection and preparation of the nursing home site. Many nursing homes would be inappropriate or unworkable locations for an interdisciplinary geriatric team for any of a number of reasons ranging from management philosophy to patient mix. This issue may be secondary, however, since those nursing homes that are receptive to teaching and research relationships with the academic community tend to be more easily recognizable. The selection of such sites and the development of an ongoing working relationship that may parallel only in part the operation of a teaching hospital require careful preparation. In the past, many of the best working relationships between well-motivated researchers and top-quality nursing homes have broken down because of a lack of careful preparation and, most notably, a failure at the outset to deal with the realistic expectations of each side.

Therefore, a necessary antecedent to establishing an interdisciplinary team in a nursing home is the following two-stage process: first, leaders for the academic team and the nursing home administration must sit down together and plan the program's goals and objectives and agree on the constraints and expectations that apply to each side. Second, the nursing home staff must be prepared for their participation—preferably through an incentive program. Similar partnerships have failed in the past (or succeeded only minimally) when the nursing home administration has not prepared the staff for participation or anticipated their concerns. Nursing home administrators often merely caution the outsider to avoid interfering with staff job performance and to be "sensitive" to their needs. Staff members, on the other hand, are often directed only with the general encouragement to "be as cooperative as possible."

To promote a TNH relationship that will really work requires the preparation of staff for new roles and for a different philosophy and style of care management within the nursing home. At a minimum, an attitude change will be required. Additionally, some sort of incentive may need to be a part of initiating team training and care. A variety of incentive programs are available from the personnel management plans of other organizations. Given the similarity in organizational structure and staff roles, the work quality incentive programs used by hospitals might be the first place to look. Fiscal bonuses, salary increases, compensatory time off, increased responsibility, and other forms of staff recognition are standard ways of approaching the motivational issue. Such incentives could become less important when positive patient care outcomes begin to affect staff morale directly. However, some form of ongoing staff recognition should be maintained.

These practical issues require careful consideration and significant investment or commitment at the outset. The selection of the nursing home site, preparation of the participants, and the orientation to group behavior and to a different style of patient care must be worked through carefully before interdisciplinary team training is begun.

Patient Care Plans as a Team Focus

Where should the interdisciplinary team begin its work? Given present staffing patterns and constraints, the patient care plan is an obvious focal point. Current regulations require the development of patient care plans by an interdisciplinary team, which should include a doctor, nurse, dietitian, social worker, and activities director. This team should be expanded beyond its regulated minimum to encompass the physical therapist, occupational or recreational therapists (if other therapists beyond the activities director are involved), the licensed practical nurse, and representation from other ancillary health staff such as mental health workers.

This broad base of participation at all staff levels in team planning of patient care will require a significant commitment from health professionals and nursing home administrators. For example, the consultant role taken by many professionals in the nursing home will need to change for the team to be truly interdisciplinary and effective. Physical therapists, social workers, and others will be required to participate actively in the consideration of the overall care plan for an individual patient in addition to making a determination of physical therapy, social work, and other health care needs. Some might argue that this level of activity is presently taking place in the development of individual care plans. However, it is more likely that its occurrence is only at a minimal level of conformity to regulations. There is generally little incentive for the active, ongoing involvement of consultants in the overall care plan beyond meeting their own specific responsibilities. Whether additional incentives can be found for increasing the team participation of such consultants is an important question for consideration. It may be that the minimal standards regulated in patient care plans need to be raised, given the inclination to accept minimal requirements as "standard procedure"—i.e., minimum requirements tend to become maximum outcomes.

Framework for Team Participation

Nearly 10 years ago, Katz and his colleagues (2) provided a useful perspective on team care of the chronically ill and disabled. With some adaptation, the design of a team-care plan is essentially the same now in a TNH context.

As suggested by Katz et al., the starting point for geriatric care is assessment. An interdisciplinary team model provides an opportunity for assessing the older patient from various important perspectives. Differences between these perspectives have significant implications for establishing care priorities and service goals. Of greater importance for training purposes, however, will be the effects of differences in assessment perspectives on the dynamics of the group's working relationship. Besdine (*this volume*) indicates that physicians tend to have a very distorted view of the nature of illness in the elderly when it is assessed only in a hospital setting. It may be necessary to go a step further and state that there is additional distortion inherent in conducting only a medical assessment. Thus, a broad-based physical and functional assessment from the perspectives of different health professionals and nursing home staff levels will be useful in establishing workable patient care plans and in training the interdisciplinary health care team. Recent improvements in assessment instrumentation and technology should greatly facilitate this process. Moreover, the opportunity to computerize the links between care needs and service goals and options increases the likelihood that the TNH and its health care team will be extended into the community.

The assessment stage leads to the establishment of patient care objectives and of the treatment and care strategies appropriate to meeting such objectives. Past experience with patient care plans would suggest that there is considerable "slippage" at this stage. Inappropriate or unreasonable goal setting, combined with little monitoring of care management, can easily turn a treatment plan into maintenance care for institutional efficiency. One of the goals of team training should be the development of individual responsibility for setting workable and measurable goals that have the consensus of the group, and for continued involvement in the overall management plan beyond the specific task or function of each individual in providing care. This form of personal commitment to the patient care plan should improve the validity of treatment goals as well as the compliance of patients. If the group dynamic is effective as a pressure or force on its individual participants, little monitoring will be required.

The geriatric patient also will need to be sensitized to a team-care process and to his/her opportunities to participate in it. With some patient education, for example, the accuracy and relevance of assessment can improve considerably. Similarly, the patients' participation in self-care activities as part of their individual care plans can be affected by training and education. Although there is likely to be wide variability among patients on this issue, patient involvement in various stages of the treatment plan is fundamental to the success of an interdisciplinary team strategy. On the one hand, the patients' consideration and involvement from the beginning will have a personalizing effect on the team and on the care plan. On the other hand, patient education and involvement at even a minimal level are essential to the development of a team relationship with the patient. To the extent that they are capable of it, geriatric patients will need to relate to the health care system at different levels and not merely to their doctors. This must be taught and reinforced by members of the health care team—especially by the physician members.

Team Leadership

Given this context and operational framework, how is team leadership established? Conventional wisdom places the physician—or sometimes the nurse—at the head of the health care team. There is no strong countervailing trend in the literature or recent practice despite recurrent observations about how poorly physicians relate to their geriatric patients. Many people believe that team care will never become successful with physicians retaining the leadership role. An incrementalist would argue that, in the absence of convincing evidence to the contrary, it is easiest to retain the physician in a leadership role. However, the dimensions and exercise of leadership may need to change considerably for an interdisciplinary care team to be effective in the nursing home setting. The leadership of the physician may eventually be focused on the medical care of acute episodes and life-threatening illnesses. In the caretaking roles of rehabilitation, maintenance of functioning, and assisting patients with personal and life-style adjustments, leadership should be shared with and delegated to other health care and ancillary professionals most appropriately qualified for the role.

The task of communicating leadership roles effectively to the patient can be a difficult one. Patients find it easier to relate to one person, typically the physician. Older patients need to have a sense that each member of their health care team understands their total health care needs and the treatment plan. The patient also needs to know who has responsibility for carrying out different aspects of the treatment.

CONCLUSION

As in earlier discussions of team care by Katz (2), Horowitz (3), and others, this chapter continues to address the ambiguities inherent in operationalizing a team-care concept. The literature and recent practice do not provide clear-cut models of team care or any tested framework for designing training to transcend traditional professional and disciplinary boundaries. Moreover, the history of interdisciplinary training and cooperation in nursing homes is quite limited. A more serious impediment, however, resides in the philosophical and fiscal contexts of nursing home care in the United States. The regulatory and reimbursement frameworks that define nursing home care and determine its outcome tend to reduce care to the lowest levels possible.

The potential benefits of interdisciplinary nursing home team care are as obvious as the limitations to its implementation. For the patient, there is the potential for improved care, comfort, and maintenance of daily functioning. Patient interactions with staff and the nursing home environment should also be more favorable. Moreover, various studies have shown that the health status of residents is likely to improve in institutions that are caring and individually focused and that do not cultivate the conforming, passive patient. The traditional paternalistic framework of care may disappear in institutions where priority is given to the healthy aspects of their residents.

For health care professionals, interdisciplinary team training should increase their knowledge of the specialized needs of the geriatric patient and their proficiencies in dealing with the chronically impaired. Staff morale, job satisfaction, and professional peer relations would also have the potential for positive change. For the long-term health care system, the teaching nursing home is in an important pivotal position between hospitals and other service options in the community. An effective team-care strategy should strengthen that linkage in the long-term care system. As in the Minnesota demonstration (1), the TNH concept brings the hospital and the medical school closer to the community for long-term care. If a comprehensive assessment process is used in a team approach to patient care plans, then the TNH will be the focal point but not the only locus of geriatric care.

Although there are numerous potential benefits to be derived from implementation of team care in the TNH, the perspective presented in this chapter suggests only cautious optimism. The obstacles are numerous. Nevertheless, interdisciplinary team care represents an important goal for geriatric care. Moreover, the training objectives for a TNH are an important component in the successful accomplishment of such a goal (4). Of greater practical significance may be the need to demonstrate the effectiveness of the concept in at least a limited manner. This would be an important first step towards addressing the overriding philosophical and fiscal constraints on nursing homes.

REFERENCES

1. Breitenbucher RB, Schultz AL: Extended care in nursing homes: A program for a county teaching medical center. *Ann Intern Med* 1983;1:96–100.
2. Katz S, Holstead L, Wierenga M: A medical perspective of team care, in Sherwood S (ed): *Long-Term Care: A Handbook for Researchers, Planners, and Providers.* New York, Spectrum, 1975, pp 213–252.
3. Horowitz JJ: *Team Practice and the Specialist.* Springfield, IL, Charles C Thomas, 1970.
4. Butler RN: The teaching nursing home. *JAMA* 1981;245:435–437.

PART VII
The Future of the Teaching Nursing Home

The Teaching Nursing Home, edited by Edward
L. Schneider et al. © 1985 The Beverly
Foundation. Raven Press, New York.

The Private View

David R. Banks

Beverly Enterprises, South Pasadena, California 91030

Widespread opportunities exist for collaborative teaching nursing home (TNH) efforts both within the private sector and between the private and public sectors. The future success of the TNH concept will depend on the effectiveness with which TNHs address critical issues facing long-term care and contribute to improvements in the quality of care and life of the elderly patient that is served. The private sector offers some unique opportunities for meeting these challenges since the overwhelming majority of nursing homes and other long-term care services are operated on a proprietary basis. It is, therefore, important that this sector directly participate and aid in the development and implementation of TNH models. As these models develop, it is also important to consider the future of nursing homes and the long-term care industry.

In viewing the future of nursing homes and long-term care, it is useful to consider the demographic changes under way in the population, the economic and reimbursement changes related to financing health care in general and long-term care in particular, as well as the regulatory environment within which nursing homes and long-term care must operate. These are less than ideal times for certain types of changes and innovations. If we can assume that nursing homes will continue to be the critical service delivery point for chronically ill elderly, the major focus for TNHs should be to address issues that will affect elderly patients and nursing homes in the future.

Certain issues facing long-term care and nursing homes point to the need for alternative thinking and new approaches, which TNHs could help develop. The private and public sectors can collaborate in helping to make TNHs successful in this regard.

FUTURE DEMAND AND SUPPLY ISSUES

Projections indicate that the United States population in general is becoming older (1–5). The percentage of persons 65 and older will by some projections double or triple over the next 30 to 40 years. This sector of the population currently accounts for the majority of nursing home patients. The supply of nursing home beds, however, is not expected to grow at the same rate during this same period. Approximately 5% of persons 65 and older are in nursing homes at any point in time (5). If there is a static or near constant supply of nursing home beds over the foreseeable future, nursing homes will be unable to continue to admit and serve this same percentage of the 65 and older population. Thus, the increasing number of elderly and the fixed supply of beds suggest that future nursing home patients will be sicker and older and the cost of their care more expensive.

The aging veteran population of this country is a special case, which has received little attention. Currently, veterans constitute approximately 27% of the older male population (6, 7). This percentage is projected to increase to 60% by 1990 and 70% by the year 2000. Demand by veterans for nursing home care should peak in the 1990s. One of the issues that confront the Veterans Administration (VA) is whether to build VA nursing homes or to use existing community nursing homes. The direction taken by the VA will have significant social, medical, and financial implications. For example, the majority of patients in community nursing homes are female. If the VA builds its own nursing homes, 99% of the patients will be male, causing a further isolation of the veteran patient. The expense to the VA of building nursing homes for a demand situation that may peak in the 1990s will, by some estimates, be much greater than that of caring for the veteran population in existing community nursing homes. However, the use of community nursing homes by veterans will limit the availability of beds for others. One advantage is that there would be a more equal mix of males and females in nursing home settings, reducing the isolation of both groups.

ECONOMIC AND FINANCING ISSUES

The introduction of prospective reimbursement for hospitals raises important issues for long-term care. Medicare, under its DRG payment system for hospitals, is the first major payer to move in this direction. The use of prospective reimbursement or DRG payments will very likely result in a general lowering of the length of stay in acute-care hospitals. It is thought that many Medicare patients will arrive at the nursing home earlier and sicker than in the past. Moreover, there is likely to be new demand for nursing home care by patients served under alternative delivery systems (e.g., HMOs). Some of these systems are beginning to view long-term care in general and nursing homes in particular as cost-effective alternatives to acute health care services. To cope with changing patient profiles, the health system must become more efficient in providing appropriate care for patients to maintain optimal functioning.

REGULATORY ENVIRONMENT

Currently, there are efforts both to increase and to reduce the regulation of nursing homes. One major reason for the heavy level of regulation related to patient abuses and poor quality of care. The industry, with the help of others, has made significant strides in correcting these problems; nevertheless, there is still room for improvement.

Regulation through health planning and the certificate of need process has placed constraints on the supply of nursing home beds. Although there are currently movements under way to eliminate certificates of need, the supply of nursing home beds will not significantly increase in the near future, in large part because of the reimbursement practices of Medicaid agencies, which account for approximately two-thirds of the industry's revenues. There is no indication that the rate of reimbursement for nursing homes by Medicaid, Medicare, or the private sector is likely to increase, although the private sector may account for an even larger share of the reimbursement in the future. The increasing competition for capital in today's economy will reduce the availability of funds for new construction unless the return on investment from producing more nursing home beds meets or exceeds returns in other areas of comparable risk.

Regardless of the future direction of regulations and reimbursements for long-term care, it will be increasingly difficult for independent nursing homes or other providers of long-term care to compete and remain viable. Thus, there will be a continued concentration of service units through the growth of chain operations. One result of the growth of chains will be an increased emphasis on operating and management objectives. The sick older patient will have limited access to the nursing home unless health professionals and the nursing home industry work closer together.

Given the complexities of these issues and the multiple constraints facing long-term care, the critical question for the private sector is: how to improve the quality of care and life of elderly patients, especially those in nursing homes. But the issues involve both the public and private sectors, and the ideal approach would be a collaborative one. Since both sectors are interested in TNHs, financially as well as operationally, the TNH provides an excellent framework within which to work together toward common goals. These issues are far more important to address together than to let past traditions and philosophical and operational status (e.g., profit versus nonprofit) stand in the way of a truly collaborative approach.

ISSUES FACING TEACHING NURSING HOMES IN THE FUTURE

The potential success of the TNH in dealing with health problems facing elderly patients will depend, in part, on the ability of its decisionmakers to plan for the future of long-term care. Since it is likely that patients served will be sicker and perhaps have more concomitant social and psychological problems, there will be a need for increased service capability at the long-term care site. This might require a redefinition or a redesign of the nursing home structure or home health care methods and procedures.

Various operators within the industry are beginning to develop special units or capabilities in and outside of nursing homes to care for the sicker patient. Terms such as "heavy care," "super skilled," or "subacute" are used to identify the higher levels of care required by sicker patients. These special units will require higher staffing levels, more highly trained personnel, some additional equipment, and in some cases, different construction, and an emphasis on rehabilitation services. The investigation and evaluation of alternative methods and procedures to care for sicker patients through the use of nursing homes and other long-term care services is an excellent arena for TNH involvement. Development of research and training agendas should include model programs, procedures, and services sites for elderly patients.

In order to provide this increased service capacity, providers must become operationally efficient. This might be partially accomplished through improved management techniques. Large chain operators have certain advantages in achieving economies of scale (e.g., bulk purchasing). However, the greatest challenge and potential for improved efficiency is through human resource development. This is an important study area for THNs. However, given the high number of nursing aides presently functioning in long-term care and higher education's lack of involvement with "non-professional" health workers, one may question the priority the TNH will place on this area. Improvements in the human resource area would be a major contribution to long-term care.

There is a real need to find better methods for improving the motivation and functioning of nursing aides and other nondegreed long-term care personnel. The training of health professionals who choose careers in long-term care should include courses and field work that would better prepare them to supervise, work with, and motivate personnel of various backgrounds and education they are likely to encounter in long-term care. Also, the development of realistic "career ladders" for long-term care personnel should be explored. Alternative staffing patterns, performance standards, long-term care competency levels, and certification for employees are subjects worthy of attention. Improving the quality and career outlook for long-term care personnel will have a positive impact on the quality of care and life of the patient.

Another major issue facing long-term care is how to attract physicians and other health professionals (e.g., the geriatric nurse practitioner) to the nursing home (8–11). Too few physicians have backgrounds or training in geriatrics or spend enough time in nursing homes. Current reimbursement practices and professional practice regulations limit the use of other specialists in nursing homes. However, as a greater proportion of sicker patients enter long-term care settings, there will be a need for an increased presence of a diverse group of health professionals trained in geriatrics.

It will be interesting to observe what occurs if and when this presence is increased. Will the nursing home move more in the direction of the medical model? Will there be an increased demand for support services such as those that generally exist at the acute-care level? Will the demands on the current work force in the nursing home increase turnover, at least initially? Over time, long-term care should improve as a result of increased professional presence. However, the transition period may result in changes that might be unsettling. The TNHs should play an important role during this transition period through assisting in improved preparation of medical and health-related professionals to function together in caring for the elderly.

OPPORTUNITIES FOR PARTNERSHIPS AND AFFILIATIONS

Innovation in long-term care will require effective working relationships between the private and public sectors. Within these sectors, there is a need to establish and improve working relationships, which will benefit elderly patients. For example, within the private sector, past practices, policies, and in some cases legal interpretations have prohibited nonprofit organizations and profit organizations from working together in areas of mutual interest. Similarly, unnecessary barriers have made it difficult or impossible for different levels and agencies of government to direct their full attention toward these activities. Notwithstanding these intra- and intersector differences and difficulties, it is patient care that will suffer if avenues of cooperation are not found.

The academic/research community, government, and foundations have more of a history of working together, especially in areas related to acute care. These traditional working relationships must be expanded to include greater roles for industry and proprietary organizations in long-term care service delivery. There have been some notable recent attempts by teaching institutions and the proprietary hospital sector to form associations and affiliations. However, skepticism remains as to the effectivenss of this type of association. Some of this skepticism may be related to the limited exposure to and lack of understanding of possible relationships between academia and for-profit hospitals and, subsequently, this may be related to the fact that the majority of teaching hospitals in the country are operated on a not-for-profit basis.

Just the opposite is the case in long-term care. The majority of nursing homes in this country are operated on a proprietary basis. Although there has been less than full communication between nursing homes and professional health schools, there has been a great deal of involvement with community and vocational colleges, particularly related to the training of personnel. The for-profit nursing home industry will welcome the opportunity to work with any groups interested in long-term care.

Reimbursement methods for nursing homes have not provided sufficient incentives or rewards for innovation, especially with respect to clinical care

(5). Nor is the cost for affiliating with academic institutions provided for in the reimbursement. As a result, proprietary and chain operators of nursing homes have mainly emphasized innovations in the management and financing areas to effectively compete and attract investment capital. Incentives and opportunities to innovate in areas of clinical care have been limited. The lack of effective working relationships and the absence of specially trained health professionals in the nursing home and other areas of long-term care have made it increasingly more difficult to innovate with respect to clinical care. The TNH can help to solve this problem by bringing together professional and industry expertise, financial resources, and research and demonstration settings to find improvements in the area of clinical care. This type of approach has worked in other areas, and it should be effective in long-term care.

Thus, several opportunities exist for the nursing home industry, foundations, government, and the university for joint ventures in TNHs. The definition of the TNH model should not be so rigid as to preclude these types of relationships and strategies. Flexible arrangements are needed that focus on specific projects aimed at improving patient care and service delivery as well as broad efforts encompassing training, research, service innovations, and education.

TRAINING, RESEARCH AND DEVELOPMENT, AND DEMONSTRATION PROJECTS

One obvious approach to joint involvement is the use of nursing homes as a resource or site for assistance in the training of health professionals. This could be accomplished through rotation programs involving medical and nursing schools as well as other schools of allied health professionals. Health administration programs should incorporate more courses and information on long-term care rather than rely on the hospital model for teaching purposes. The more information obtained during student training on the operational realities and constraints facing long-term care, the better the health professionals will be prepared to face those realities when they begin their careers. Also, researchers will be better able to investigate or evaluate industry practices toward this goal of achieving excellence in patient care within the realities of financial and human constraints.

If the academic community and industry are to collaborate in research and development, there must be both short- and long-term rewards. Research topics should be selected that address short-term payoffs in the form of improvements in the clinical care of patients as well as in operational efficiency and/or managment of facilities. A balance between short- and long-term successes will allow industry to justify more adequately the use of industry resources for research and development activities. Industry and the universities are involved in research together, but only to a small degree in long-term care. An increased effort must occur. This effort might begin by joint sponsorship of educational programs and research projects in long-term care.

Demonstration projects also offer opportunities for collaboration. For example, the nursing home can be used as a base to deliver and manage a broad range of long-term care services. Since the nursing home currently provides or arranges for certain professional and support services, organizing and extending this base to provide a broader range of long-term care services to both institutionalized and noninstitutionalized patients would appear logical, viable, and efficient. By packaging a full set of long-term care services and reimbursing them on a *per capita*, per case, or other risk basis, nursing homes would have appropriate incentives to place the patient at the preferred level of care. Of course, this assumes that issues of case mix, resource use, reimbursement methods and rates, and appropriateness of care can be resolved. This is a big assumption; however, private and public sector initiatives could determine whether this approach is feasible.

Collaboration to demonstrate alternative reimbursement policies and procedures should be encouraged. Current methods and amounts of funding may very well be inadequate, especially in light of "the graying of America." Since there obviously are differing opinions regarding how to address reimbursement, perhaps this too is an appropriate subject for the TNHs to make a contribution. Long-term care demonstrations could be sponsored jointly by the public and private sectors and used to examine and propose new policies and procedures in this area.

SUMMARY

Some long-term care providers have health delivery system networks that cover large geographic areas and, in some cases, span the country. These systems represent a vast resource for research and demonstration projects in terms of patient population, geographic and economic distribution, size of facility, financing methods, and management styles. Many previous studies of long-term care have been of limited use because of their narrow scope and lack of demonstrated widespread applicability. The network systems that have developed would appear to be able to address some of the past limitations if reasonable arrangements for thier use could be made.

Viable TNH models for the future should avoid the acute-care model. Although there will be an increase in sicker and older patients, long-term care can be improved without imposing the significant cost and supporting services that are involved in acute care. Although long-term care cannot substitute for acute care, long-term care in general and nursing homes in particular have achieved a modicum of success under severely limited circumstances. The private and public sectors can collaborate through the TNH to enhance and expand these earlier successes and together help advance the quality of life for the elderly patient.

REFERENCES

1. US General Accounting Office: *Medicaid and Nursing Home Care: Cost Increases and the Need for Services are Creating Problems for the States and the Elderly*. Ser. No. GAO/PE-8. Washington, DC, General Accounting Office, October 21, 1983, pp 33–36.

2. Office of Technology Assessment: *Technology and Aging in America*, Study Plan, Washington, Government Printing Office 1982, p 9.

3. Siegel JS: Prospective trends in the size and structure of the elderly population, impact on mortality trends, and some implications. *Curr Pop Rep* 1979;78:7–13.

4. Fries JF: Aging, natural death and the compression of morbidity. *N Engl J Med* 1980;303:130–135.

5. National Center for Health Statistics: *The National Nursing Home Survey: 1977 Summary for the United States*. Hyattsville, MD, DHHS, 1980, p 31.

6. Wallace C: VA plans to double nursing home beds as number of elderly veterans triples. *Mod Healthcare* 1983;7:61–62.

7. Rice DP, Feldman JJ: Tables and charts for demographic changes and the health needs of the elderly. Distributed at the Institute of Medicine Annual Meeting on Aging and Health: New Perspectives in Science and Policy, 1982.

8. Johnson MD III, Bennett JE, Ruth B, et al: *Undergraduate Medical Education Preparation for Improved Geriatric Care, a Guideline for Curriculum Assessment*. *J Med Educ* 1983;28:7–8.

9. Libow LS, Sherman FT: *The Core of Geriatric Medicine: A Guide for Students and Practitioners*. St. Louis, CV Mosby, 1981.

10. Steel K: *Geriatric Education*. Lexington, MA, Cullamore Press, 1981.

11. Kane RL, Solomon DH, Beck JC: The future need for geriatric manpower in the United States. *N Engl J Med* 1980;302:1327–1331.

The Teaching Nursing Home, edited by Edward
L. Schneider et al. © 1985 The Beverly
Foundation. Raven Press, New York.

The Public View

T. Franklin Williams

National Institute on Aging, National Institutes of Health, Bethesda, Maryland 20205

The public view of the future of teaching nursing homes (TNH) should
cover two perspectives: the local community level and the national level.
First, a public view of the future of TNH needs to be assessed in the context
of the local community in which it must exist. This opinion reflects my 15
years' experience, from 1968 to 1983, in the initiation and development of
one of the first TNHs in this country in a setting in which there were the
essential ingredients of the solid marriage of a university, the University of
Rochester, with a public facility, Monroe Community Hospital, and close
ties with the entire panoply of community services for older people.

The initiation of a TNH in Rochester and Monroe County, New York,
came from the combined leadership of the business community, represented
most importantly by the Honorable Marion B. Folsom, executive of Kodak
and Secretary of Health, Education, and Welfare in the Eisenhower Administration, together with political leaders responsible for the public long-
term care facility, Monroe Community Hospital, and university leadership
responsible for medical education and research.

There was agreement that the community needed better long-term care
(to help avoid inappropriate use of acute hospital beds), that the public long-
term care facility needed high-quality medical staffing, which the university
could provide, and that the medical school needed to be involved in long-
term care activities for sound teaching of medical students and house staff
and for research. These goals and principles sound self-evident now, but
15 to 20 years ago they were only beginning to be thought about in most
settings. In the Rochester environment the commitments led to a formal
affiliation agreement, which in turn led to a major development of academic
medical staff in the nursing home environment from 1970 on; the regular
rotation of students and house staff through this environment and the undertaking of a wide range of research in geriatrics, in chronic diseases, and
in delivery of services to elderly and chronically ill people. Extensive teaching was also developed for undergraduate and graduate nursing students,
geriatric nurse practitioners, and students in social work, in physical, occupational, speech, and recreational therapy, and in health administration
(1).

The development of many facets of this program also required and led to the development of a comprehensive assessment service (2) and to continuing close working relationships with providers of the full range of long-term care services in the community, including both nonprofit and proprietary nursing homes, home-care services, and regulatory and reimbursement agencies. It meant participation by the university medical leadership and by the administrative and nursing leadership of the long-term care facility in the chronic-care aspects of the health planning council (Health Systems Agency) and to medical staff participation in board activities and in consulting roles with many long-term care facilities. Similar public and community activities would be necessary for the successful operation of a TNH program in any community.

In that particular community, the extent of the interrelationships can perhaps best be epitomized in the officers and board membership of the ACCESS Long-Term Care Program, a model county-wide comprehensive assessment and placement program, which evolved from services initially developed at Monroe Community Hospital. The sustained leadership of this program has included the chairman of community medicine and associate dean of the medical school, the director of the university's program at the Monroe Community Hospital, the director of the County Department of Health, the director of the County Department of Social Services, the owner of the largest proprietary nursing home, the president of a manufacturing company, the president of the League of Women Voters, the director of the antipoverty organization, the director of the Visiting Nurses Association, the director of the County Office for the Aging, and others. The involvement of these individuals, with their ties and constituencies in the community, illustrates that long-term care is a very public and community enterprise and will increasingly involve multifaceted relationships in every community.

An academic medical center and a nursing home, proprietary, nonprofit, or public, might start a TNH arrangement on simple one-to-one terms, but the realities of the continuum of long-term care, including hospital, nursing home, and home support resources, and the realities of the pressures of payment and regulation will quickly require understanding and workable arrangements with the community as a whole. These relationships are as important for the achievement of the academic goals of teaching and research as they are for the operation of the participating nursing home. Older people, as they become frail, are likely to move back and forth among these various services and settings; medical students, residents, fellows, nursing and social work students, and those in other health-related professions need to be involved during their training in the care of such patients in all settings. The research opportunities and challenges that exist among the problems common in patients in nursing homes are also common in frail older persons anywhere, and the latter should be involved in the research in ways similar to nursing home patients.

Ties between academic medical centers and nursing homes are inevitably going to include ties with the entire range of community long-term care services. In this sense, the TNH must be considered a "public" undertaking no matter whether the background or ownership of any of the individual components is private or public.

To proceed to consider the future of TNHs from a national perspective, it would seem that within a relatively short time, i.e., 5 to 10 years, essentially every medical school, nursing school, and other relevant professional school in this country will have an affiliation with one or more nursing homes for required experience for students and house staff and with varying degrees of involvement in research. And, as indicated above, these arrangements would rapidly, and preferably from the beginning, also involve teaching and research ties with the entire range of community long-term care services.

This development in every academic medical center will be dictated by several factors. First, its logic for adequate medical education is unassailable: the heart of medical education is to take the student to the patient. In Osler's day, the dramatic innovative step was to take the student to the bedside of the acutely ill patient, in the hospital for the most part. The major problems and challenges in medicine at that time were the innumerable life-threatening acute illnesses. Today, as Fries (3), Schneider and Brody (4), and others point out, our most pressing challenges, in terms of numbers and burden, are the functional losses and multiple chronic diseases among our rapidly growing numbers of older people and the interrelation of these problems with the available support systems wherever the older people may be living. Thus, "to take the student to the bedside" means to go to the private home, to the nursing home, to the retirement home, to the hospital at times, to wherever the older person may be. Virtually every doctor will be caring for many old and very old people. In almost any specialty, doctors will need to learn the basic clinical facts about older patients by going to the person wherever he or she may be.

Anyone conducting responsible planning for medical curricula should see the necessity for including the long-term care component or, more specifically, the TNH in the curriculum. The same will apply in nursing, social work, and other health-related professions.

A second factor, related to the first, that will hasten the development of TNHs is the requirement by licensing and certifying boards of geriatric knowledge and experience. The National Board of Medical Examiners, the American Board of Internal Medicine, and the American Board of Family Practice are among those who have added such requirements. Academic centers must provide the settings for such learning.

A third factor that will influence academic medical centers and teaching hospitals to develop TNH relationships is the rapidly increasing economic pressure on teaching hospitals, as on all hospitals, to have readily available arrangements for prompt discharge of patients to nursing homes or into home-care services. The DRG approach to hospital payment and the steady and rapid growth of HMO arrangements by teaching hospitals and their medical staffs, including Medicare–HMO arrangements, will be powerful economic incentives to have close ties with one or more nursing homes and home-care services.

Similarly, with chronic diseases and disabilities becoming our major health problems and the recognition of the need to understand aging, the direction of research has turned more and more to these problems. Investigators in most fields related to health—biomedical, behavioral, social, categorical disease-oriented as well as functionally oriented—find that they need access to older persons, both those who are healthy and those who have chronic diseases and disabilities.

From the perspective of the nation as a whole, there is the need for the development of TNHs and related community teaching activities to provide for the proper training of future practitioners nationwide, to provide for research in gerontology and geriatrics, and to develop and serve as models for better care for older and chronically disabled people. Some of these settings should have a sufficient group of academic leaders—investigators and teachers—to train needed faculties and investigators for this field.

The interest among nursing homes in becoming involved in such affiliations is growing, and information to date indicates that many nursing homes do and will continue to find it greatly to their advantage to have such affiliations. Therefore, there will be more than enough opportunities to provide such affiliations for every medical and nursing school. The participating nursing home acquires assured medical staff of high quality, access to specialty consultants, participation by medical, nursing, and other faculty for in-service education for nursing home staff, access to hospital beds for the nursing home patients when needed, and a source of patients for the nursing home. There is also the stimulation of new ideas and the latest findings.

The rights and preferences of patients must be respected; this has been true in the TNHs that I know, and the vast majority of patients welcome and benefit from the increased interest and attention from students, house staff, and faculty. Many are eager to take part in research that may benefit themselves or other older people; their participation in itself adds interest to their lives as well as to those of the staff of the nursing home.

The costs of the TNH arrangement must be carefully weighed for the nursing home as well as for the medical or nursing school, in terms of time consumed by staff of both institutions and portions of salaries of participating house staff. It seems justifiable to seek an arrangement in which payment for the portion of house staff time spent in a required rotation in the TNH would be compensable in the same way as house staff salaries in teaching hospitals. The issue of how to pay for house staff salaries in teaching hospitals is currently under review; it would be appropriate for whatever arrangement is developed in TNHs to parallel that employed in teaching hospitals.

In relation to payment of the cost of faculty members participating in TNH care and teaching, given the generally modest salaries of medical faculty compared to the general medical marketplace, payment for their patient care services in the TNH may be covered by available third-party reimbursements.

What about external sources of support for research in TNHs? The commitment of the National Institute on Aging to relatively large support of a limited number of ambitious and exciting research programs in teaching TNHs is described in this volume. Each of these programs involves several individual research projects. Six research Teaching Nursing Home Programs have now been funded by the NIA. More will be added, a few at a time, depending on the quality of applications and funds available. But the development of teaching nursing home relationships by academic medical centers offers far more opportunities for a wide variety of research efforts than can or should be supported by these NIA-funded TNH research programs. Academic medical centers and nursing schools can find in these affiliations opportunities to develop and apply for individual research projects in the entire range of functional disabilities affecting older people, in the chronic diseases commonly present, and in approaches to improved care. All of the funding mechanisms of the NIA as well as those of the other Institutes in the National Institutes of Health, of the National Institute of Mental Health, of the Administration on Aging, of the Veterans Administration, and of many private foundations should be available and are appropriate for support of research related to TNHs.

From a national perspective, there should evolve a rapid development of TNHs for teaching and research by essentially all academic medical centers and nursing schools in the country. There will be close integration of the teaching of all aspects of long-term care and of the chronic functional disabilities and diseases affecting older people throughout the full range of long-term settings. The research that will continue to develop around such TNHs will be integrated into the overall research activities of academic medical centers and will use essentially the same range of funding sources as used by teaching hospitals as well as a limited number of special resources targeted specifically at the TNH development.

How may the advances in knowledge and in quality of care that we expect to be achieved by TNH be spread throughout our long-term care services? New knowledge and new discoveries will become known by and large through the normal channels of presentation at meetings and publications. To achieve more prompt and effective incorporation of better care in nursing home and community settings by participating in TNH programs, we should explore the development of a network, a guiding consortium of organizations involved with nursing homes and other aspects of care for older people. This consortium would have the mission of encouraging and assisting in the introduction of new findings, better approaches to long-term care, in all nursing homes and community services. The type of groups that might be represented in such a consortium include the American Health Care Association, the American Association of Homes for the Aging, the organizations represented in their Leadership Council of Aging Organizations, the Coalition for Nursing Home Reforms, and others.

A few of the issues raised in other chapters merit special comment. First, in relation to the portentous demographic and epidemiologic characteristics and projections about older persons, the most important additional information we need concerns the trends in morbidity and burden of care among older people, trends over the past 10 years and on into the next 5 to 10 years. Is the period of "active life expectancy," the term used by Katz, Branch, and Jette (5), extended or not, coming closer to the total life expectancy? My own experience suggests that it is, with the result that the extent of functional disability is declining per population age group. Studies of successive cohorts of older people are needed over time in order to shed clear light on this question. The answer to this question would be of great assistance in planning for future care and services.

Second, Brody, C. Williams, Pastalan, Maddox, and Eisdorfer in their chapters in this volume address the issue of the institutional nature of nursing homes and raise the question of how to recast our views of nursing homes and our ways of building as well as operating them to give more meaning to the fact that they are, first of all, homes to people. Various efforts have been and are being made to address this question, but there is much more that can and should be done. Most importantly, we need to put the resident (whom we change into a patient in most of our thinking by calling him/her that) and his/her family in a central position in controlling and determining his/her living environment while a resident in the nursing home building. This might be approached in a number of different ways and various experiments undertaken. The issues range from participation in the governance and even ownership of the facility to control of one's own private living space to individualization of institutional services including the times of services.

REFERENCES

1. Williams TF, Izzo AJ, Steel RK: Innovations in teaching about chronic illness and aging in a chronic disease hospital, in Clark DW, Williams TF (eds): *The Teaching of Chronic Illness and Aging*, Bethesda, Fogarty International Center, National Institutes of Health, 1976, pp 21–30.
2. Williams TF, Hill JG, Fairbank ME, et al: Appropriate placement of the chronically ill and aged. *JAMA* 1973;226:1332–1335.

3. Fries J, Crapo LM: *Vitality and Aging.* San Francisco. WH Freeman, 1981.
4. Schneider EL, Brody JA: Aging, natural death, and the compression of morbidity: Another view. *N Engl J Med* 1983;854–855.
5. Katz S, Branch LG, Branson MH, et al: Active life expectancy. *N Engl J Med* 1983;309:1218–1224.

Subject Index